T0296590

HOW PEOPLE CHANGE

HOW PEOPLE CHANGE

The Short Story as Case History

William Tucker, M.D.

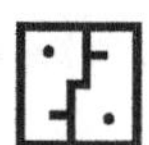

Other Press • New York

Copyright © 2007 William M. Tucker

Production Editor: Robert D. Hack

This book was set in Goudy and Ocean Sans MT by Alpha Graphics of Pittsfield, New Hampshire.

All rights reserved. No part of this publication may be reproduced or transmitted in any form or by any means, electronic or mechanical, including photocopying, recording, or by any information storage and retrieval system, without written permission from Other Press LLC, except in the case of brief quotations in reviews for inclusion in a magazine, newspaper, or broadcast. For information write to Other Press LLC, 267 Fifth Avenue, 6th Floor, New York, NY 10016. Or visit our Web site: www.otherpress.com.

Library of Congress Cataloging-in-Publication Data

Tucker, William M.
How people change : the short story as case history / William M. Tucker
p. cm.
ISBN-13: 978-1-59051-212-8 (alk. paper)
ISBN-10: 1-59051-212-X (alk. paper)
1. Psychotherapy. 2. Psychotherapy in literature. I. Title.
[DNLM: 1. Patients—psychology. 2. Literature. 3. Life Change Events. 4. Physician—Patient Relations. W 85 T895h 2007]
RC480.T83 2007
616.89'14—dc22

2006024221

For Sheila,
who changed me

Contents

Foreword

It was not until I was in graduate school in the humanities that I realized poems had meaning, and that poets were trying to communicate to readers or listeners what they felt, passionately, about ways of seeing or feeling. That is, poems were worth reading closely, for their content. The poet Wordsworth said they arose from "emotion recollected in tranquility." As an undergraduate all I had recognized was that their words had music to them and made for beautiful images. Much later, after medical school and fifteen years or so of clinical practice, I came back to another version of that split between life and literature, between experience and structured experience. I stumbled upon short stories as a form of poetry attenuated, revealed, and ready for use. Patients began to seem to me like characters in a handful of these stories, which were applicable to one clinical situation after another. I started teaching these stories to residents and colleagues as if they were clinical cases. Later, I began to offer them to patients as ways of looking at their own experiences. This book discusses the impact that skillful writers have on us through the plots, characters, and situations they present in their stories.

Acknowledgments

The author gratefully acknowledges permission to reprint the following material:

"Grisha," "Oysters," and "Gooseberries" from *Tales of Chekhov* by Anton Chekhov, translated by Constance Garnett. Published by The Ecco Press, 1984. Copyright © 1917, 1944, 1972 by Macmillan Company (now in the public domain).

"The Rocking-Horse Winner," copyright 1933 by the estate of D. H. Lawrence, renewed © 1961 by Angelo Ravagli and C. M. Weekley, executors of the estate of Frieda Lawrence, from *Complete Short Stories of D. H. Lawrence* by D. H. Lawrence. Used by permission of Viking Penguin, a division of Penguin Group (USA) Inc.

"Good-bye Marcus, Good-bye Rose" and "Sleep It Off, Lady" from *Jean Rhys: The Collected Short Stories*, W.W. Norton & Company, Inc. New York. Copyright © 1976, 1987 by Jean Rhys. Used by permission of the Wallace Literary Agency, Inc.

"Araby" and "The Dead" from *Dubliners* by James Joyce, copyright © 1916 by B. W. Heubsch. Definitive text copyright © 1967 by the estate of James Joyce. Used by permission of Viking Penguin, a division of Penguin Group (USA) Inc.

"Her First Ball" from *The Short Stories of Katherine Mansfield* by Katherine Mansfield, copyright © 1923 by Alfred A. Knopf, a division of Random House, Inc. and renewed 1951 by John Middleton Murry. Used by permission of Alfred A. Knopf, a division of Random House, Inc.

"The Man Who Was Almost a Man" from *Eight Men* by Richard Wright. Copyright © 1961 Richard Wright. Reprinted by permission of John Hawkins & Associates, Inc.

"In Dreams Begin Responsibilities" by Delmore Schwartz, from *In Dreams Begin Responsibilities*, copyright © 1937, 1978 by New Directions Publishing. Reprinted by permission of New Directions Publishing Corporation.

"My First Marriage" taken from *Out of India* by Ruth Prawer Jhabvala. Copyright © Ruth Prawer Jhabvala. Reproduced by permission of John Murray (Publishers) Limited.

"Good Country People" from *A Good Man is Hard to Find and Other Stories*, copyright © 1955 by Flannery O'Connor and renewed 1983 by Regina O'Connor, reprinted by permission of Harcourt, Inc.

"The Adulterous Woman" from *Exile and the Kingdom* by Albert Camus, translated by Justin O'Brien, copyright © 1957, 1958 by Alfred A. Knopf, a division of Random House, Inc. Used by permission of Alfred A. Knopf, a division of Random House, Inc.

"He" from *Flowering Judas and Other Stories*, copyright © 1930 and renewed 1958 by Katherine Anne Porter, reprinted by permission of Harcourt, Inc.

"The Overcoat" from *The Overcoat & Other Tales of Good and Evil* by Nicolai Gogol, translated by David Magarshack, copyright © 1957 by David Magarshack. Used by permission of Doubleday, a division of Random House, Inc.

Colleagues too numerous to mention have contributed suggestions to the analyses of the stories presented here, doing their best to help me avoid idiosyncrasies of interpretation. Among the most persistent have been Suzanne Flater, R.N., Jane Fried, M.D., Kathleen Ibrahim, R.N., David Joseph, M.D., Clarice Kestenbaum, M.D., Randall Marshall, M.D., Lawrence Maayan, M.D., Gerald Segal, M.A., Gretchen Seirmarco, R.N., Steven Simring, M.D., Helle Thorning, Ph.D., Donna Vermes, R.N., and Joseph Youngerman, M.D.

Introduction

The purpose of this book is to show practitioners and teachers of medicine how to use short stories to illustrate change at different phases of life. It draws on the richness and drama that great writers use in short stories to illustrate their insights into character, growth, and the process of change. It offers a simple, systematic way to use short stories to highlight these elements for physicians-in-training and practicing physicians who desire to expand their scope of knowledge about people and about how they change.

Goal

The goal of this book is to encourage practitioners and teachers of medicine to use the characters in these stories and the changes they undergo to understand more fully what their patients may be experiencing. Patients expect their physicians not merely to listen to them and to be curious, but also to know what is important in life: how relationships develop, how people of different ages can change and grow, and how, given their particular strengths and weaknesses, they can do so. That is, patients expect their physicians to pass on a certain amount of wisdom. Wisdom is precisely what no amount of training in medicine confers. It comes only out of an accumulation of experience and reflection, and even then, only by chance and in fragments, and to those with a talent for picking it up. Thus, we feel at least a little fraudulent at the beginning of our medical careers, and even later on, when confronted with a patient whose problem we have not encountered, we feel similarly so. Patients tend to forget that we have our limitations when it comes to empathy and understanding, limitations that the insights and power of great writers can help us overcome.

The Tradition of Medical Humanities

I have long wanted to bridge this gap in knowledge and experience through practical and accessible ways that respect the exigencies of our training and clinical commitments. For most people, regardless of cultural background or educational level, the quickest route to wisdom, other than the hard way (that is, through experience), is through anecdotal stories. Children grow up on stories in the form of fairy tales; adolescents regale one another with stories of their favorite heroes, sports or otherwise; and adults convey their most important feelings and experiences to one another by presenting them in the form of stories. Stories condense and heighten experience and make it memorable; more importantly, they give it meaning. "Stories" in this sense are anecdotes. Robert Coles, M.D., a child psychiatrist at Harvard, in *The Call of Stories: Teaching and the Moral Imagination* (Houghton Mifflin, Boston, 1989) offered brief, poignant accounts of patients' and doctors' experiences of illness.

Many teachers of medicine have recognized the potential of narrative, which is an extended and more formalized form of anecdote, to help both patients and trainees in medicine better understand their experiences of suffering and illness. A refinement within this tradition is the practice of regarding psychotherapy itself as the construction of personal narrative, giving form and meaning to the patient's experience. The function of narrative in psychotherapy has been explored in depth, most notably by Donald Spence, Ph.D., and by Roy Schafer, Ph.D.

More recently, medical schools have recognized the importance of humane education and have drawn on the construction of narrative as an approach to better understanding both their trainees' and their patients' experiences. At least one medical school has established a program in narrative medicine, and its director, Rita Charon, M.D., Ph.D., founded and edits a journal, *Literature and Medicine,* devoted to these issues. She has argued forcibly that attentive reading is akin to good listening and that both help bridge the gap between "the molecules and the metaphors." These noteworthy efforts are focused on the notion of stories as developed anecdotes. The oral tale, as Joyce Carol Oates reminds us in her introduction to her anthology, *The Oxford Book of American Short Stories* (Oxford University Press, New York, 1992), is the "ancestor" of the literary short story.

In the therapeutic realm, this approach has recently been applied to the treatment of victims of severe trauma, where it has been conceptualized as the attempt to make their terrible experience "only" a story, one of many in their past. Otherwise, victims of repeated abuse in childhood, for example, risk remaining mired in the reliving of their traumata and precluded from engagement in their current lives. Phoebe, in "Good-bye Marcus, Good-bye Rose," decides she will accept the altered trajectory forced on her by her own traumatic experience and use it, perhaps, to her advantage.

Freud himself, of course, used works by great writers—notably Sophocles, Shakespeare, and Goethe—to buttress his arguments for the universality of his concepts of the unconscious and of internal conflict. Following him, there is a long tradition of using literature and other artistic forms to validate psychoanalytic theory. This is one goal of the psychoanalytic studies of art by Lawrence Kubie, M.D. Residency training programs in psychiatry have borrowed from this tradition by considering works of literature to illustrate pathology, for example, Alan Stone's *Abnormal Personality Through Literature* (Prentice-Hall, Englewood Cliffs, 1966). That both this and Coles's books remain in print attests to the usefulness of providing literary references for the training of residents in psychiatry and other medical specialties.

Doctors' Limited Experience of Life

Why is empathy not enough in itself to understand our patients? In theory it should be, but in reality, most of us physicians simply have not had many of these life experiences, and even when we have, in our lives or through those of people close to us, there are limits to our comprehension, limits that the great writers have transcended. They simply have understood more about life than the rest of us, and they know how to elevate experience to the level of meaning. The ability to write case histories that work symbolically and convey the sense of life in all its richness is something that even experienced psychiatrists, with the exception of Freud and of D. W. Winnicott, have not possessed. Furthermore, there are a host of important clinical issues—deformity, spirituality, disability, ethnicity and culture, and abuse, just to name a few—with which we often have less familiarity than our patients do. Finally, most of us realized early on that we would have to develop extensive study skills in order to compete for admission to medical school. Therefore, many of us gave up the kind of experimentation with life that other adolescents pursued, and as a result, we are likely to have a narrower range of experiences than many of our patients.

There is a characterological issue in this for us as well, cloaked in our professional demeanor. By necessity, we distance ourselves from our patients' suffering. "Isolation of affect," the technical term for this distancing, can be an asset in our daily work. On the other hand, how are we to know what our patients are experiencing if we lack an emotional connection? For me, from an early age, literature was the window through which I could see what others felt. It helped me to become, in John Donne's words, "involved in mankind."

Short Stories

This book sets out to extend the efforts of those medical humanists in a practical way, with the premise that the insights of great writers may be used in the service of teaching doctors about life. Here, "stories" are literary productions and are fictional. Since the time of Homer, the best storytellers, at least in the West, have been writers of fiction. To some extent through skill and technique, but also certainly through gift and inspiration, writers have been able to do more with stories than condense, heighten, and instruct: they have been able to convey the richness of life with all its dazzle and possibility. Each piece of great fiction conveys not only a sense of the reality of the particular situation and characters it describes, but also of all of life. That is, it is convincing—not only on the intellectual but also on the emotional level, on the conscious and the unconscious. Great writers know how to make each situation and each detail work as a symbol, uniting the idea with the feeling. And they make the events and characters they describe memorable. We come away from literary stories with the sense that we know the characters, often better than our patients and even better than the people in our own lives.

It is possible to target stories to the interests and needs of various groups of trainees. Stories fill gaps in their life experiences. Reading a story such as James Joyce's "Araby" helps us to recapture elements of our own lost adolescence and thus better assess normality in this confusing developmental phase. Similarly, a story such as Anton Chekhov's "Gooseberries" helps us understand some of the despair and unresolved longings that even relatively well-adjusted older adults might feel at moments of heightened awareness, when they regret having missed out on or failed to pursue possibilities earlier in their lives. Young physicians who withdraw from involvement with elderly people facing deterioration and death may understand their own fears better by reading Jean Rhys's "Sleep It Off, Lady," a story that depicts in graphic detail an elderly alcoholic woman's withdrawal from her familiar surroundings.

It is not only trainees who may forget earlier life experiences. Teachers of medical students and residents also find stories help them reexperience some of the difficulties they may have forgotten in their own learning process. A story such as D. H. Lawrence's "The Rocking-Horse Winner" helped a group of teachers of child psychiatry recall the difficulty in planning the treatment of a case. They had to decide whether to approach the child's problems directly or through treatment of the mother. Katherine Mansfield's "Her First Ball" provides an example of intergenerational competition. This story helped a group of teachers of psychotherapy experience afresh some of the intensity of their difficult teaching experiences, when some of them identified with the adolescent girl, and some with the middle-aged man who tries to ruin her excitement.

Great stories speak not only across generational lines but also across cultures. Stories by their nature emphasize the commonality of human experience in a way that helps trainees overcome deficiencies in cultural knowledge. Certain stories break down cultural bias and stereotype. Ruth Prawer Jhabvala's "My First Marriage" illustrates the kind of play and freedom that a traditional Hindu family permits. In discussions of this story a group of Asian physicians acknowledged their own cultural biases against the role of the guru and of animism. Even the highly problematic issue of race yields something to this approach. Ralph Ellison's "Flying Home" provides insight into the ineluctable and regressive forces of racism that draw the main character, a black pilot, down to earth and to humiliation. He has crash-landed in a field in the South and because of his color is taken for insane rather than injured, since neither black nor white rescuers believe a black man could be a pilot. After discussion of this story a black medical student introduced several other stories relevant to racial issues, written by the first well-known black American fiction writer, Charles Chesnutt. This experience is typical: trainees and teachers bring in stories that have had a particular impact on them.

Stories offer insight into the psychological issues involved in certain specialized and unfamiliar situations, issues whose understanding is often counterintuitive. Flannery O'Connor's "Good Country People" illustrates the investment a deformed person has in the deformity. Katherine Anne Porter's "He" illustrates the consequences of denying the limitations of a retarded child.

Teachers of young physicians may also use stories in case discussion. When a resident reported that a patient had asked how he might take charge of this life, the teacher suggested that the trainee formulate an answer by reading Joseph Conrad's "The Secret Sharer," which depicts a young sea captain taking command by embracing and integrating the aggressive aspects of his personality.

As Freud knew and used so well, stories can illustrate psychoanalytic concepts that had not even been articulated when the stories were written. When asked to find the source of the downtrodden hero's inspiration to buy himself a new overcoat in Nikolai Gogol's "The Overcoat," trainees correctly recognized that Gogol was inadvertently illustrating the comforting and inspiring effects of a so-called transitional object.

In responding to stories, one is both close to the events and characters and also able to stand back from them. Strong negative reactions to characters in stories help trainees understand what would be too painful to acknowledge with an actual patient, where negative reactions and fear of failure might cloud their awareness of the problem. Responding to

Herman Melville's "Bartleby, the Scrivener" one resident became impatient with the narrator, announcing that the narrator's indulgence of Bartleby in his increasing withdrawal was not credible and that the story, therefore, did not hold together. Later in the discussion he revealed that during his childhood his parents had taken in an uncommunicative old sailor, pampering him and insisting that their children cede a place to him in the family. This revelation was instrumental in promoting self-awareness that, in turn, improved his clinical skills.

Points of view vary with the age and life experience of the trainees, demonstrating that there is no single interpretation of a story, any more than of a clinical case. Nevertheless, trainees are able to maintain a more consistent view of a character than they usually do with their actual patients; they even see characters as more human and, paradoxically, less objectified and pathological. Stories tend to de-pathologize; they make it easier for trainees to engage on both an emotional and an intellectual level. Trainees speak more freely about characters in stories than they dare to about their own or colleagues' cases.

Why is the short-story format particularly serviceable for this purpose? A short story takes no longer to read than a typical case write-up, 30 to 45 minutes. Therefore, it fits naturally into the format often used for case conferences in many medical specialties. Residents or medical students can, and frequently do, read it over lunch, just prior to showing up for the conference. They are used to a standard format for case write-ups, so the simple set of questions laid out for the analysis of each story seems familiar. More important even than these elements of preparation, however, is the serviceability of the short-story format for discussion. Since the case write-up is the story itself, and since it can be counted on to hold together so well, each participant has the same information as the teacher, and no lesser claim to authority. This contrasts with the usual case discussion, where the treating physician or student always has more clinical information than she or he has written in the summary, and where the teacher's greater knowledge of medicine always lends a greater authority to her or his clinical impressions.

Longer literary formats, by contrast, require that considerable time be devoted outside the usual clinical setting; furthermore, they present the difficulty of locating specific passages quickly in the course of discussion. Readers cannot hold an entire novel in their minds, as they can a short story. Other formats, such as film, may be even more accessible to those brought up in the current popular culture, but they also require more time than the typical case write-up and also impose difficulties finding the specific segments a participant may choose to focus on in discussions. Given the presently available technology, only the preceptor would have the prerogative of preselecting favorite or illustrative film segments. To the degree that the approach to creative works such as these has remained unsystematic, their use tends for the most part to be relegated to after-hours discussions at the homes of faculty members and is regarded as outside the core curriculum—an enjoyable and stimulating exercise, but hardly central to preparation for clinical work. By contrast, the approach to short stories proposed here assumes that their study is as relevant to medical practice as any other body of knowledge.

CHANGE

Even among the skeptical there are at least two widely accepted models of change: (1) growth and development from childhood to maturity, and (2) religious awakening. The former includes not only the unfolding or acquisition of new age-appropriate skills and abilities, but more importantly, greater flexibility and self-awareness, based on experience and learning of all kinds, that permit individuals to adapt to demands that they could not have managed earlier in life. The latter, taken either narrowly in the sense of a specific religious tradition or broadly in a general, spiritual sense, and emerging either from within, as from the impact of experience, or from without, as through "grace" or meditation, refers to an awakening in which individuals see the larger picture or context of their actions. "The scales fell from my eyes," as the saying goes. James Joyce called such a moment of awakening an "epiphany," a term combining both literary and religious perspectives. Wordsworth called this experience "see[ing] into the heart of things." Since it is central to the human experience, it should not be surprising that the process of change would be an appropriate subject for literature.

What about change through psychotherapy? Some patients deliberately seek it out, while others fear it will happen to them. In *How People Change* (Harper & Row, New York, 1973) the psychoanalyst Allen Wheelis takes the view that "personality change follows change in behavior. Since we are what we do, if we want to change what we are we must begin by changing what we do. . . . Change will occur only if such action is maintained over a long period of time." More broadly, we physicians may be regarded as change agents every time we attempt to bring about healthier lifestyles in our patients.

Change as illustrated and reflected in these stories encompasses both the common notions of this process—compromised growth and development (as in "Grisha," "Oysters," "Good-bye Marcus, Good-bye Rose," "Her First Ball," and "The Man Who Was Almost a Man"), and religious awakening (as in a possible reading of "Good Country People," "The Dead," or perhaps "Gooseberries")—as well as a range of examples following the Eriksonian models (see next section), including both failed attempts at change (Paul's efforts in "The Rocking-Horse Winner," Akaky's in "The Overcoat," or the soldier's in "The Kiss") or even change for the worse (as in "Sleep It Off, Lady"). Some stories explicitly announce at the end that things are different, such as the transformation Leila has undergone with the loss of her naïveté by the end of "Her First Ball," or the expectation that life has many more possibilities, as Phoebe recognizes at the end of "Good-bye Marcus, Good-bye Rose," but these are exceptions.

Change for the better, in literature as in life, generally follows a whole succession of failures. These have resulted from the inadequate repertoire of actions and responses that real people or fictional characters bring to the problems they face in loving or working. The inevitable response of each of us to such failures is to rationalize them somehow and then to try again, only harder. We cannot see beyond our habitual perspectives and, except under unusually favorable circumstances, we cannot accept constructive advice. But eventually, the cascade of failures wears us down, and we become open to a new way of approaching old problems. We step onto uncertain ground, sometimes emerging with more than we could have bargained for. Each of these stories illustrating change presents just such a cascade of events, leading up to the climax that offers a new resolution.

To show change and growth is a difficult feat in a literary work of any length, let alone in a short story. Each of these stories shows a character caught off-guard and suddenly vulnerable in the course of a situation that is not in itself extraordinary for the character. That is, it is a moment not brought about by external circumstances, but rather by the character's own desire to make something more of an ordinary event. Often the climactic moment occurs when the expected event fails to occur, as when the pubescent boy in "Araby" fails to find an appropriate gift for his first love at the fair, or when Gabriel Conroy's wife fails to share his fantasies for the evening in "The Dead," or when the veterinarian Ivan's story of how his brother has found happiness fails to have the desired effect upon his friend, the schoolteacher, in "Gooseberries." It is the character's reaction to this failed expectation that reveals all the preparation for the moment, all the anguish and creative tension that have gone before. Here again, as is typical, the nature of the change is left unsaid, implicit, yet suggested by the rush of events, up for grabs, and open for discussion.

Even those who accept that change is possible, however, differ as to their notions of how it comes about. Is it anything beyond simple unfolding? Can it be actively sought, or does it come as a gift from outside? What is the role of cognitive processes, such as education, including self-education through reading or through examination of experience? Once change has occurred, can the individual regress to prior, less adaptive modes of functioning? Classical Freudian theory is not explicit on these points, in part because it generally implies that character is set by age 5, when psychosexual development—the oral, anal, and genital stages—is complete. But the psychoanalyst Erik Erikson, though certainly a Freudian at heart, was in fact explicit about this possibility. He elaborated a notion that he called "epigenesis," or ongoing development.

Erikson's Framework for Defining Change

Although he does not mention change explicitly in this context, Erikson provides us with an ideal framework for defining it. In everyday language he presents the terms that measure its dimensions, positively and negatively, at each stage of life. He describes what he calls the "life cycle," which he divides into eight "ages," each characterized by its own specific, age-appropriate conflict. At each of these ages there is an opportunity to resolve the conflict more—or less—successfully than during the preceding one, so that change in either direction should be possible, from birth to death. These conflicts are (1) basic trust vs. basic mistrust (0 to 18 months of age), (2) autonomy vs. shame and doubt (18 to 36 months), (3) initiative vs. guilt (3 to 5 years), (4) industry vs. inferiority (6 to 10 years), (5) ego identity vs. role confusion (11 to 17 years), (6) intimacy vs. isolation (18 to 40 years), (7) generativity vs. stagnation (40 to 60 years), and (8) ego integrity vs. despair (60 years to the end of life).

I have grouped the stories included in this book according to these ages. Thus one focus for the issue of change in each of them will include the conflict Erikson has identified for any person of that age, in addition to the specific issues that the particular character faces in the course of the story. You, the reader, are asked to consider whether a character in a story has changed, that is, whether that character has successfully resolved her or his age-appropriate conflict. For example, has Gabriel Conroy, the central character in Joyce's "The Dead," not only given up some of his narcissism in favor of an appreciation of his wife as a person in her own right but also moved toward generativity, that is, regeneration, and away from stagnation, that is, the danger of only repeating interactions and activities he has developed up to that time in his life?

Another important issue about the succession of these stages is that, either at the beginning or during the course of each one, it is necessary to relinquish the gains achieved at the previous stage. Thus, for example, it is critical to consolidate identity during adolescence, in order to be able to give it up in critical situations faced by the young adult that require merger, such as the achievement of intimacy. This necessary abandonment of previous gains creates a new risk, and there is no guarantee based on earlier successes that the next resolution will succeed.

What follows are excerpts from Erikson's descriptions of the defining conflicts for each of the "Eight Ages of Man" (*Childhood and Society*, W.W. Norton, New York, 1950). Readers may want to refer back to them before reading the stories in each successive section. His terms—trust, initiative, industry, identity, etc.—have both broadly understood as well as narrower technical meanings, and thus serve to link the literary and clinical worlds.

1. Basic Trust vs. Basic Mistrust

"The infant's first social achievement, then, is his willingness to let the mother out of sight without undue anxiety or rage, because she has become an inner certainty as well as an outer predictability. Such consistency, continuity, and sameness of experience provide a rudimentary sense of ego identity which depends, I think, on the recognition that there is an inner population of remembered and anticipated sensations and images which are firmly correlated with the outer population of familiar and predictable things and people."

2. Autonomy vs. Shame and Doubt

"This stage becomes decisive, therefore, for the ratio of love and hate, cooperation and willfulness, freedom of self-expression and its suppression. From a sense of self-control without loss of self-esteem comes a lasting sense of good will and pride; from a sense of loss of self-control and of foreign overcontrol comes a lasting propensity for doubt and shame."

3. Initiative vs. Guilt

"Initiative adds to autonomy the quality of undertaking, planning and 'attacking' a task for the sake of being active and on the move, where before self-will, more often than not, inspired acts of defiance or, at any rate, protested independence. . . . The danger of this stage is a sense of guilt over the goals contemplated and the acts initiated in one's exuberant enjoyment of new locomotor and mental power: acts of aggressive manipulation and coercion which soon go far beyond the executive capacity of organism and mind and therefore call for an energetic halt on one's contemplated initiative."

4. Industry vs. Inferiority

"With the oncoming latency period, the normally advanced child forgets, or rather sublimates, the necessity to 'make' people by direct attack or to become papa and mama in a hurry: he now learns to win recognition by producing things. . . . He has experienced a sense of finality regarding the fact that there is no workable future within the womb of his family, and thus becomes ready to apply himself to given skills and tasks, which go far beyond the mere playful expression of his organ modes [i.e., oral, anal, or genital] or the pleasure in the function of his limbs. He develops a sense of industry—i.e., he adjusts himself to the inorganic laws of the tool world. . . . If he despairs of his tools and skills or of his status among his tool partners, he may be discouraged from identification with them and with a section of the tool world."

5. Ego Identity vs. Role Confusion

"In their search for a new sense of continuity and sameness, adolescents have to refight many of the battles of earlier years, even though to do so they must artificially appoint perfectly well-meaning people to play the roles of adversaries; and they are ever ready to install lasting idols and ideals as guardians of a final identity. . . . The integration of ego identity is more than the sum of the childhood identifications. It is the accrued experience of the ego's ability to integrate all identifications with the vicissitudes of the libido, with the aptitudes developed out of endowment, and with the opportunities offered in social roles. The sense of ego identity, then, is the accrued confidence that the inner sameness and continuity prepared in the past are matched by the sameness and continuity of one's meaning for others, as evidenced in the tangible promise of a 'career.'"

6. Intimacy vs. Isolation

"Intimacy is the capacity to commit oneself to concrete affiliations and partnerships and to develop the ethical strength to abide by such commitments, even though they may call for significant sacrifices and compromises. Body and ego must now be masters of the organ modes and of the nuclear conflicts, in order to be able to face the fear of ego loss in situations which call for self-abandon: in the solidarity of close affiliations, in orgasm and sexual unions, in close friendships and in physical combat, in experiences of inspiration by teachers and of intuition from the recesses of the self. The avoidance of such experiences because of a fear of ego loss may lead to a deep sense of isolation and consequent self-absorption."

7. Generativity vs. Stagnation

"This term encompasses the evolutionary development which has made man the teaching and instituting as well as the learning animal. . . . Mature man needs to be needed, and maturity needs guidance as well as encouragement from what had been produced and must be taken care of. . . . [It] is primarily the concern in establishing and guiding the next generation. Where such enrichment fails altogether, regression to an obsessive need for pseudo-intimacy takes place, often with a pervading sense of stagnation and personal impoverishment."

8. Ego Integrity vs. Despair

"It is the ego's accrued assurance of its proclivity for order and meaning. It is a post-narcissistic love of the human ego—not of the self—as an experience which conveys some world order and spiritual sense, no matter how dearly paid for. It is the acceptance of one's one and only life cycle as something that had to be and that, by necessity, permitted of no substitutions. It is a comradeship with the ordering ways of distant times and different pursuits, as expressed in the simple products and sayings of such times and pursuits. Although aware of the relativity of all the various life styles which have given meaning to human striving, the possessor of integrity is ready to defend the dignity of his own life style against all physical and economic threats."

Case Histories

The medical case history is the formalized summary, presented orally at the bedside or in written form in the chart, of the relevant findings on which treatment is to be based. It begins with the immediate precipitant bringing the patient to treatment, proceeds through a review of recent and earlier symptoms and possible contributing factors, and ends with a limited number of likely underlying causes—the so-called differential diagnosis. Ideally, the presenter or writer has sifted, gleaned, and mixed the elements so successfully that they form a consistent pattern in the listener's or reader's mind, even before the presentation is complete. It aims at "economy" of etiological factors, such that one etiology from the traditional categories—genetic, developmental, infectious, traumatic, or neoplastic—can usually explain all aspects of the current pathology.

Students of medicine spend hours with the patient and from months to years learning to formulate such summaries before they are able to deliver them in a succinct and meaningful way to their teachers and peers. Some medical schools lay more emphasis on executing this process expertly than others, and as a result not all summaries are equally useful for the formulation of treatment; indeed, the advent of more exhaustive diagnostic tests has at times excused a more cursory rendition of the case history. But the history is critical, for starters, to the establishment of the doctor–patient relationship, to say nothing of the planning of the trajectory of treatment beyond the immediate intervention. Later reviews allow for open-ended discussion as to whether the treatment was successful or is likely to require further intervention. Such reviews are far from routine and ordinarily occur only if initial treatment is unsuccessful, or at the time of a recurrence of symptoms, or in the highly useful if sometimes painful setting of the postmortem conference that is a routine feature of good clinical departments.

Psychiatric case histories modify the general medical format to some extent with their greater emphasis on the psychosocial and, often to their loss, a more cursory review of the general systemic, but include the same categories and aim. Their main contribution to the process of formulating case histories may be in taking a generally longer time frame as their point of reference.

Medicine derives from science, which, proceeding from statistically expectable and replicable observations, applies them to the individual case. Literature proceeds in the opposite direction, creating the individualized situation that, when successful, is recognized by the observer as universally "true." In the approach that follows, I have selected five questions that are roughly analogous to those included in the typical medical case history, including course of treatment and prognosis, but they are couched in language that allows their application to the fictional situation.

1

A Method for Discussing Short Stories as Case Histories

I will show how stories illustrate change by using them to do so. Medical students learning about the process of change are able to relate particularly well to stories, since stories do not depend on familiarity with specialized psychiatric or literary terminology. The sixteen stories selected for analysis here follow the course of the human life cycle as defined by Erikson. Each is by someone widely considered to be a great writer, and each deliberately presents, convincingly or not, a process of change. For heuristic purposes a story may be compared to a course of medical treatment, to a crucial visit in its course, or, more narrowly, to an intense encounter with a physician. Taken in this way, stories offer a whole catalogue of treatment summaries, which are easy to recall and to apply to ongoing cases.

I propose five questions to frame an analysis of each of the sixteen stories. They highlight the elements of change in the characters and relate them to potential clinical situations, that is, those that might arise if a patient resembling one of these characters came to one of us for issues similar to those in the story itself. Each character and situation then becomes part of the repertoire of our treated cases.

I make no claim for the originality of this approach but only for its simplicity and predictability. Thus, it allows physicians and trainees reading stories as case histories to anticipate what to focus on in their readings of each story, and what to anticipate in discussions of them. These questions attempt to bridge the gap between the events of the story and the clinical realm. They do not depend on familiarity with literary history or theory, even less with psychoanalytic theory. Other versions of these questions or another set altogether might be just as serviceable. The five questions are as follows:

(1) *Whose story is it, that is, who, if anyone, changes? (Who is the patient?)*

This question seems equivalent to asking who is the principal character, who is usually the one most likely to change. Such is not always the case, however. Sometimes the subject of change is a kind of unit, such as the mother and son together in "The Rocking-Horse Winner." Sometimes it is the narrator, as in "Bartleby." Sometimes it may be a somewhat fluid group of onlookers and peripheral characters, as in "The Overcoat." This question is akin to identifying the patient. Like the initial description in a good case history, it requires the presenter to sum up how this character strikes her or him as a person in a few words—for example, "this favorite nephew, married and with children, in his early to mid-40's, who supports himself as a teacher and freelance journalist," to describe Gabriel Conroy, the principal character in "The Dead."

(2) *What is the nature of this character's problem as the story opens? (What is the chief complaint and the history of the present illness?)*

This question asks for the patient's history from the physician's perspective. It asks what is wrong with this character, even if he or she would not necessarily acknowledge having this problem, any more than some patients will acknowledge, beyond a perfunctory dismissal, the unhealthy lifestyle that has eventuated in their symptoms. It should include Erikson's stage-appropriate conflict—in the example of Gabriel, this would be the signs of his beginning to stagnate rather than regenerate himself. But it must be specific to the character. The physician might see him as a well-intentioned but mildly pompous man with very limited self-awareness who is consequently vulnerable to repeated bouts of self-doubt and anxiety.

(3) *What is the nature of the change that this character undergoes? (The treatment summary)*

This question refers to the details of the course of treatment. The event that grips the reader's attention is the crisis, usually inevitable, that is now occurring in the character's life. Everything that has gone before, and that is revealed only in the most abbreviated form in such a brief format, has been leading up to it. Usually many factors combine to provide the impact, and untangling the particular ones responsible for the change will necessarily remain subjective. In Gabriel's case each of the discomfiting encounters and recollections stirred up in him by the party, as well as its general stimulation, repeated in highly intensified form during the encounter with his wife thereafter, contributes to the dissolving and reconstituting process he undergoes.

(4) *Will this character be likely to maintain this change in the face of future challenges, and in particular, how is he or she likely to develop in the future or to respond to crises of a similar nature? (The prognosis)*

This question, of course, refers to the prognosis for this character. Though the brief, vertical slice we have been given may have been critical, it is hardly likely to be unique for this character's life. Even if the special circumstances do not recur, confronting the next stage of life will necessarily require at least a relinquishment and reformulation of the current gains. As with a clinical case review, this is perhaps the most subjective element, as it is for the fictional character, because the suggestion about the future is usually relegated to no more than a final image or few words. Has Gabriel's surrender to the powerful image of the snow, "general over Ireland," indeed brought him in touch with his cultural and affective heritage, such that he can finally be whole and strong enough to accept and love his wife as a separate and distinct person?

(5) *What would it be like to encounter an actual patient similar to this character in a clinical situation, and what approaches would be most likely to help—or to hinder—this character's change in a positive direction? (The relationship to the physician)*

This question invites you to accept the character into your practice, at least hypothetically. Though you may not have encountered such a person before, surely there have been similar or analogous ones. The story itself, where such a change-agent has necessarily been described in some detail, frequently suggests an effective model. Sometimes this agent has been quite harsh, as with the painful encounters with the three women, Lily, Molly, and finally Gretta, who may be said finally to have brought Gabriel around. Though experienced physicians are well aware of the necessity of causing pain in order to promote healing, younger ones may be overly fearful of confronting this necessity and thus retreat behind the shibboleth of the neutral, professional stance.

While these five questions frame the approach, the process involves fitting each piece of the plot and characterization together, word by word, image by image, and step by step. If any new bit of information does not seem to fit, you will have to pause and figure out what you have missed or misunderstood, since in these stories everything fits seamlessly.

Uses of Group Discussion

Both residents and colleagues endeavoring to discuss short stories in this way tend to respond fairly predictably. Even after considerable experience with this method, most are skeptical, on first reading, that the story has illustrated change. Almost invariably, first readings lead to pessimistic conclusions about the possibility of change. Readers react with confusion or disappointment to the absence of any clear evidence that change has occurred. They are likely to come away with the impression that more questions about change have been raised than answered. Asked their first impressions of "The Dead," for example, many readers will recall a melancholy sense of loss, rather than new possibility. In my experience, something happens to this initial response, however, in the process of group discussion, independent of the discussion leader's influence, who, in any event, has no more claim to authority in her or his interpretations than does any other reader. As individual participants see their views reflected and refined through the group discussion, they tend toward more positive interpretations of change.

I would not discount my influence on moving interpretations in this direction, but I believe I am only following the lead of these authors in exerting it. Not only their individual stories, but also their gifts of structuring experience in the first place, show how to take a step back and establish distance from our experience, so as to learn from it and see how to use it to do better. The act of structuring the chaotic material of life, intrinsic to writing a story, is itself a comforting, reassuring, and even hopeful exercise.

Like group learning in clinical situations (the tradition of "see one, do one, teach one"), this approach becomes familiar through practice. It is better than self- or individualized teaching in being able to convey a multiplicity of views that remain, nevertheless, consistent across the five questions. It is useful to have male medical students learn about women's psychology by analyzing stories in a group together with women and vice versa, and to compare responses to a given story by participants of different age groups and life experiences.

Stories depicting change in a credible way do not necessarily beat the reader over the head with what has happened; that is, they do not have the character announce how or whether she or he has changed. Indeed, many end in disappointment or failure or at least sound a melancholy note. This is a subtle process, one where we do not see the authors manipulate us to hammer home the point. They do not insist that change has occurred, a rather pretentious claim, after all. So, Gabriel Conroy in "The Dead" has taken the necessary "journey westward," in his mind, at least, and seems to have achieved a measure of peace, for the first time. But is he only suffering from a sense of loss, or has he also embarked on a more satisfactory and satisfying life?

It is, therefore, frequently on rereading—or, as often happens, during class discussion—that the impression of opening up to something new arises. I have found that the experience of learning from the accumulation of examples and illustrations gradually overcomes resistance to the method. So lively is the discussion format, in fact, that I have found it a formidable challenge to render the effect of this process on the silent page.

In these discussions it is essential to stay with the data the story presents, rather than drifting off into a discussion of the writer's possible intent, whether that be based on literary history or theory, or on familiarity with the author, her or his contemporaries, or any literary tradition. It is essential that each question be answered by reference to a specific item in the text itself, whether explicit or implied. No single reader's analysis—certainly not mine—has any more validity than anyone else's.

I probably absorbed this approach during my undergraduate days, when I was exposed to the emerging school of New Criticism, where the work was presumed to stand alone, independent of its author. Each of these short stories reflects, of course, the time and place in which it was written. Nevertheless, if it reflected only its time and place, it would not have survived over time and spread across cultures. We identify with its characters and their travails, and this identification enables us to interpret each of the stories as if it were taken out of time and away from its author. This does not result, of course, in a balanced view, from a literary-historical perspective, but it is helpful in avoiding over-intellectualization and, in workshops, unproductive competition among participants.

What happens in a group discussion that leads to a different outcome regarding the possibility of change from mere individual reading occurs so regularly that it demands at least some tentative explanation. Why should groups be more optimistic about the possibility of change than individuals, after all? Group members speak to each other through the story, and they learn to be more objective. There may be something of the sense of support, of peers guiding each other through a difficult situation, even if no single participant knows the way, precisely, through it. Perhaps our shared experiences provide a greater range of solutions than anyone's alone. Physicians discussing difficult cases have such experiences not infrequently. Even if neither colleague has treated a given case previously, we can often help each other through it to a viable plan of treatment. Indeed, the mere process of formulating the case in order to present it to a colleague is frequently enough to provide the desired solution. So it is with the discussion of stories in a group format: one hears one's thoughts aloud as they are spoken, by oneself as well as by others, as if for the first time.

Lest this sound too personal, however, let me bring it around to an experience many of us have had in the course of our nonprofessional work. The common life experience probably closest to what the reader is being asked to bring to this way of analyzing short stories is that of serving on a jury. There the judge charges jury members, after the evidence has been summarized by the opposing attorneys, just prior to beginning jury deliberations, in reaching their verdict to consider only (1) the evidence presented, (2) their experience of life, and (3) common sense. That is, they are to discount any outside influences, whether extraneous information they may have acquired or any specialized or expert knowledge they may bring to the issues before them. Similarly here, readers are enjoined not to bring theoretical knowledge, particularly of the psychoanalytic or literary-historical variety, into their formulations, but rather to rely on the evidence presented by the story, by their clinical and life experience, and by their common sense and good judgment.

Caveats and Limitations

Beyond the adage—often an excuse for lack of precision—that medicine is an art as well as a science, there is the reality that the two worlds must intersect in the practitioner's mind, even though they are difficult to reconcile conceptually. Diagnosis and effective treatments emerge from objective and replicable observations; not all approaches are equally effective. Literary interpretations, by contrast, are subjective, and reasonable scholars will differ, although this fact does not mean that one interpretation is as good as another: skill and experience still count. Where literature presents the particular for consideration as universal, medicine presents the general and tries to apply it to the individual, with the result that the patient sometimes gets the feeling of lying on the Procrustean bed. But the patient, one way or another, will have a say in the process. The approach here offers a framework or tool for busy practitioners to use in increasing their understanding of the patients' experience of that process. Engaging in it requires a leap of faith or willing suspension of disbelief, in order to take in every detail and interpret it as a whole with definite meaning, just as an actual case history would ideally, though frequently not in practice, present a unified clinical picture.

I want to say one thing more about the discussions of the stories that follow. They are not interpretations, much less do they attempt to explain what the stories mean. The stories mean what they say, after all, and are readily available to anyone who will read them closely. Rather, these discussions are attempts at appreciations of the stories, in both senses of that word, and applications of the stories to clinical situations. Archibald MacLeish wrote, "A poem should not mean but be" (*Ars Poetica*, 1926). In her collection of essays, *Against Interpretation* (Farrar, Straus, & Giroux, New York, 1966), Susan Sontag wrote, "The aim of all commentary on art now should be to make works of art—and, by analogy, our own experience—more, rather than less, real to us. This function of criticism should be to show how it is what it is, even that it is what it is, rather than to show what it means." It is in this sense that I present these discussions.

Each of the stories discussed here has been the subject of class discussion in workshop format, and I have included a range of interpretations around many of the issues. However, as any teacher using this format will quickly discover, these stories, which have survived the test of time and frequently the translation across cultures, are open to a range of interpretations, depending on the life experiences and the particular skills and interests of each group of students or practitioners. Thus, as in the workshop discussions themselves, there is no claim for correctness of interpretation. Especially the conviction as to whether the presentation of change has been convincing or not will vary considerably. The only requirement for any given assertion is that it be carried through all five of the questions in a consistent fashion. Indeed, those utilizing this format will quickly discover that such a requirement is hardly necessary, since readers will tend on their own to develop internally consistent interpretations.

Because each story speaks to us so personally, it will necessarily evoke some of our most deeply held views of life, not to mention many of our intensely personal experiences. These associations will necessarily color each reader's responses. In psychoanalytic terms, each reader will be influenced by her or his countertransference reactions. (Whether these are disruptive distortions, as classical theory taught, or in fact useful to each person's understanding of interpersonal situations, is beyond the scope of this discussion.) Nevertheless, it is critical for group discussion that the instructor or discussion leader not denigrate what could be called a personalized or idiosyncratic reaction, because this will necessarily cause discussion participants to become self-conscious and pull back. It is much more useful for the development of meaningful discussion to focus on the generally relevant aspect that is contained in the personalized response.

Typically, a group of eight to ten participants will produce two or three distinct sets of interpretations, each internally consistent. Consensus is not the goal and would not even be desirable; in this respect, the stories more closely resemble living patients with ongoing issues rather than deceased ones with postmortem findings, for whom a single, final diagnosis usually emerges. Such a result is helpful, incidentally, in convincing students that there may be a range of defensible formulations of a differential diagnosis, of the effectiveness of a brief course of treatment, and, especially, of the prognosis for a case. Readers—especially groups of them in discussions together—will not fail to come up with refinements and extensions of the interpretations offered here. Be careful: students will continue to improve on whatever the instructor offers them, just as mine have.

Since this method depends on close reading, some interpretations of stories will be closer to the text than others, and thus more useful for promoting and expanding the discussion. It would be unrealistic to deny that some readers have more of a knack for this or simply more experience at doing it than others. But the method does not depend upon arriving at the best interpretation, since its focus, ultimately, is not the elucidation of the story but rather the issues in the lives of patients that require deeper understanding. When the discussion stimulates participants to rethink issues in their own lives or in those of particular patients, they find new ways to introduce change. Teachers in all clinical specialties should feel encouraged to use stories in this way to help structure the trajectory of personally challenging cases their trainees encounter.

Sixteen Stories Illustrating Change

There are two reasons why I have had to include the texts themselves in this book, even though most of the stories are well known and readily available in various editions and collections. The first is that this is intended as a textbook for workshops, where the method outlined in the previous section requires that the exact phrase or image under discussion must be readily retrievable. Thus students and teacher need the same edition and pagination. The second is that the discussions are most useful and convincing immediately upon completing the reading of a story; general familiarity is inadequate to support an argument for an interpretation, since everything is in the details. The discussions presented in what follows are not independent of the texts they refer to and do not stand alone.

The reader will note that there are stories for each of Erikson's eight stages except the first, "basic trust vs. basic mistrust (0 to 18 months)." I have not been able to find a story dealing with this stage and would be surprised to find one, since at this stage it would be difficult to conceive of a change in the infant, who is not yet differentiated as an individual, however much experienced neonatal care nurses may be able to decipher their temperaments.

I have selected each of these stories as an example of the process of change. I do not believe that most stories, even those by great authors, attempt to show change, nor do I believe that all readers will agree with me that all of these reprinted here do. I believe all of Shakespeare's tragedies and comedies show change, though not all of his so-called history plays—*Henry V*, for example—do, so this effort is not necessarily the marker of greatness. But since it is my subject, I look for it in every short story I read, and I am always disappointed when an otherwise fine story—in terms of character, plot, liveliness, and clarity of vision—turns out to be the more common variety, which is content merely to unfold a sequence of events without leading to change.

I have introduced the analysis of each story with a brief summary of the plot. This is intended simply as a refresher for the reader who has just finished the story. It is necessarily subjective and should not be taken as a substitute for the actual words of the story. (Note: some references are to stories not reprinted or discussed here but are included in the Appendix.)

2

The Short Stories

Anton Chekhov

GRISHA

Grisha, a chubby little boy, born two years and eight months ago, is walking on the boulevard with his nurse. He is wearing a long, wadded pelisse, a scarf, a big cap with a fluffy pom-pom, and warm over-boots. He feels hot and stifled, and now, too, the rollicking April sunshine is beating straight in his face, and making his eyelids tingle. The whole of his clumsy, timidly and uncertainly stepping little figure expresses the utmost bewilderment.

Hitherto Grisha has known only a rectangular world, where in one corner stands his bed, in the other nurse's trunk, in the third a chair, while in the fourth there is a little lamp burning. If one looks under the bed, one sees a doll with a broken arm and a drum; and behind nurse's trunk, there are a great many things of all sorts: cotton reels, boxes without lids, and a broken Jack-a-dandy. In that world, besides nurse and Grisha, there are often mamma and the cat. Mamma is like a doll, and puss is like papa's fur-coat, only the coat hasn't got eyes and a tail. From the world which is called the nursery a door leads to a great expanse where they have dinner and tea. There stands Grisha's chair on high legs, and on the wall hangs a clock which exists to swing its pendulum and chime. From the dining-room, one can go into a room where there are red arm-chairs. Here, there is a dark patch on the carpet, concerning which fingers are still shaken at Grisha. Beyond that room is still another, to which one is not admitted, and where one sees glimpses of papa—an extremely enigmatical person! Nurse and mamma are comprehensible: they dress Grisha, feed him, and put him to bed, but what papa exists for is unknown. There is another enigmatical person, auntie, who presented Grisha with a drum. She appears and disappears. Where does she disappear to? Grisha has more than once looked under the bed, behind the trunk, and under the sofa, but she was not there.

In this new world, where the sun hurts one's eyes, there are so many papas and mammas and aunties, that there is no knowing to whom to run. But what is stranger and more absurd than anything is the horses. Grisha gazes at their moving legs, and can make nothing of it. He looks at his nurse for her to solve the mystery, but she does not speak.

All at once he hears a fearful tramping. . . . A crowd of soldiers, with red faces and bath brooms under their arms, move in step along the boulevard straight upon him. Grisha turns cold all over with terror, and looks inquiringly at nurse to know whether it is dangerous. But nurse neither weeps nor runs away, so there is no danger. Grisha looks after the soldiers, and begins to move his feet in step with them himself.

Two big cats with long faces run after each other across the boulevard, with their tongues out, and their tails in the air. Grisha thinks that he must run too, and runs after the cats.

"Stop!" cries nurse, seizing him roughly by the shoulder. "Where are you off to? Haven't you been told not to be naughty?"

Here there is a nurse sitting holding a tray of oranges. Grisha passes by her, and, without saying anything, takes an orange.

"What are you doing that for?" cries the companion of his travels, slapping his hand and snatching away the orange. "Silly!"

Now Grisha would have liked to pick up a bit of glass that was lying at his feet and gleaming like a lamp, but he is afraid that his hand will be slapped again.

"My respects to you!" Grisha hears suddenly, almost above his ear, a loud thick voice, and he sees a tall man with bright buttons.

To his great delight, this man gives nurse his hand, stops, and begins talking to her. The brightness of the sun, the noise of the carriages, the horses, the bright buttons are all so impressively new and not dreadful, that Grisha's soul is filled with a feeling of enjoyment and he begins to laugh.

"Come along! Come along!" he cries to the man with the bright buttons, tugging at his coattails.

"Come along where?" asks the man.

"Come along!" Grisha insists.

He wants to say that it would be just as well to take with them papa, mamma, and the cat, but his tongue does not say what he wants to.

A little later, nurse turns out of the boulevard, and leads Grisha into a big courtyard where there is still snow; and the man with the bright buttons comes with them too. They carefully avoid the lumps of snow and the puddles, then, by a dark and dirty staircase, they go into a room. Here there is a great deal of smoke, there is a smell of roast meat, and a woman is standing by the stove frying cutlets. The cook and the nurse kiss each other, and sit down on the bench together with the man, and begin talking in a low voice. Grisha, wrapped up as he is, feels insufferably hot and stifled.

"Why is this?" he wonders, looking about him.

He sees the dark ceiling, the oven fork with two horns, the stove which looks like a great black hole.

"Mam-ma," he drawls.

"Come, come, come!" cries the nurse. "Wait a bit!"

The cook puts a bottle on the table, two wine-glasses, and a pie. The two women and the man with the bright buttons clink glasses and empty them several times, and, the man puts his arm round first the cook and then the nurse. And then all three begin singing in an undertone.

Grisha stretches out his hand towards the pie, and they give him a piece of it. He eats it and watches nurse drinking. . . . He wants to drink too.

"Give me some, nurse!" he begs.

The cook gives him a sip out of her glass. He rolls his eyes, blinks, coughs, and waves his hands for a long time afterwards, while the cook looks at him and laughs.

When he gets home Grisha begins to tell mamma, the walls, and the bed where he has been, and what he has seen. He talks not so much with his tongue, as with his face and his hands. He shows how the sun shines, how the horses run, how the terrible stove looks, and how the cook drinks. . . .

In the evening he cannot get to sleep. The soldiers with the brooms, the big cats, the horses, the bit of glass, the tray of oranges, the bright buttons, all gathered together, weigh on his brain. He tosses from side to side, babbles, and, at last, unable to endure his excitement, begins crying.

"You are feverish," says mamma, putting her open hand on his forehead. "What can have caused it?"

"Stove!" wails Grisha. "Go away, stove!"

"He must have eaten too much . . ." mamma decides.

And Grisha, shattered by the impressions of the new life he has just experienced, receives a spoonful of castor-oil from mamma.

D. H. Lawrence

The Rocking-Horse Winner

There was a woman who was beautiful, who started with all the advantages, yet she had no luck. She married for love, and the love turned to dust. She had bonny children, yet she felt they had been thrust upon her, and she could not love them. They looked at her coldly, as if they were finding fault with her. And hurriedly she felt she must cover up some fault in herself. Yet what it was that she must cover up she never knew. Nevertheless, when her children were present, she always felt the centre of her heart go hard. This troubled her, and in her manner she was all the more gentle and anxious for her children, as if she loved them very much. Only she herself knew that at the centre of her heart was a hard little place that could not feel love, no, not for anybody. Everybody else said of her: "She is such a good mother. She adores her children." Only she herself, and her children themselves, knew it was not so. They read it in each other's eyes.

There were a boy and two little girls. They lived in a pleasant house, with a garden, and they had discreet servants, and felt themselves superior to anyone in the neighbourhood.

Although they lived in style, they felt always an anxiety in the house. There was never enough money. The mother had a small income, and the father had a small income, but not nearly enough for the social position which they had to keep up. The father went in to town to some office. But though he had good prospects, these prospects never materialized. There was always the grinding sense of the shortage of money, though the style was always kept up.

At last the mother said: "I will see if I can't make something." But she did not know where to begin. She racked her brains, and tried this thing and the other, but could not find anything successful. The failure made deep lines come into her face. Her children were growing up, they would have to go to school. There must be more money, there must be more money. The father, who was always very handsome and expensive in his tastes, seemed as if he never *would* be able to do anything worth doing. And the mother, who had a great belief in herself, did not succeed any better, and her tastes were just as expensive.

And so the house came to be haunted by the unspoken phrase: There must be more money! There must be more money! The children could hear it at Christmas, when the expensive and splendid toys filled the nursery. Behind the shining modern rocking-horse, behind the smart doll's-house, a voice would start whispering: "*There must be more money! There must be more money!*"

It came whispering from the springs of the still-swaying rocking-horse, and even the horse, bending his wooden, champing head, heard it. The big doll, sitting so pink and smirking in her new pram, could hear it quite plainly, and seemed to be smirking all the more self-consciously because of it. The foolish puppy, too, that took the place of the teddy-bear, he was looking so extraordinarily foolish for no other reason but that he heard the secret whisper all over the house: "There *must* be more money!"

Yet nobody ever said it aloud. The whisper was everywhere, and therefore no one spoke it. Just as no one ever says: "We are breathing!" in spite of the fact that breath is coming and going all the time.

"Mother," said the boy Paul one day, "why don't we keep a car of our own? Why do we always use uncle's or else a taxi?"

"Because we're the poor members of the family," said the mother.

"But why *are* we, mother?"

"Well—I suppose," she said slowly and bitterly, "it's because your father has no luck."

The boy was silent for some time.

"Is luck money, mother?" he asked, rather timidly.

"No, Paul. Not quite. It's what causes you to have money."

"Oh!" said Paul vaguely. "I thought when Uncle Oscar said *filthy lucker*, it meant money."

"*Filthy lucre* does mean money," said the mother, "But it's lucre, not luck."

"Oh!" said the boy. "Then what is luck, mother?"

"It's what causes you to have money. If you're lucky you have money. That's why it's better to be born lucky than rich. If you're rich, you may lose your money. But if you're lucky, you will always get more money."

"Oh! Will you? And is father not lucky?"

"Very unlucky, I should say," she said bitterly.

The boy watched her with unsure eyes.

"Why?" he asked.

"I don't know. Nobody ever knows why one person is lucky and another unlucky."

"Don't they? Nobody at all? Does *nobody* know?"

"Perhaps God. But He never tells."

"He ought to, then. And aren't you lucky either, mother?"

"I can't be, if I married an unlucky husband."

"But by yourself, aren't you?"

"I used to think I was, before I married. Now I think I am very unlucky indeed."

"Why?"

"Well—never mind! Perhaps I'm not really," she said.

The child looked at her, to see if she meant it. But he saw, by the lines of her mouth, that she was only trying to hide something from him.

"Well, anyhow," he said stoutly, "I'm a lucky person."

"Why?" said his mother, with a sudden laugh.

He stared at her. He didn't even know why he had said it.

"God told me," he asserted, brazening it out.

"I hope He did, dear!"

"He did, mother!"

"Excellent!" said the mother, using one of her husband's exclamations.

The boy saw she did not believe him; or, rather, that she paid no attention to his assertion. This angered him somewhat, and made him want to compel her attention.

He went off by himself, vaguely, in a childish way, seeking for the clue to "luck." Absorbed, taking no heed of other people, he went about with a sort of stealth, seeking inwardly for luck. He wanted luck, he wanted it, he wanted it. When the two girls were playing dolls in the nursery, he would sit on his big rocking-horse, charging madly into space, with a frenzy that made the little girls peer at him uneasily. Wildly the horse careered, the waving dark hair of the boy tossed, his eyes had a strange glare in them. The little girls dared not speak to him.

When he had ridden to the end of his mad little journey, he climbed down and stood in front of his rocking-horse, staring fixedly into its lowered face. Its red mouth was slightly open, its big eye was wide and glassy-bright.

"Now!" he would silently command the snorting steed, "Now, take me to where there is luck! Now take me!"

And he would slash the horse on the neck with the little whip he had asked Uncle Oscar for. He knew the horse could take him to where there was luck, if only he forced it. So he would mount again, and start on his furious ride, hoping at last to get there. He knew he could get there.

"You'll break your horse, Paul!" said the nurse.

"He's always riding like that! I wish he'd leave off!" said his elder sister Joan.

But he only glared down on them in silence. Nurse gave him up. She could make nothing of him. Anyhow he was growing beyond her.

One day his mother and his Uncle Oscar came in when he was on one of his furious rides. He did not speak to them.

"Hallo, you young jockey! Riding a winner?" said his uncle.

"Aren't you growing too big for a rocking-horse? You're not a very little boy any longer, you know," said his mother.

But Paul only gave a blue glare from his big, rather close-set eyes. He would speak to nobody when he was in full tilt. His mother watched him with an anxious expression on her face.

At last he suddenly stopped forcing his horse into the mechanical gallop, and slid down.

"Well, I got there!" he announced fiercely, his blue eyes still flaring, and his sturdy long legs straddling apart.

"Where did you get to?" asked his mother.

"Where I wanted to go," he flared back at her.

"That's right, son!" said Uncle Oscar. "Don't you stop till you get there. What's the horse's name?"

"He doesn't have a name," said the boy.

"Gets on without all right?" asked the uncle.

"Well, he has different names. He was called Sansovino last week."

"Sansovino, eh? Won the Ascot. How did you know his name?"

"He always talks about horse-races with Bassett," said Joan.

The uncle was delighted to find that his small nephew was posted with all the racing news. Bassett, the young gardener, who had been wounded in the left foot in the war and got his present job through Oscar Cresswell, whose batman he had been, was a perfect blade of the "turf." He lived in the racing events, and the small boy lived with him.

Oscar Cresswell got it all from Bassett.

"Master Paul comes and asks me, so I can't do more than tell him, sir," said Bassett, his face terribly serious, as if he were speaking of religious matters.

"And does he ever put anything on a horse he fancies?"

"Well—I don't want to give him away—he's a young sport, a fine sport, sir. Would you mind asking him himself? He sort of takes a pleasure in it, and perhaps he'd feel I was giving him away, sir, if you don't mind."

Bassett was serious as a church.

The uncle went back to his nephew, and took him off for a ride in the car.

"Say, Paul, old man, do you ever put anything on a horse?" the uncle asked.

The boy watched the handsome man closely.

"Why, do you think I oughtn't to?" he parried.

"Not a bit of it! I thought perhaps you might give me a tip for the Lincoln."

The car sped on into the country, going down to Uncle Oscar's place in Hampshire.

"Honour bright?" said the nephew.

"Honour bright, son!" said the uncle.

"Well, then, Daffodil."

"Daffodil! I doubt it, sonny. What about Mirza?"

"I only know the winner," said the boy. "That's Daffodil."

"Daffodil, eh?"

There was a pause. Daffodil was an obscure horse comparatively.

"Uncle!"

"Yes, son?"

"You won't let it go any further, will you? I promised Bassett."

"Bassett be damned, old man! What's he got to do with it?"

"We're partners. We've been partners from the first, Uncle, he lent me my first five shillings, which I lost. I promised him, honour bright, it was only between me and him; only you gave me that ten-shilling note I started winning with, so I thought you were lucky. You won't let it go any further, will you?"

The boy gazed at his uncle from those big, hot, blue eyes, set rather close together. The uncle stirred and laughed uneasily.

"Right you are, son! I'll keep your tip private. Daffodil, eh? How much are you putting on him?"

"All except twenty pounds," said the boy. "I keep that in reserve."

The uncle thought it a good joke.

"You keep twenty pounds in reserve, do you, you young romancer? What are you betting, then?"

"I'm betting three hundred," said the boy gravely. "But it's between you and me, Uncle Oscar! Honour bright?"

The uncle burst into a roar of laughter.

"It's between you and me all right, you young Nat Gould," he said, laughing. "But where's your three hundred?"

"Bassett keeps it for me. We're partners."

"You are, are you! And what is Bassett putting on Daffodil?"

"He won't go quite as high as I do, I expect. Perhaps he'll go a hundred and fifty."

"What, pennies?" laughed the uncle.

"Pounds," said the child, with a surprised look at his uncle. "Bassett keeps a bigger reserve than I do."

Between wonder and amusement Uncle Oscar was silent. He pursued the matter no further, but he determined to take his nephew with him to the Lincoln races.

"Now, son," he said, "I'm putting twenty on Mirza, and I'll put five for you on any horse you fancy. "What's your pick?"

"Daffodil, uncle."

"No, not the fiver on Daffodil!"

"I should if it was my own fiver," said the child.

"Good! Good! Right you are! A fiver for me and a fiver for you on Daffodil."

The child had never been to a race-meeting before, and his eyes were blue fire. He pursed his mouth tight, and watched. A Frenchman just in front had put his money on Lancelot. Wild with excitement, he flayed his arms up and down, yelling "*Lancelot! Lancelot!*" in his French accent.

Daffodil came in first, Lancelot second, Mirza third.

The child, flushed and with eyes blazing, was curiously serene. His uncle brought him four five-pound notes, four to one.

"What am I to do with these?" he cried, waving them before the boy's eyes.

"I suppose we'll talk to Bassett," said the boy. "I expect I have fifteen hundred now; and twenty in reserve; and this twenty."

His uncle studied him for some moments.

"Look here, son!" he said. "You're not serious about Bassett and that fifteen hundred, are you?"

"Yes, I am. But it's between you and me, uncle. Honour bright!"

"Honour bright all right, son! But I must talk to Bassett."

"If you'd like to be a partner, uncle, with Bassett and me, we could all be partners. Only, you'd have to promise, honour bright, uncle, not to let it go beyond us three. Bassett and I are lucky, and you must be lucky, because it was your ten shillings I started winning with . . ."

Uncle Oscar took both Bassett and Paul into Richmond Park for an afternoon, and there they talked.

"It's like this, you see, sir. Master Paul would get me talking about racing events, spinning yarns, you know, sir. And he was always keen on knowing if I'd made or if I'd lost. It's about a year since, now, that I put five shilling on Blush of Dawn for him—and we lost. Then the luck turned, with that ten shillings he had from you, that we put on Singhalese. And since that time, it's been pretty steady, all things considering. What do you say, Master Paul?"

"We're all right when we're sure," said Paul. "It's when we're not quite so sure that we go down."

"Oh, but we're careful then," said Bassett.

"But when are you *sure*?" smiled Uncle Oscar.

"It's Master Paul, sir," said Bassett in a secret, religious voice. "It's as if he had it from heaven. Like Daffodil, now, for the Lincoln. That was as sure as eggs."

"Did you put anything on Daffodil?" asked Oscar Cresswell.

"Yes, sir. I made my bit."

"And my nephew?"

Bassett was obstinately silent, looking at Paul.

"I made twelve hundred, didn't I, Bassett? I told uncle I was putting three hundred on Daffodil."

"That's right," said Bassett, nodding.

"But where's the money?" asked the uncle.

"I keep it safe locked up, sir. Master Paul he can have it any minute he likes to ask for it."

"What, fifteen hundred pounds?"

"And twenty! And *forty*, that is, with the twenty he made on the course."

"It's amazing!" said the uncle.

"If Master Paul offers you to be partners, sir, I would, if I were you; if you'll excuse me," said Bassett.

Oscar Cresswell thought about it.

"I'll see the money," he said.

They drove home again, and sure enough, Bassett came round to the garden-house with fifteen hundred pounds in notes. The twenty pounds reserve was left with Joe Glee, in the Turf Commission deposit.

"You see, it's all right, uncle, when I'm sure! Then we go strong, for all we're worth. Don't we Bassett?"

"We do that, Master Paul."

"And when are you sure?" said the uncle, laughing.

"Oh, well, sometimes I'm *absolutely* sure, like about Daffodil," said the boy; "and sometimes I have an idea; and sometimes I haven't even an idea, have I, Bassett? Then we're careful, because we mostly go down."

"You do, do you! And when you're sure, like about Daffodil, what makes you sure, sonny?"

"Oh, well, I don't know," said the boy uneasily. "I'm sure, you know, uncle; that's all."

"It's as if he had it from heaven, sir," Bassett reiterated.

"I should say so!" said his uncle.

But he became a partner. And when the Leger was coming on, Paul was "sure" about Lively Spark, which was a quite inconsiderable horse. The boy insisted on putting a thousand on the horse, Bassett went for five hundred, and Oscar Cresswell two hundred. Lively Spark came in first, and the betting had been ten to one against him. Paul had made ten thousand.

"You see," he said, "I was absolutely sure of him."

Even Oscar Cresswell had cleared two thousand.

"Look here, son," he said, "this sort of thing makes me nervous."

"It needn't, uncle! Perhaps I shan't be sure again for a long time."

"But what are you going to do with your money?" asked the uncle.

"Of course," said the boy, "I started it for mother. She said she had no luck, because father is unlucky, so I thought if *I* was lucky, it might stop whispering."

"What might stop whispering?"

"Our house. I *hate* our house for whispering."

"What does it whisper?"

"Why—why"—the boy fidgeted—"why, I don't know. But it's always short of money, you know, uncle."

"I know it son, I know it."

"You know people send mother writs, don't you, uncle?"

"I'm afraid I do," said the uncle.

"And then the house whispers, like people laughing at you behind your back. It's awful, that is! I thought if I was lucky . . ."

"You might stop it," added the uncle.

The boy watched him with big blue eyes, that had an uncanny cold fire in them, and he said never a word.

"Well, then!" said the uncle. "What are we doing?"

"I shouldn't like mother to know I was lucky," said the boy.

"Why not, son?"

"She'd stop me."

"I don't think she would."

"Oh!"—and the boy writhed in an odd way—"I *don't* want her to know, uncle."

"All right, son! We'll manage it without her knowing."

They managed it very easily. Paul, at the other's suggestion, handed over five thousand pounds to his uncle, who deposited it with the family lawyer, who was then to inform Paul's mother that a relative had put five thousand pounds into his hands, which sum was to be paid out a thousand pounds at a time, on the mother's birthday, for the next five years.

"So she'll have a birthday present of a thousand pounds for five successive years," said Uncle Oscar. "I hope it won't make it all the harder for her later."

Paul's mother had her birthday in November. The house had been "whispering" worse than ever lately, and, even in spite of his luck, Paul could not bear up against it. He was very anxious to see the effect of the birthday letter, telling his mother about the thousand pounds.

When there were no visitors, Paul now took his meals with his parents, as he was beyond the nursery control. His mother went into town nearly every day. She had discovered that she had an odd knack of sketching furs and dress materials, so she worked secretly in the studio of a friend who was the chief "artist" for the leading drapers. She drew the figures of ladies in furs and ladies in silk and sequins for the newspaper advertisements. This young woman artist earned several thousand pounds a year, but Paul's mother only made several hundred, and she was again dissatisfied. She so wanted to be first in something, and she did not succeed, even in making sketches for drapery advertisements.

She was down to breakfast on the morning of her birthday. Paul watched her face as she read her letters. He knew the lawyer's letter. As his mother read it, her face hardened and became more expressionless. Then a cold, determined look came on her mouth. She hid the letter under the pile of others, and said not a word about it.

"Didn't you have anything nice in the post for your birthday, mother?" said Paul.

"Quite moderately nice," she said, her voice cold and absent.

She went away to town without saying more. But in the afternoon Uncle Oscar appeared. He said Paul's mother had had a long interview with the lawyer, asking if the whole five thousand could not be advanced at once, as she was in debt.

"What do you think, uncle?" said the boy.

"I leave it to you, son."

"Oh, let her have it, then! We can get some more with the other," said the boy.

"A bird in the hand is worth two in the bush, laddie!" said Uncle Oscar.

"But I'm sure to *know* for the Grand National; or the Lincolnshire; or else the Derby. I'm sure to know for *one* of them," said Paul.

So Uncle Oscar signed the agreement, and Paul's mother touched the whole five thousand. Then something very curious happened. The voices in the house suddenly went mad, like a chorus of frogs on a spring evening. There were certain new furnishings, and Paul had a tutor. He was *really* going to Eton, his father's school, in the following autumn. There were flowers in the winter, and a blossoming of the luxury Paul's mother had been used to. And yet the voices in the house, behind the sprays of mimosa and almond blossom, and from under the piles of iridescent cushions, simply trilled and screamed in a sort of ecstasy: "There must be more money! Oh-h-h; there *must* be more money. Oh, now, now-w! Now-w-w—there *must* be more money!—more than ever! More than ever!"

It frightened Paul terribly. He studied away at his Latin and Greek with his tutors. But his intense hours were spent with Bassett. The Grand National had gone by: he had not "known," and had lost a hundred pounds. Summer was at hand. He was in agony for the Lincoln. But even for the Lincoln he didn't "know," and he lost fifty pounds. He became wild-eyed and strange, as if something were going to explode in him.

"Let it alone, son! Don't you bother about it!" urged Uncle Oscar. But it was as if the boy couldn't really hear what his uncle was saying.

"I've got to know for the Derby! I've got to know for the Derby!" the child reiterated, his big blue eyes blazing with a sort of madness.

His mother noticed how overwrought he was.

"You'd better go the seaside. Wouldn't you like to go now to the seaside, instead of waiting? I think you'd better," she said, looking down at him anxiously, her heart curiously heavy because of him.

But the child lifted his uncanny blue eyes.

"I couldn't possibly go before the Derby, mother!" he said. "I couldn't possibly!"

"Why not?" she said, her voice becoming heavy when she was opposed. "Why not? You can still go from the seaside to see the Derby with your Uncle Oscar, if that's what you wish. No need for you to wait here. Besides, I think you care too much about these races. It's a bad sign. My family has been a gambling family, and you won't know till you grow up how much damage it has done. But it has done damage. I shall have to send Bassett away, and ask Uncle Oscar not to talk racing to you unless you promise to be reasonable about it; go away to the seaside and forget it. You're all nerves!"

"I'll do what you like, mother, so long as you don't send me away till after the Derby," the boy said.

"Send you away from where? Just from this house?"

"Yes," he said gazing at her.

"Why, you curious child, what makes you care about this house so much, suddenly? I never knew you loved it."

He gazed at her without speaking. He had a secret within a secret, something he had not divulged, even to Bassett or to his Uncle Oscar.

But his mother, after standing undecided and a little bit sullen for some moments, said:

"Very well, then! Don't go to the seaside till after the Derby, if you don't wish it. But promise me you won't let your nerves go to pieces. Promise you won't think so much about horse-racing and *events*, as you call them!"

"Oh, no," said the boy casually. "I won't think much about them, mother. You needn't worry. I wouldn't worry, mother, if I were you."

"If you were me and I were you," said his mother, "I wonder what we *should* do!"

"But you know you needn't worry, mother, don't you?" the boy repeated.

"I should be awfully glad to know it," she said wearily.

"Oh, well, you *can*, you know. I mean, you *ought* to know you needn't worry," he insisted.

"Ought I? Then I'll see about it," she said.

Paul's secret of secrets was his wooden horse, that which had no name. Since he was emancipated from a nurse and a nursery-governess, he had had his rocking-horse removed to his own bedroom at the top of the house.

"Surely, you're too big for a rocking-horse!" his mother had remonstrated.

"Well, you see, mother, till I can have a *real* horse, I like to have *some* sort of animal about," had been his quaint answer.

"Do you feel he keeps you company?" she laughed.

"Oh, yes! He's very good, he always keeps me company, when I'm there," said Paul.

So the horse, rather shabby, stood in an arrested prance in the boy's bedroom.

The Derby was drawing near, and the boy grew more and more tense. He hardly heard what was spoken to him, he was very frail, and his eyes were really uncanny. His mother had sudden strange seizures of uneasiness about him. Sometimes, for half-an-hour, she would feel a sudden anxiety about him that was almost anguish. She wanted to rush to him at once, and know he was safe.

Two nights before the Derby, she was at a big party in town, when one of her rushes of anxiety about her boy, her first-born, gripped her heart till she could hardly speak. She fought with the feeling, might and main, for she believed in common-sense. But it was too strong. She had to leave the dance and go downstairs to telephone to the country. The children's nursery-governess was terribly surprised and startled at being rung up in the night.

"Are the children all right, Miss Wilmot?"

"Oh, yes, they are quite all right."

"Master Paul? Is he all right?"

"He went to bed as right as a trivet. Shall I run up and look at him?"

"No," said Paul's mother reluctantly. "No! Don't trouble. It's all right. Don't sit up. We shall be home fairly soon." She did not want her son's privacy intruded upon.

"Very good," said the governess.

It was about one o'clock when Paul's mother and father drove up to their house. All was still. Paul's mother went to her room and slipped off her white fur cloak. She had told her maid not to wait up for her. She heard her husband downstairs, mixing a whisky-and-soda.

And then, because of the strange anxiety at her heart, she stole upstairs to her son's room. Noiselessly she went along the upper corridor. Was there a faint noise? What was it?

She stood, with arrested muscles, outside his door, listening. There was a strange, heavy, and yet not loud noise. Her heart stood still. It was a soundless noise, yet rushing and powerful. Something huge, in violent, hushed motion. What was it? What in God's name was it? She ought to know. She felt that she knew the noise. She knew what it was.

Yet she could not place it. She couldn't say what it was. And on and on it went, like a madness.

Softly, frozen with anxiety and fear, she turned the door-handle.

The room was dark. Yet in the space near the window, she heard and saw something plunging to and fro. She gazed in fear and amazement.

Then suddenly she switched on the light, and saw her son, in his green pyjamas, madly surging on the rocking-horse. The blaze of light suddenly lit him up, as he urged the wooden horse, and lit her up, as she stood, blonde, in her dress of pale green and crystal, in the doorway.

"Paul!" she cried. "Whatever are you doing?"

"It's Malabar!" he screamed, in a powerful, strange voice. "It's Malabar!"

His eyes blazed at her for one strange and senseless second, as he ceased urging his wooden horse. Then he fell with a crash to the ground, and she, all her tormented motherhood flooding upon her, rushed to gather him up.

But he was unconscious, and unconscious he remained, with some brain-fever. He talked and tossed, and his mother sat stonily by his side.

"Malabar! It's Malabar! Bassett, Bassett, I *know*! It's Malabar!"

So the child cried, trying to get up and urge the rocking-horse that gave him his inspiration.

"What does he mean by Malabar?" asked the heart-frozen mother.

"I don't know," said the father stonily.

"What does he mean by Malabar?" she asked her brother Oscar.

"It's one of the horses running for the Derby," was the answer.

And, in spite of himself, Oscar Cresswell spoke to Bassett, and himself put a thousand on Malabar, at fourteen to one.

The third day of the illness was critical: they were waiting for a change. The boy, with his rather long, curly hair, was tossing ceaselessly on the pillow. He neither slept nor regained consciousness, and his eyes were like blue stones. His mother sat, feeling her heart had gone, turned actually into a stone.

In the evening, Oscar Cresswell did not come, but Bassett sent a message, saying could he come up for one moment, just one moment? Paul's mother was very angry at the intrusion, but on second thought she agreed. The boy was the same. Perhaps Bassett might bring him to consciousness.

The gardener, a shortish fellow with a little brown moustache, and sharp little brown eyes, tiptoed into the room, touched his imaginary cap to Paul's mother, and stole to the bedside, staring with glittering, smallish eyes, at the tossing, dying child.

"Master Paul!" he whispered. "Master Paul! Malabar came in first all right, a clean win. I did as you told me. You've made over seventy thousand pounds, you have; you've got over eighty thousand. Malabar came in all right, Master Paul."

"Malabar! Malabar! Did I say Malabar, mother? Did I say Malabar? Do you think I'm lucky, mother? I knew Malabar, didn't I? Over eighty thousand pounds! I call that lucky, don't you, mother? Over eighty thousand pounds! I knew, didn't I know I knew? Malabar came in all right. If I ride my horse till I'm sure, then I tell you, Bassett, you can go as high as you like. Did you go for all you were worth, Bassett?"

"I went a thousand on it, Master Paul."

"I never told you, mother, that if I can ride my horse, and *get there*, then I'm absolutely sure—oh, absolutely! Mother, did I ever tell you? I *am* lucky!"

"No, you never did," said the mother.

But the boy died in the night.

And even as he lay dead, his mother heard her brother's voice saying to her:

"My God, Hester, you're eighty thousand to the good, and a poor devil of a son to the bad. But, poor devil, poor devil, he's best gone out of a life where he rides his rocking-horse to find a winner."

Anton Chekhov

Oysters

I need no great effort of memory to recall, in every detail, the rainy autumn evening when I stood with my father in one of the more frequented streets of Moscow, and felt that I was gradually being overcome by a strange illness. I had no pain at all, but my legs were giving way under me, the words stuck in my throat, my head slipped weakly on one side . . . It seemed as though, in a moment, I must fall down and lose consciousness.

If I had been taken into a hospital at that minute, the doctors would have had to write over my bed: *fames*, a disease which is not in the manuals of medicine.

Beside me on the pavement stood my father in a shabby summer overcoat and a serge cap, from which a bit of white wadding was sticking out. On his feet he had big heavy goloshes. Afraid, vain man, that people would see that his feet were bare under his goloshes, he had drawn the tops of some old boots up round the calves of his legs.

This poor, foolish, queer creature, whom I loved the more warmly the more ragged and dirty his smart summer overcoat became, had come to Moscow, five months before, to look for a job as copying-clerk. For those five months he had been trudging about Moscow looking for work, and it was only on that day that he had brought himself to go into the street to beg for alms.

Before us was a big house of three storeys, adorned with a blue signboard with the word "Restaurant" on it. My head was drooping feebly backwards and on one side, and I could not help looking upwards at the lighted windows of the restaurant. Human figures were flitting about at the windows. I could see the right side of the orchestrion, two oleographs, hanging lamps . . . Staring into one window, I saw a patch of white. The patch was motionless, and its rectangular outlines stood out sharply against the dark, brown background. I looked intently and made out of the patch a white placard on the wall. Something was written on it, but what it was, I could not see . . .

For half an hour I kept my eyes on the placard. Its white attracted my eyes, and, as it were, hypnotised my brain. I tried to read it, but my efforts were in vain.

At last the strange disease got the upper hand.

The rumble of the carriages began to seem like thunder, in the stench of the street I distinguished a thousand smells. The restaurant lights and the lamps dazzled my eyes like lightning. My five senses were overstrained and sensitive beyond the normal. I began to see what I had not seen before.

"Oysters . . ." I made out on the placard.

A strange word! I had lived in the world eight years and three months, but had never come across that word. What did it mean? Surely it was not the name of the restaurant-keeper? But signboards with names on them always hang outside, not on the walls indoors!

"Papa, what does 'oysters' mean?" I asked in a husky voice, making an effort to turn my face towards my father.

My father did not hear. He was keeping a watch on the movements of the crowd, and following every passer-by with his eyes . . . From his eyes I saw that he wanted to say something to the passers-by, but the fatal word hung like a heavy weight on his trembling lips and could not be flung off. He even took a step after one passer-by and touched him on the sleeve, but when he turned round, he said, "I beg your pardon," was overcome with confusion, and staggered back.

"Papa, what does 'oysters' mean?" I repeated.

"It is an animal . . . that lives in the sea."

I instantly pictured to myself this unknown marine animal . . . I thought it must be something midway between a fish and a crab. As it was from the sea they made of it, of course, a very nice hot fish soup with savoury pepper and laurel leaves, or broth with vinegar and fricassee of fish and cabbage, or crayfish sauce, or served it cold with horse-radish . . . I vividly imagined it being brought from the market, quickly cleaned, quickly put in the pot, quickly, quickly, for everyone was hungry . . . awfully hungry! From the kitchen rose the smell of hot fish and crayfish soup.

I felt that this smell was tickling my palate and nostrils, that it was gradually taking possession of my whole body . . . The restaurant, my father, the white placard, my sleeves were all smelling of it, smelling so strongly that I began to chew. I moved my jaws and swallowed as though I really had a piece of this marine animal in my mouth . . .

My legs gave way from the blissful sensation I was feeling, and I clutched at my father's arm to keep myself from falling, and leant against his wet summer overcoat. My father was trembling and shivering. He was cold . . .

"Papa, are oysters a Lenten dish?" I asked.

"They are eaten alive . . ." said my father. "They are in shells like tortoises, but . . . in two halves."

The delicious smell instantly left off affecting me, and the illusion vanished. . . . Now I understood it all!

"How nasty," I whispered, "how nasty!"

So that's what "oysters" meant! I imagined to myself a creature like a frog. A frog sitting in a shell, peeping out from it with big, glittering eyes, and moving its revolting jaws. I imagined this creature in a shell with claws, glittering eyes, and a slimy skin, being brought from the market . . . The children would all hide while the cook, frowning with an air of disgust, would take the creature by its claw, put it on a plate, and carry it into the dining-room. The grown-ups would take it and eat it, eat it alive with its eyes, its teeth, its legs! While it squeaked and tried to bite their lips . . .

I frowned, but . . . but why did my teeth move as though I were munching? The creature was loathsome, disgusting, terrible, but I ate it, ate it greedily, afraid of distinguishing its taste or smell. As soon as I had eaten one, I saw the glittering eyes of a second, a third . . . I ate them too. . . . At last I ate the table-napkin, the plate, my father's goloshes, the white placard . . . I ate everything that caught my eye, because I felt that nothing but eating would take away my illness. The oysters had a terrible look in their eyes and were loathsome. I shuddered at the thought of them, but I wanted to eat! To eat!

"Oysters! Give me some oysters!" was the cry that broke from me and I stretched out my hand.

"Help us, gentlemen!" I heard at that moment my father say, in a hollow and shaking voice. "I am ashamed to ask but—my God!—I can bear no more!"

"Oysters!" I cried, pulling my father by the skirts of his coat.

"Do you mean to say you eat oysters? A little chap like you!" I heard laughter close to me.

Two gentlemen in top hats were standing before us, looking into my face and laughing.

"Do you really eat oysters, youngster? That's interesting! How do you eat them?"

I remember that a strong hand dragged me into the lighted restaurant. A minute later there was a crowd round me, watching me with curiosity and amusement. I sat at a table and ate something slimy, salt with a flavour of dampness and mouldiness. I ate greedily without chewing, without looking and trying to discover what I was eating. I fancied that if I opened my eyes I should see glittering eyes, claws, and sharp teeth.

All at once I began biting something hard, there was a sound of a scrunching.

"Ha, ha! He is eating the shells," laughed the crowd. "Little silly, do you suppose you can eat that?"

After that I remember a terrible thirst. I was lying in my bed, and could not sleep for heartburn and the strange taste in my parched mouth. My father was walking up and down, gesticulating with his hands.

"I believe I have caught cold," he was muttering. "I've a feeling in my head as though someone were sitting on it . . . Perhaps it is because I have not . . . er . . . eaten anything to-day. . . . I really am a queer, stupid creature . . . I saw those gentlemen pay ten roubles for the oysters. Why didn't I go up to them and ask them . . . to lend me something? They would have given something."

Towards morning, I fell asleep and dreamt of a frog sitting in a shell, moving its eyes. At midday I was awakened by thirst, and looked for my father: he was still walking up and down and gesticulating.

Jean Rhys

GOOD-BYE MARCUS, GOOD-BYE ROSE

"When first I wore my old shako," sang Captain Cardew, "ten, twenty, thirty, forty, fifty years ago . . ." and Phoebe thought what a wonderful bass voice he had. This was the second time he had called to take her for a walk, and again he had brought her a large box of chocolates.

Captain Cardew and his wife were spending the winter in Jamaica when they visited the small island where she lived and found it so attractive and unspoilt that they decided to stay. They even talked of buying a house and settling there for good.

He was not only a very handsome old man but a hero who had fought bravely in some long ago war which she thought you only read about in history books. He'd been wounded and had a serious operation without an anaesthetic. Anaesthetics weren't invented in those days. (Better not think too much about that.)

It had been impressed on her how kind it was of him to bother with a little girl like herself. Anyway she liked him, he was always so carefully polite to her, treating her as though she were a grown-up girl. A calm unruffled man, he only grew annoyed if people called him "Captain" too often. Sometimes he lost his temper and would say loudly things like: "What d'you think I'm Captain of now—a Penny a Liner." What was a Penny a Liner? She never found out.

It was a lovely afternoon and they set out. She was wearing a white blouse with a sailor collar, a long full white skirt, black stockings, black buttoned boots and a large wide-brimmed white hat anchored firmly with elastic under her chin.

When they reached the Botanical Gardens she offered to take him to a shady bench and they walked slowly to the secluded part of the Gardens that she'd spoken of and sat under a large tree. Beyond its shadow they could see the yellow dancing patches of sunlight.

"Do you mind if I take off my hat? The elastic is hurting me," Phoebe said.

"Then take it off, take it off," said the Captain.

Phoebe took off her hat and began to talk in what she hoped was a grown-up way about the curator, Mr. Harcourt-Smith, who'd really made the Gardens as beautiful as they were. He'd come from a place in England called the Kew. Had he ever heard of it? Yes he had heard of it. He added: "How old are you, Phoebe?"

"I'm twelve," said Phoebe, "—and a bit."

"Hah!" said the Captain. "Then soon you'll be old enough to have a lover!" His hand, which had been lying quietly by his side, darted towards her, dived inside her blouse and clamped itself around one very small breast. "Quite old enough," he remarked.

Phoebe remained perfectly still. "He's making a great mistake, a great mistake," she thought. "If I don't move he'll take his hand away without really noticing what he'd done."

However the Captain showed no sign of that at all. He was breathing rather heavily when a couple came strolling round the corner. Calmly, without hurry, he withdrew his hand and after a while said: "Perhaps we ought to be going home now."

Phoebe, who was in a ferment, said nothing. They walked out of the shade into the sun and as they walked she looked up at him as though at some aged but ageless god. He talked of usual things in a usual voice and she made up her mind that she would tell nobody of what had happened. Nobody. It was not a thing you could possibly talk about. Also no one would believe exactly how it happened, and whether they believed her or not she would be blamed.

If he was as absentminded as all that—for surely it could be nothing but absentmindedness—perhaps there oughtn't to be any more walks. She could excuse herself by saying that she had a headache. But that would only do for once. The walks continued. They'd go into the Gardens or up the Morne, a hill overlooking the town. There were benches and seats there but few houses and hardly anybody about.

He never touched her again but all through the long bright afternoons Captain Cardew talked of love and Phoebe listened, shocked and fascinated. Sometimes she doubted what he said: surely it was impossible, horrifyingly impossible. Sometimes she was on the point of saying, not "You oughtn't to talk to me like this," but babyishly "I want to go home." He always knew when she felt this and would at once change the subject and tell her amusing stories of his life when he was a young man and a subaltern in India. "Hot?" he'd say. "This isn't hot. India's hot. Sometimes the only thing to do is take off your clothes and see that the punkah's going."

Or he'd talk about London long ago. Someone—was it Byron?—had said that women were never so unattractive as when they were eating and it was still most unfashionable for them to eat heartily. He'd watch in wonder as the ethereal creatures pecked daintily, then send away almost untouched plates. One day he had seen a maid taking a tray laden with food up to the bedrooms and the mystery was explained.

But these stories were only intervals in the ceaseless talk of love, various ways of making love, various sorts of love. He'd explain that love was not kind and gentle, as she had imagined, but violent. Violence, even cruelty, was an essential part of it. He would expand on this, it seemed to be his favorite subject.

The walks had gone on for some time when the Captain's wife, Edith, who was a good deal younger than her husband, became suspicious and began making very sarcastic remarks. Early one evening when the entire party had gone up the Morne to watch the sunset, she'd said to her husband, after a long look at Phoebe: "Do you really find the game worth the candle?" Captain Cardew said nothing. He watched the sun going down without expression, then remarked that it was quite true that the only way to get rid of a temptation was to yield to it.

Phoebe had never liked Edith very much. Now she began to dislike her. One afternoon they were in a room together and she said: "Do you see how white my hair's becoming? It's all because of you." And when Phoebe answered truthfully that she didn't notice any white hairs: "What a really dreadful little liar you are!"

After this she must have spoken to Phoebe's mother, a silent, reserved woman, who said nothing to her daughter but began to watch her in a puzzled, incredulous, even faintly suspicious way. Phoebe knew that very soon she would be questioned, she'd have to explain.

So she was more than half relieved when Edith Cardew announced that they'd quite given up their first idea of spending the rest of the winter on the island and were going back to England by the next boat. When Captain Cardew said "Good-bye" formally, the evening before they left, she had smiled and shaken hands, not quite realizing that she was very unlikely ever to seen him again.

There was a flat roof outside her bedroom window. On hot fine nights she'd often lie there in her nightgown looking up at the huge brilliant stars. She'd once tried to write a poem about them but had not got beyond the first line: "My stars. Familiar jewels." But that night she knew that she would never finish it. They were not jewels. They were not familiar. They were cold, infinitely far away, quite indifferent.

The roof looked onto the yard and she could hear Victoria and Joseph talking and laughing outside the pantry, then they must have gone away and it was quite silent. She was alone in the house for she'd not gone with the others to see the Cardews off. She was sure that now they had gone her mother would be very unlikely to question her, and then began to wonder how he had been so sure, not only that she'd never tell anybody but that she'd make no effort at all to stop him talking. That could only mean that he'd seen at once that she was not a good girl—who could object—but a wicked one—who would listen. He must know. He knew. It was so.

It was so and she felt not so much unhappy about this as uncomfortable, even dismayed. It was like wearing a dress that was much too big for her, a dress that swallowed her up.

Wasn't it quite difficult being a wicked girl? Even more difficult than being a good one? Besides, didn't the nuns say that Chastity, in Thought, Word, and Deed was your most precious possession? She remembered Mother Sacred Heart, her second favorite, reciting in her lovely English voice:

"*So dear to Heaven is saintly chastity . . .*"

How did it go on? Something about "a thousand livered angels lackey her . . ."

"A thousand liveried angels" now no more. The thought of some vague irreparable loss saddened her. Then she told herself that anyway she needn't bother any longer about whether she'd get married or not. The older girls that she knew talked a great deal about marriage, some of them talked about very little else. And they seemed so sure. No sooner had they put their hair up and begun going to dances, than they'd marry someone handsome (and rich). Then the fun of being grown-up and important, of doing what you wanted instead of what you were told to do, would start. And go on for a long long time.

But she'd always doubted if this would happen to her. Even if numbers of rich and handsome young men suddenly appeared, would she be one of the chosen?

If no one ever marries me
And I don't see why they should
For nurse says I'm not pretty
And I'm seldom very good . . .

That was it exactly.

Well there was one thing. Now she felt very wise, very grown-up, she could forget these childish worries. She could hardly believe that only a few weeks ago she, like all the others, had secretly made lists of her trousseau, decided on the names of her three children, Jack, Marcus. And Rose.

Now good-bye Marcus. Good-bye Rose. The prospect before her might be difficult and uncertain but it was far more exciting.

James Joyce

ARABY

North Richmond Street, being blind, was a quiet street except at the hour when the Christian Brothers' School set the boys free. An uninhabited house of two storeys stood at the blind end, detached from its neighbours in a square ground. The other houses of the street, conscious of decent lives within them, gazed at one another with brown imperturbable faces.

The former tenant of our house, a priest, had died in the back drawing-room. Air, musty from having been long enclosed, hung in all the rooms, and the waste room behind the kitchen was littered with old useless papers. Among these I found a few paper-covered books, the pages of which were curled and damp: *The Abbot*, by Walter Scott, *The Devout Communicant*, and *The Memoirs of Vidocq*. I liked the last best because its leaves were yellow. The wild garden behind the house contained a central apple-tree and a few straggling bushes, under one of which I found the late tenant's rusty bicycle-pump. He had been a very charitable priest; in his will he had left all his money to institutions and the furniture of his house to his sister.

When the short days of winter came, dusk fell before we had well eaten our dinners. When we met in the street the houses had grown sombre. The space of sky above us was the colour of ever-changing violet and towards it the lamps of the street lifted their feeble lanterns. The cold air stung us and we played till our bodies glowed. Our shouts echoed in the silent street. The career of our play brought us through the dark muddy lanes behind the houses, where we ran the gauntlet of the rough tribes from the cottages, to the back doors of the dark dripping gardens where odours arose from the ashpits, to the dark odorous stables where a coachman smoothed and combed the horse or shook music from the buckled harness. When we returned to the street, light from the kitchen windows had filled the areas. If my uncle was seen turning the corner, we hid in the shadow until we had seen him safely housed. Or if Mangan's sister came out on the doorstep to call her brother in to his tea, we watched her from our shadow peer up and down the street. We waited to see whether she would remain or go in and, if she remained, we left our shadow and walked up to Mangan's steps resignedly. She was waiting for us, her figure defined by the light from the half-opened door. Her brother always teased her before he obeyed, and I stood by the railings looking at her. Her dress swung as she moved her body, and the soft rope of her hair tossed from side to side.

Every morning I lay on the floor in the front parlour watching her door. The blind was pulled down to within an inch of the sash so that I could not be seen. When she came out on the doorstep my heart leaped. I ran to the hall, seized my books and followed her. I kept her brown figure always in my eye and, when we came near the point at which our ways diverged, I quickened my pace and passed her. This happened morning after morning. I had never spoken to her, except for a few casual words, and yet her name was like a summons to all my foolish blood.

Her image accompanied me even in places the most hostile to romance. On Saturday evenings when my aunt went marketing I had to go to carry some of the parcels. We walked through the flaring streets, jostled by drunken men and bargaining women, amid the curses of labourers, the shrill litanies of shop-boys who stood on guard by the barrels of pigs' cheeks, the nasal chanting of street-singers, who sang a come-all-you about O'Donovan Rossa, or a ballad about the troubles in our native land. These noises converged in a single sensation of life for me: I imagined that I bore my chalice safely through a throng of foes. Her name sprang to my lips at moments in strange prayers and praises which I myself did not understand. My eyes were often full of tears (I could not tell why) and at times a flood from my heart seemed to pour itself out into my bosom. I thought little of the future. I did not know whether I would ever speak to her or not or, if I spoke to her, how I could tell her of my confused adoration. But my body was like a harp and her words and gestures were like fingers running upon the wires.

One evening I went into the back drawing-room in which the priest had died. It was a dark rainy evening and there was no sound in the house. Through one of the broken panes I heard the rain impinge upon the earth, the fine incessant needles of water playing in the sodden beds. Some distant lamp or lighted window gleamed below me. I was thankful that I could see so little. All my senses seemed to desire to veil themselves and, feeling that I was about to slip from them, I pressed the palms of my hands together until they trembled, murmuring: '*O love! O love!*' many times.

At last she spoke to me. When she addressed the first words to me I was so confused that I did not know what to answer. She asked me was I going to Araby. I forgot whether I answered yes or no. It would be a splendid bazaar; she said she would love to go.

'And why can't you?' I asked.

While she spoke she turned a silver bracelet round and round her wrist. She could not go, she said, because there would be a retreat that week in her convent. Her brother and two other boys were fighting for their caps, and I was alone at the railings. She held one of the spikes, bowing her head towards me. The light from the lamp opposite our door caught the white curve of her neck, lit up her hair that rested there and, falling, lit up the hand upon the railing. It fell over one side of her dress and caught the white border of a petticoat, just visible as she stood at ease.

'It's well for you,' she said.

'If I go,' I said, 'I will bring you something.'

What innumerable follies laid waste my waking and sleeping thoughts after that evening! I wished to annihilate the tedious intervening days. I chafed against the work of school. At night in my bedroom and by day in the classroom her image came between me and the page I strove to read. The syllables of the word Araby were called to me through the silence in which my soul luxuriated and cast an Eastern enchantment over me. I asked for leave to go to the bazaar on Saturday night. My aunt was surprised, and hoped it was not some Freemason affair. I answered few questions in class. I watched my master's face pass from amiability to sternness; he hoped I was not beginning to idle. I could not call my wandering thoughts together. I had hardly any patience with the serious work of life which, now that it stood between me and my desire, seemed to me child's play, ugly monotonous child's play.

On Saturday morning I reminded my uncle that I wished to go to the bazaar in the evening. He was fussing at the hallstand, looking for the hat-brush, and answered me curtly:

'Yes, boy, I know.'

As he was in the hall I could not go into the front parlour and lie at the window. I felt the house in bad humour and walked slowly towards the school. The air was pitilessly raw and already my heart misgave me.

When I came home to dinner my uncle had not yet been home. Still it was early. I sat staring at the clock for some time and, when its ticking began to irritate me, I left the room. I mounted the staircase and gained the upper part of the house. The high, cold, empty, gloomy rooms liberated me and I went from room to room singing. From the front window I saw my companions playing below in the street. Their cries reached me weakened and indistinct and, leaning my forehead against the cool glass, I looked over at the dark house where she lived. I may have stood there for an hour, seeing nothing but the brown-clad figure cast by my imagination, touched discreetly by the lamplight at the curved neck, at the hand upon the railings and at the border below the dress.

When I came downstairs again I found Mrs Mercer sitting at the fire. She was an old, garrulous woman, a pawnbroker's widow, who collected used stamps for some pious purpose. I had to endure the gossip of the tea-table. The meal was prolonged beyond an hour and still my uncle did not come. Mrs Mercer stood up to go: she was sorry she couldn't wait any longer, but it was after eight o'clock and she did not like to be out late, as the night air was bad for her. When she had gone I began to walk up and down the room, clenching my fists. My aunt said:

'I'm afraid you may put off your bazaar for this night of Our Lord.'

At nine o'clock I heard my uncle's latchkey in the hall door. I heard him talking to himself and heard the hallstand rocking when it had received the weight of his overcoat. I could interpret these signs. When he was midway through his dinner I asked him to give me the money to go to the bazaar. He had forgotten.

'The people are in bed and after their first sleep now,' he said.

I did not smile. My aunt said to him energetically:

'Can't you give him the money and let him go? You've kept him late enough as it is.'

My uncle said he was very sorry he had forgotten. He said he believed in the old saying: 'All work and no play makes Jack a dull boy.' He asked me where I was going and, when I told him a second time, he asked me did I know *The Arab's Farewell to His Steed*. When I left the kitchen he was about to recite the opening lines of the piece to my aunt.

I held a florin tightly in my hand as I strode down Buckingham Street towards the station. The sight of the streets thronged with buyers and glaring with gas recalled to me the purpose of my journey. I took my seat in a third-class carriage of a deserted train. After an intolerable delay the train moved out of the station slowly. It crept onward among ruinous houses and over the twinkling river. At Westland Row Station a crowd of people pressed to the carriage doors; but the porters moved them back, saying that it was a special train for the bazaar. I remained alone in the bare carriage. In a few minutes the train drew up beside an improvised wooden platform. I passed out on to the road and saw by the lighted dial of a clock that it was ten minutes to ten. In front of me was a large building which displayed the magical name.

I could not find any sixpenny entrance and, fearing that the bazaar would be closed, I passed in quickly through a turnstile, handing a shilling to a weary-looking man. I found myself in a big hall girded at half its height by a gallery. Nearly all the stalls were closed and the greater part of the hall was in darkness. I recognized a silence like that which pervades a church after a service. I walked into the centre of the bazaar timidly. A few people were gathered about the stalls which were still open. Before a curtain, over which the words Café Chantant were written in coloured lamps, two men were counting money on a salver. I listened to the fall of the coins.

Remembering with difficulty why I had come, I went over to one of the stalls and examined porcelain vases and flowered tea-sets. At the door of the stall a young lady was talking and laughing with two young gentlemen. I remarked their English accents and listened vaguely to their conversation.

'O, I never said such a thing!'

'O, but you did!'

'O, but I didn't!'

'Didn't she say that?'

'Yes. I heard her.'

'O, there's a . . . fib!'

Observing me, the young lady came over and asked me did I wish to buy anything. The tone of her voice was not encouraging; she seemed to have spoken to me out of a sense of duty. I looked humbly at the great jars that stood like eastern guards at either side of the dark entrance to the stall and murmured:

'No, thank you.'

The young lady changed the position of one of the vases and went back to the two young men. They began to talk of the same subject. Once or twice the young lady glanced at me over her shoulder.

I lingered before her stall, though I knew my stay was useless, to make my interest in her wares seem the more real. Then I turned away slowly and walked down the middle of the bazaar. I allowed the two pennies to fall against the sixpence in my pocket. I heard a voice call from one end of the gallery that the light was out. The upper part of the hall was now completely dark.

Gazing up into the darkness I saw myself as a creature driven and derided by vanity; and my eyes burned with anguish and anger.

Richard Wright

The Man Who Was Almost a Man

Dave struck out across the fields, looking homeward through paling light. Whut's the use talking wid em niggers in the field? Anyhow, his mother was putting supper on the table. Them niggers can't understand nothing. One of these days he was going to get a gun and practice shooting, then they couldn't talk to him as though he were a little boy. He slowed, looking at the ground. Shucks, Ah ain scareda them even ef they are biggern me! Aw, Ah know whut Ahma do. Ahm going by ol Joe's sto n git that Sears Roebuck catlog n look at them guns. Mebbe Ma will lemme buy one when she gits ma pay from ol man Hawkins. Ahma beg her t gimme some money. Ahm ol enough to hava gun. Ahm seventeen. Almos a man. He strode, feeling his long loose-jointed limbs. Shucks, a man oughta hava little gun aftah he done worked hard all day.

He came in sight of Joe's store. A yellow lantern glowed on the front porch. He mounted steps and went through the screen door, hearing it bang behind him. There was a strong smell of coal oil and mackerel fish. He felt very confident until he saw fat Joe walk in through the rear door, then his courage began to ooze.

"Howdy, Dave! Whutcha want?"

"How yuh, Mistah Joe? Aw, Ah don wanna buy nothing. Ah jus wanted t see ef yuhd lemme look at tha catlog erwhile."

"Sure! You wanna see it here?"

"Nawsuh. Ah wants t take it home wid me. Ah'll bring it back termorrow when Ah come in from the fiels."

"You planning on buying something?"

"Yessuh."

"Your ma letting you have your own money now?"

"Shucks. Mistah Joe, Ahm gittin t be a man like anybody else!"

Joe laughed and wiped his greasy white face with a red bandanna.

"What you planning on buyin?"

Dave looked at the floor, scratched his head, scratched his thigh, and smiled. Then he looked up shyly.

"Ah'll tell yuh, Mistah Joe, ef yuh promise yuh won't tell."

"I promise."

"Waal, Ahma buy a gun."

"A gun? What you want with a gun?"

"Ah wanna keep it."

"You ain't nothing but a boy. You don't need a gun."

"Aw, lemme have the catlog, Mistah Joe. Ah'll bring it back."

Joe walked through the rear door. Dave was elated. He looked around at barrels of sugar and flour. He heard Joe coming back. He craned his neck to see if he were bringing the book. Yeah, he's got it. Gawddog, he's got it!

"Here, but be sure you bring it back. It's the only one I got."

"Sho, Mistah Joe."

"Say, if you wanna buy a gun, why don't you buy one from me? I gotta gun to sell."

"Will it shoot?"

"Sure it'll shoot."

"Whut kind is it?"

"Oh, it's kinda old . . . a left-hand Wheeler. A pistol. A big one."

"Is it got bullets in it?"

"It's loaded."

"Kin Ah see it?"

"Where's your money?"

"What yuh wan fer it?"

"I'll let you have it for two dollars."

"Just two dollahs? Shucks, Ah could buy tha when Ah git mah pay."

"I'll have it here when you want it."

"Awright, suh. Ah be in fer it."

He went through the door, hearing it slam again behind him. Ahma git some money from Ma n buy me a gun! Only two dollahs! He tucked the thick catalogue under his arm and hurried.

"Where yuh been, boy?" His mother held a steaming dish of black-eyed peas.

"Aw, Ma, Ah just stopped down the road t talk wid the boys."

"Yuh know bettah t keep suppah waiting."

He sat down, resting the catalogue on the edge of the table.

"Yuh git up from there and git to the well n wash yosef! Ah ain feedin no hogs in mah house!"

She grabbed his shoulder and pushed him. He stumbled out of the room, then came back to get the catalogue.

"Whut this?"

"Aw, Ma, it's jusa catlog."

"Who yuh git it from?"

"From Joe, down at the sto."

"Waal, thas good. We kin use it in the outhouse."

"Naw, Ma." He grabbed for it. "Gimme ma catlog, Ma."

She held onto it and glared at him.

"Quit hollerin at me! Whut's wrong wid yuh? Yuh crazy?"

"But Ma, please. It ain mine! It's Joe's! He tol me t bring it back t im termorow."

She gave up the book. He stumbled down the back steps, hugging the thick book under his arm. When he had splashed water on his face and hands, he groped back to the kitchen and fumbled in a corner for the towel. He bumped into a chair; it clattered to the floor. The catalogue sprawled at his feet. When he had dried his eyes he snatched up the book and held it again under his arms. His mother stood watching him.

"Now, ef yuh gonna act a fool over that ol book, Ah'll take it n burn it up."

"Naw, Ma, please."

"Waal, set down n be still!"

He sat down and drew the oil lamp close. He thumbed page after page, unaware of the food his mother set on the table. His father came in. Then his small brother.

"Whutcha got there, Dave?" His father asked.

"Jusa catlog," he answered, not looking up.

"Yeah, here they is!" His eyes glowed at blue-and-black revolvers. He glanced up, feeling sudden guilt. His father was watching him. He eased the book under the table and rested it on his knees. After the blessing was asked, he ate. He scooped up peas and swallowed fat meat without chewing. Buttermilk helped to wash it down. He did not want to mention money before his father. He would do much better by cornering his mother when she was alone. He looked at his father uneasily out of the edge of his eye.

"Boy, how come yah don quit foolin wid tha book n eat yo suppah?"

"Yessuh."

"How you n ol man Hawkins gitten erlong?"

"Suh?"

"Can't yuh hear? Why don yuh listen? Ah ast you how wuz yuh n ol man Hawkins gittin erlong?"

"Oh, swell, Pa. Ah plows mo lan than anybody over there."

"Waal, yuh oughta keep you mind on whut yuh doin."

"Yessuh."

He poured his plate full of molasses and sopped it up slowly with a chunk of cornbread. When his father and brother had left the kitchen, he still sat and looked again at the guns in the catalogue, longing to muster courage enough to present his case to his mother. Lawd, ef Ah only had tha pretty one! He could almost feel the slickness of the weapon with his fingers. If he had a gun like that he would polish it and keep it shining so it would never rust. N Ah'd keep it loaded, by Gawd!

"Ma?" His voice was hesitant.

"Hunh?"

"Ol man Hawkins give yuh mah money yit?"

"Yeah, but ain no usa yuh thinking about throwin nona it erway. Ahm keeping tha money sos yuh kin have cloes t go to school this winter."

He rose and went to her side with the open catalogue in his palms. She was washing dishes, her head bent low over a pan. Shyly he raised the book. When he spoke, his voice was husky, faint.

"Ma, Gawd knows Ah wans one of these."

"One of whut?" she asked, not raising her eyes.

"One of these," he said again, not daring even to point. She glanced up at the page, then at him with wide eyes.

"Nigger, is yuh gone plumb crazy?"

"Aw, Ma—"

"Git outta here! Don yuh talk talk t me bout no gun! Yuh a fool!"

"Ma, Ah kin buy one fer two dollahs."

"Not ef Ah knows it, yuh ain!"

"But yuh promised me one—"

"Ah don care what Ah promised! Yuh ain gonna toucha penny of tha money for no gun! Thas how come Ah has Mistah Hawkins t pay yu wages t me, cause Ah knows yuh ain got no sense."

"But, Ma, we needa gun. Pa ain got no gun. We needa gun in the house. Yuh kin never tell whut might happen."

"Now don yuh try to maka fool outta me, boy! Ef we did hava gun, yuh wouldn't have it!"

He laid the catalogue down and slipped his arm around her waist.

"Aw, Ma, Ah done worked hard all summer n ain ast yuh fer nothing, is Ah, now?"

"Thas whut yuh spose t do!"

"But Ma, Ah wans a gun. Yuh kin lemme have two dollahs outta mah money. Please, Ma. I kin give it to Pa . . . Please, Ma! Ah loves yuh, Ma."

When she spoke her voice came soft and low.

"What yu wan wida gun, Dave? Yuh don need no gun. Yuh'll git in trouble. N ef yo pa just thought Ah let yuh have money t buy a gun he'd hava fit."

"Ah'll hide it, Ma. It ain but two dollahs."

"Lawd, chil, whut's wrong wid yuh?"

"Ain nothing wrong, Ma. Ahm almos a man now. Ah wans a gun."

"Who gonna sell yuh a gun?"

"Ol Joe at the sto."

"N it don cos but two dollahs?"

"Thas all, Ma. Jus two dollahs. Please, Ma."

She was stacking the plates away; her hands moved slowly, reflectively. Dave kept an anxious silence. Finally, she turned to him.

"Ah'll let yuh git tha gun ef yuh promise me one thing."

"Whut's tha, Ma?"

"Yuh bring it straight back t me, yuh hear? It be fer Pa."

"Yessum! Lemme go now, Ma."

She stooped, turned slightly to one side, raised the hem of her dress, rolled down the top of her stocking, and came up with a slender wad of bills.

"Here," she said. "Lawd knows yuh don need no gun. But yer pa does. Yuh bring it right back t me, yuh hear? Ahma put it up. Now ef yuh don, Ahma have yuh pa lick yuh so hard yuh won fergit it."

"Yessum."

He took the money, ran down the steps, and across the yard.

"Dave! Yuuuuu Daaaaave!"

He heard, but he was not going to stop now. "Naw, Lawd!"

The first movement he made the following morning was to reach under his pillow for the gun. In the gray light of dawn he held it loosely, feeling a sense of power. Could kill a man with a gun like this. Kill anybody, black or white. And if he were holding his gun in his hand, nobody could run over him; they would have to respect him. It was a big gun, with a long barrel and a heavy handle. He raised and lowered it in his hand, marveling at its weight.

He had not come straight home with it as his mother had asked; instead he had stayed out in the fields, holding the weapon in his hand, aiming it now and then at some imaginary foe. But he had not fired it; he had been afraid that his father might hear. Also he was not sure he knew how to fire it.

To avoid surrendering the pistol he had not come into the house until he knew that they were all asleep. When his mother had tiptoed to his bedside late that night and demanded the gun, he had first played possum; then he had told her that the gun was hidden outdoors, that he would bring it to her in the morning. Now he lay turning it slowing in his hands. He broke it, took out the cartridges, felt them, and then put them back.

He slid out of bed, got a long strip of old flannel from a trunk, wrapped the gun in it, and tied it to his naked thigh while it was still loaded. He did not go in to breakfast. Even though it was not yet daylight, he started for Jim Hawkins' plantation. Just as the sun was rising he reached the barns where the mules and plows were kept.

"Hey! That you, Dave?"

He turned. Jim Hawkins stood eying him suspiciously.

"What're yuh doing here so early?"

"Ah didn't know Ah wuz gittin up so early, Mistah Hawkins. Ah was fixin t hitch up ol Jenny n take her t the fiels."

"Good. Since you're so early, how about plowing that stretch down by the woods?"

"Suits me, Mistah Hawkins."

"O.K. Go to it!"

He hitched Jenny to a plow and started across the fields. Hot dog! This was just what he wanted. If he could get down by the woods, he could shoot his gun and nobody would hear. He walked behind the plow, hearing the traces creaking, feeling the gun tied tight to his thigh.

When he reached the woods, he plowed two whole rows before he decided to take out the gun. Finally, he stopped, looked in all directions, then untied the gun and held it in his hand. He turned to the mule and smiled.

"Know whut this is, Jenny? Naw, yuh wouldn know! Yuhs jusa ol mule! Anyhow, this is a gun, n it kin shoot, by Gawd!"

He held the gun at arm's length. Whut t hell, Ahma shoot this thing! He looked at Jenny again.

"Lissen here, Jenny! When Ah pull this ol trigger, Ah don wan yuh to run n acka fool now!"

Jenny stood with head down, her short ears pricked straight. Dave walked off about twenty feet, held the gun far out from him at arm's length, and turned his head. Hell, he told himself, Ah ain afraid. The gun felt loose in his fingers; he waved it wildly for a moment. Then he shut his eyes and tightened his forefinger. *Bloom*! A report half deafened him and he thought his right hand was torn from his arm. He heard Jenny whinnying and galloping over the field, and he found himself on his knees, squeezing his fingers hard between his legs. His hand was numb; he jammed it into his mouth, trying to warm it, trying to stop the pain. The gun lay at his feet. He did not quite know what had happened. He stood up and stared at the gun as though it were a living thing. He gritted his teeth and kicked the gun. Yuh almos broke mah arm! He turned to look for Jenny; she was far over the fields, tossing her head and kicking wildly.

"Hol on there, ol mule!"

When he caught up with her she stood trembling, walling her big white eyes at him. The plow was far away; the traces had broken. Then Dave stopped short, looking, not believing. Jenny was bleeding. Her left side was red and wet with blood. He went closer. Lawd, have mercy! Wondah did Ah shoot this mule? He grabbed for Jenny's mane. She flinched, snorted, whirled, tossing her head.

"Hol on now! Hol on."

Then he saw the hole in Jenny's side, right between the ribs. It was round, wet, red. A crimson stream streaked down the front leg, flowing fast. Good Gawd! Ah wuzn't shootin at tha mule. He felt panic. He knew he had to stop that blood, or Jenny would bleed to death. He had never seen so much blood in all his life. He chased the mule for half a mile, trying to catch her. Finally she stopped, breathing hard, stumpy tail half arched. He caught her mane and led her back to where the plow and gun lay. Then he stooped and grabbed handfuls of damp black earth and tried to plug the bullet hole. Jenny shuddered, whinnied, and broke from him.

"Hol on! Hol on now!"

He tried to plug it again, but blood came anyhow. His fingers were hot and sticky. He rubbed dirt into his palms, trying to dry them. Then again he attempted to plug the bullet hole, but Jenny shied away, kicking her heels high. He stood helpless. He had to do something. He ran at Jenny; she dodged him. He watched a red stream of blood flow down Jenny's leg and form a bright pool at her feet.

"Jenny . . . Jenny," he called weakly.

His lips trembled. She's bleeding t death! He looked in the direction of home, wanting to go back, wanting to get help. But he saw the pistol lying in the damp black clay. He had a queer feeling that if he only did something, this would not be; Jenny would not be there bleeding to death.

When he went to her this time, she did not move. She stood with sleepy, dreamy eyes; and when he touched her she gave a low-pitched whinny and knelt to the ground, her front knees slopping in blood.

"Jenny . . . Jenny . . ." he whispered.

For a long time she held her neck erect; then her head sank, slowly. Her ribs swelled with a mighty heave and she went over.

Dave's stomach felt empty, very empty. He picked up the gun and held it gingerly between his thumb and forefinger. He buried it at the foot of a tree. He took a stick and tried to cover the pool of blood with dirt—but what was the use? There was Jenny lying with her mouth open and her eyes walled and glassy. He could not tell Jim Hawkins he had shot his mule. But he had to tell something. Yeah, Ah'll tell em Jenny started gittin ill n fell on the point of the plow . . . But that would hardly happen to a mule. He walked across the field slowly, head down.

It was sunset. Two of Jim Hawkins' men were over near the edge of the woods digging a hole in which to bury Jenny. Dave was surrounded by a knot of people, all of whom were looking down at the dead mule.

"I don't see how in the world it happened," said Jim Hawkins for the tenth time.

The crowd parted and Dave's mother, father, and small brother pushed into the center.

"Where Dave?" his mother called.

"There he is," said Jim Hawkins.

His mother grabbed him.

"Whut happened, Dave? Whut yuh done?"

"Nothin."

"C'mon, boy, talk," his father said.

Dave took a deep breath and told the story he knew nobody believed.

"Waal," he drawled. "Ah brung ol Jenny down here sos Ah could do mah plowin. Ah plowed bout two rows, just like yuh see." He stopped and pointed at the long rows of upturned earth. "Then something musta been wrong wid ol Jenny. She wouldn ack right a-tall. She started snortin n kickin her heels. Ah tried t hol her, but she pulled erway, rearin n goin in. Then when the point of the plow was stickin up in the air, she swung erroun n twisted herself back on it . . . She stuck herself n started t bleed. N fo Ah could do anyting, she wuz dead."

"Did you ever hear of anything like that in all your life?" asked Jim Hawkins.

There were white and black standing in the crowd. They murmured. Dave's mother came close to him and looked hard into his face. "Tell the truth, Dave," she said.

"Looks like a bullet hole to me," said one man.

"Dave, whut yuh do wid tha gun?" his mother asked.

The crowd surged in, looking at him. He jammed his hands into his pockets, shook his head slowly from left to right, and backed away. His eyes were wide and painful.

"Did he hava gun?" asked Jim Hawkins.

"By Gawd, Ah tol yuh tha wuz a gun wound," said a man, slapping his thigh.

His father caught his shoulders and shook him till his teeth rattled.

"Tell whut happened, yuh rascal! Tell whut . . ."

Dave looked at Jenny's stiff legs and began to cry.

"Whut yuh do wid tha gun?" his mother asked.

"Whut wuz he doin wida gun?" his father asked.

"Come on and tell the truth," said Hawkins. "Ain't nobody going to hurt you . . ."

His mother crowded close to him.

"Did yuh shoot tha mule, Dave?"

Dave cried, seeing blurred white and black faces.

"Ahh ddinn gggo tt sshooot hher . . . Ah sswear tt Gawd Ahh ddin . . . Ah wuz a-tryin t sssee ef the ggun would sshoot—"

"Where yuh git the gun from?" his father asked.

"Ah got it from Joe, at the sto."

"Where yuh git the money?"

"Ma give it t me."

"He kept worrying me, Bob. Ah had t. Ah tol im t bring the gun right back t me . . . It was fer yuh, the gun."

"But how yuh happen to shoot that mule?" asked Jim Hawkins.

"Ah wuzn shootin at the mule, Mistah Hawkins! The gun jumped when Ah pulled the trigger . . . N fo Ah knowed anything Jenny was there a-bleedin."

Somebody in the crowd laughed. Jim Hawkins walked close to Dave and looked into his face.

"Well, looks like you have bought you a mule, Dave."

"Ah swear fo Gawd. Ah didn go t kill the mule, Mistah Hawkins!"

"But you killed her!"

All the crowd was laughing now. They stood on tiptoe and poked heads over one another's shoulders.

"Well, boy, looks like yuh done bought a dead mule! Hahaha!"

"Ain tha ershame."

"Hohohohoho."

Dave stood, head down, twisting his feet in the dirt.

"Well, you needn't worry about it, Bob," said Jim Hawkins to Dave's father.

"Just let the boy keep on working and pay me two dollars a month."

"What yuh wan fer yo mule, Mistah Hawkins?"

Jim Hawkins screwed up his eyes.

"Fifty dollars."

"Whut yuh do wid tha gun?" Dave's father demanded.

Dave said nothing.

"Yuh wan me t take a tree n beat yuh till yuh talk!"

"Nawsuh!"

"Whut yuh do wid it?"

"Ah throwed it erway."

"Where?"

"Ah . . . Ah throwed it in the creek."

"Wall, c'mon home. N firs thing in the mawnin git to tha creek n fin tha gun."

"Yessuh."

"Whut yuh pay fer it?"

"Two dollahs."

"Take tha gun n git yo money back n carry it t Mistah Hawkins, yuh hear? N don fergit Ahma lam you black bottom good fer this! Now march yoself on home, suh!"

Dave turned and walked slowly. He heard people laughing. Dave glared, his eyes welling with tears. Hot anger bubbled in him. Then he swallowed and stumbled on.

That night Dave did not sleep. He was glad that he had gotten out of killing the mule so easily, but he was hurt. Something hot seemed to turn over inside him each time he remembered how they had laughed. He tossed on his bed, feeling his hard pillow. N Pa says he's gonna beat me . . . He remembered other beatings, and his back quivered. Naw, naw, Ah sho don wan im t beat me tha way no mo. Dam em all! Nobody ever gave him anything. All he did was work. They treat me like a mule, n then they beat me. He gritted his teeth. N Ma had t tell on me.

Well, if he had to, he would take old man Hawkins that two dollars. But that meant selling the gun. And he wanted to keep that gun. Fifty dollars for a dead mule.

He turned over, thinking how he had fired the gun. He had an itch to fire it again. Ef other men kin shoota gun, by Gawd, Ah kin! He was still, listening. Mebbe they all sleepin now. The house was still. He heard the soft breathing of his brother. Yes, now! He would go down and get that gun and see if he could fire it! He eased out of bed and slipped into overalls.

The moon was bright. He ran almost all the way to the edge of the woods. He stumbled over the ground, looking for the spot where he had buried the gun. Yeah, here it is. Like a hungry dog scratching for a bone, he pawed it up. He puffed his black cheeks and blew dirt from the trigger and barrel. He broke it and found four cartridges unshot. He looked around; the fields were filled with silence and moonlight. He clutched the gun stiff and hard in his fingers. But, as soon as he wanted to pull the trigger, he shut his eyes and turned his head. Naw, Ah can't shoot wid mah eyes closed n mah head turned. With effort he held his eyes open; then he squeezed. *Blooooom!* He was stiff, not breathing. The gun was still in his hands. Dammit, he'd done it! He fired again. *Blooooom!*

He smiled. *Blooooom! Blooooom! Click, click.* There! It was empty. If anybody could shoot a gun, he could. He put the gun into his hip pocket and started across the fields.

When he reached the top of a ridge he stood straight and proud in the moonlight, looking at Jim Hawkins' big white house, feeling the gun sagging in his pocket. Lawd, ef Ah had just one mo bullet Ah'd taka shot at tha house. Ah'd like t scare ol man Hawkins jusa little . . . Jusa enough t let im know Dave Saunders is a man.

To his left the road curved, running to the tracks of the Illinois Central. He jerked his head, listening. From far off came a faint *hoooof-hooof; hoooof-hoooof* . . . He stood rigid. Two dollahs a mont. Les see now . . . Tha mean it'll take bout two years. Shucks! Ah'll be dam!

He started down the road, toward the tracks. Yeah, here she comes! He stood beside the track and held himself stiffly. Here she comes, erroun the ben . . . C'mon, yuh slow poke! C'mon! He had his hand on his gun; something quivered in his stomach. Then the train thundered past, the gray and brown box cars rumbling and clinking. He gripped the gun tightly; then he jerked his hand out of his pocket. Ah betcha Bill wouldn't do it! Ah betcha . . . The cars slid past, steel grinding upon steel. Ahm ridin yuh ternight, so hep me Gawd! He was hot all over. He hesitated just a moment; then he grabbed, pulled atop a car, and lay flat. He felt his pocket; the gun was still there. Ahead the long rails were glinting in the moonlight, stretching away, away to somewhere, somewhere where he could be a man . . .

Katherine Mansfield

Her First Ball

Exactly when the ball began Leila would have found it hard to say. Perhaps her first real partner was the cab. It did not matter that she shared the cab with the Sheridan girls and their brother. She sat back in her own little corner of it, and the bolster on which her hand rested felt like the sleeve of an unknown young man's dress suit; and away they bowled, past waltzing lamp-posts and houses and fences and trees.

"Have you really never been to a ball before, Leila? But, my child, how too weird—" cried the Sheridan girls.

"Our nearest neighbour was fifteen miles," said Leila softly, gently opening and shutting her fan.

Oh dear, how hard it was to be indifferent like the others! She tried not to smile too much; she tried not to care. But every single thing was so new and exciting . . . Meg's tuberoses, Jose's long loop of amber, Laura's little dark head, pushing above her white fur like a flower through snow. She would remember for ever. It even gave her a pang to see her cousin Laurie throw away the wisps of tissue paper he pulled from the fastenings of his new gloves. She would like to have kept those wisps as a keepsake, as a remembrance. Laurie leaned forward and put his hand on Laura's knee.

"Look here, darling," he said. "The third and the ninth as usual. Twig?"

Oh, how marvellous to have a brother! In her excitement Leila felt that if there had been time, if it hadn't been impossible, she couldn't have helped crying because she was an only child, and no brother had ever said "Twig?" to her; no sister would ever say, as Meg said to Jose that moment, "I've never known your hair go up more successfully than it has to-night!"

But, of course, there was no time. They were at the drill hall already; there were cabs in front of them and cabs behind. The road was bright on either side with moving fan-like lights, and on the pavement gay couples seemed to float through the air; little satin shoes chased each other like birds.

"Hold on to me, Leila; you'll get lost," said Laura.

"Come on, girls, let's make a dash for it," said Laurie.

Leila put two fingers on Laura's pink velvet cloak, and they were somehow lifted past the big golden lantern, carried along the passage, and pushed into the little room marked "Ladies." Here the crowd was so great there was hardly space to take off their things; the noise was deafening. Two benches on either side were stacked high with wraps. Two old women in white aprons ran up and down tossing fresh armfuls. And everybody was pressing forward trying to get at the little dressing-table and mirror at the far end.

A great quivering jet of gas lighted the ladies' room. It couldn't wait; it was dancing already. When the door opened again and there came a burst of tuning from the drill hall, it leaped almost to the ceiling.

Dark girls, fair girls were patting their hair, tying ribbons again, tucking handkerchiefs down the fronts of their bodices, smoothing marble-white gloves. And because they were all laughing it seemed to Leila that they were all lovely.

"Aren't there any invisible hair-pins?" cried a voice. "How most extraordinary! I can't see a single invisible hair-pin."

"Powder my back, there's a darling," cried some one else.

"But I must have a needle and cotton. I've torn simply miles and miles of the frill," wailed a third.

Then, "Pass them along, pass them along!" The straw basket of programmes was tossed from arm to arm. Darling little pink-and-silver programmes, with pink pencils and fluffy tassels. Leila's fingers shook as she took one out of the basket. She wanted to ask some one, "Am I meant to have one too?" but she had just time to read: "Waltz 3. 'Two, Two in a Canoe.' Polka 4. 'Making the Feathers Fly,'" when Meg cried, "Ready, Leila?" and they pressed their way through the crush in the passage towards the big double doors of the drill hall.

Dancing had not begun yet, but the band had stopped tuning, and the noise was so great it seemed that when it did begin to play it would never be heard. Leila, pressing close to Meg, looking over Meg's shoulder, felt that even the little quivering coloured flags strung across the ceiling were talking. She quite forgot to be shy; she forgot how in the middle of dressing she had sat down on the bed with one shoe off and one shoe on and begged her mother to ring up her cousins and say she couldn't go after all. And the rush of longing she had had to be sitting on the veranda of their forsaken up-country home, listening to the baby owls crying "More pork" in the moonlight, was changed to a rush of joy so sweet that it was hard to bear alone. She clutched her fan, and, gazing at the gleaming, golden floor, the azaleas, the lanterns, the stage at one end with its red carpet and gilt chairs and the band in a corner, she thought breathlessly, "How heavenly; how simply heavenly!"

All the girls stood grouped together at one side of the doors, the men at the other, and the chaperones in dark dresses, smiling rather foolishly, walked with little careful steps over the polished floor towards the stage.

"This is my little country cousin Leila. Be nice to her. Find her partners; she's under my wing," said Meg, going up to one girl after another.

Strange faces smiled at Leila—sweetly, vaguely. Strange voices answered, "Of course, my dear." But Leila felt the girls didn't really see her. They were looking towards the men. Why didn't the men begin? What were they waiting for? There they stood, smoothing their gloves, patting their glossy hair and smiling among themselves. Then, quite suddenly, as if they had only just made up their minds that that was what they had to do, the men came gliding over the parquet. There was a joyful flutter among the girls. A tall, fair man flew up to Meg, seized her programme, scribbled something; Meg passed him on to Leila. "May I have the pleasure?" He ducked and smiled. There came a dark man wearing an eyeglass, then cousin Laurie with a friend, and Laura with a little freckled fellow whose tie was crooked. Then quite an old man—fat, with a big bald patch on his head—took her programme and murmured,

"Let me see, let me see!" And he was a long time comparing his programme, which looked black with names, with hers. It seemed to give him so much trouble that Leila was ashamed. "Oh, please don't bother," she said eagerly. But instead of replying the fat man wrote something, glanced at her again. "Do I remember this bright little face?" he said softly. "Is it known to me of yore?" At that moment the band began playing; the fat man disappeared. He was tossed away on a great wave of music that came flying over the gleaming floor, breaking the groups up into couples, scattering them, sending them spinning . . .

Leila had learned to dance at boarding school. Every Saturday afternoon the boarders were hurried off to a little corrugated iron mission hall where Miss Eccles (of London) held her "select" classes. But the difference between that dusty-smelling hall—with calico texts on the walls, the poor terrified little woman in a brown velvet toque with rabbit's ears thumping the cold piano, Miss Eccles poking the girls' feet with her long white wand—and this was so tremendous that Leila was sure if her partner didn't come and she had to listen to that marvellous music and to watch the others sliding, gliding over the golden floor, she would die at least, or faint, or lift her arms and fly out of one of those dark windows that showed the stars.

"Ours, I think—" Some one bowed, smiled, and offered her his arm; she hadn't to die after all. Some one's hand pressed her waist, and she floated away like a flower that is tossed into a pool.

"Quite a good floor, isn't it?" drawled a faint voice close to her ear.

"I think it's most beautifully slippery," said Leila.

"Pardon!" The faint voice sounded surprised. Leila said it again. And there was a tiny pause before the voice echoed, "Oh, quite!" and she was swung round again.

He steered so beautifully. That was the great difference between dancing with girls and men, Leila decided. Girls banged into each other, and stamped on each other's feet; the girl who was gentleman always clutched you so.

The azaleas were separate flowers no longer; they were pink and white flags streaming by.

"Were you at the Bells' last week?" the voice came again. It sounded tired. Leila wondered whether she ought to ask him if he would like to stop.

"No, this is my first dance," said she.

Her partner gave a little gasping laugh. "Oh, I say," he protested.

"Yes, it is really the first dance I've ever been to." Leila was most fervent. It was such a relief to be able to tell somebody. "You see, I've lived in the country all my life up till now . . ."

At that moment the music stopped, and they went to sit on two chairs against the wall. Leila tucked her pink satin feet under and fanned herself, while she blissfully watched the other couples passing and disappearing through the swing doors.

"Enjoying yourself, Leila?" asked Jose, nodding her golden head.

Laura passed and gave her the faintest little wink; it made Leila wonder for a moment whether she was quite grown up after all. Certainly her partner did not say very much. He coughed, tucked his handkerchief away, pulled down his waistcoat, took a minute thread off his sleeve. But it didn't matter. Almost immediately the band started and her second partner seemed to spring from the ceiling.

"Floor's not bad," said the new voice. Did one always begin with the floor? And then, "Were you at the Neaves' on Tuesday?" And again Leila explained. Perhaps it was a little strange that her partners were not more interested. For it was thrilling. Her first ball! She was only at the beginning of everything. It seemed to her that she had never known what the night was like before. Up till now it had been dark, silent, beautiful very often—oh yes—but mournful somehow. Solemn. And now it would never be like that again—it had opened dazzling bright.

"Care for an ice?" said her partner. And they went through the swing doors, down the passage, to the supper room. Her cheeks burned, she was fearfully thirsty. How sweet the ices looked on little glass plates and how cold the frosted spoon was, iced too! And when they came back to the hall there was the fat man waiting for her by the door. It gave her quite a shock again to see how old he was; he ought to have been on the stage with the fathers and mothers. And when Leila compared him with her other partners he looked shabby. His waistcoat was creased, there was a button off his glove, his coat looked as if it was dusty with French chalk.

"Come along, little lady," said the fat man. He scarcely troubled to clasp her, and they moved away so gently, it was more like walking than dancing. But he said not a word about the floor. "Your first dance, isn't it?" he murmured.

"How did you know?"

"Ah," said the fat man, "that's what it is to be old!" He wheezed faintly as he steered her past an awkward couple. "You see, I've been doing this kind of thing for the last thirty years."

"Thirty years?" cried Leila. Twelve years before she was born!

"It hardly bears thinking about, does it?" said the fat man gloomily. Leila looked at his bald head, and she felt quite sorry for him.

"I think it's marvellous to be still going on," she said kindly.

"Kind little lady," said the fat man, and he pressed her a little closer, and hummed a bar of the waltz. "Of course," he said, "you can't hope to last anything like as long as that. No-o," said the fat man, "long before that you'll be sitting up there on the stage, looking on, in your nice black velvet. And these pretty arms will have turned into little short fat ones, and you'll beat time with such a different kind of fan—a black bony one." The fat man seemed to shudder. "And you'll smile away like the poor old dears up there, and point to your daughter, and tell the elderly lady next to you how some dreadful man tried to kiss her at the club ball. And your heart will ache, ache"—the fat man squeezed her closer still, as if he really was sorry for that poor heart—"because no one wants to kiss you now. And you'll say how unpleasant these polished floors are to walk on, how dangerous they are. Eh, Mademoiselle Twinkletoes?" said the fat man softly.

Leila gave a light little laugh, but she did not feel like laughing. Was it—could it all be true? It sounded terribly true. Was this first ball only the beginning of her last ball, after all? At that the music seemed to change; it sounded sad, sad; it rose upon a great sigh. Oh, how quickly things changed! Why didn't happiness last for ever? For ever wasn't a bit too long.

"I want to stop," she said in a breathless voice. The fat man led her to the door.

"No," she said, "I won't go outside. I won't sit down. I'll just stand here, thank you." She leaned against the wall, tapping with her foot, pulling up her gloves and trying to smile. But deep inside her a little girl threw her pinafore over her head and sobbed. Why had he spoiled it all?

"I say, you know," said the fat man, "you mustn't take me seriously, little lady."

"As if I should!" said Leila, tossing her small dark head and sucking her underlip . . .

Again the couples paraded. The swing doors opened and shut. Now new music was given out by the bandmaster. But Leila didn't want to dance any more. She wanted to be home, or sitting on the veranda listening to those baby owls. When she looked through the dark windows at the stars, they had long beams like wings . . .

But presently a soft, melting, ravishing tune began, and a young man with curly hair bowed before her. She would have to dance, out of politeness, until she could find Meg. Very stiffly she walked into the middle; very haughtily she put her hand on his sleeve. But in one minute, in one turn, her feet glided, glided. The lights, the azaleas, the dresses, the pink faces, the velvet chairs, all became one beautiful flying wheel. And when her next partner bumped her into the fat man and he said, "Pardon," she smiled at him more radiantly than ever. She didn't even recognise him again.

Delmore Schwartz

In Dreams Begin Responsibilities

I

I think it is the year 1909. I feel as if I were in a motion picture theatre, the long arm of light crossing the darkness and spinning, my eyes fixed on the screen. This is a silent picture as if an old Biograph one, in which the actors are dressed in ridiculously old-fashioned clothes, and one flash succeeds another with sudden jumps. The actors too seem to jump about and walk too fast. The shots themselves are full of dots and rays, as if it were raining when the picture was photographed. The light is bad.

It is Sunday afternoon, June 12th, 1909, and my father is walking down the quiet streets of Brooklyn on his way to visit my mother. His clothes are newly pressed and his tie is too tight in his high collar. He jingles the coins in his pockets, thinking of the witty things he will say. I feel as if I had by now relaxed entirely in the soft darkness of the theatre; the organist peals out the obvious and approximate emotions on which the audience rocks unknowingly. I am anonymous, and

I have forgotten myself. It is always so when one goes to the movies, it is, as they say, a drug.

My father walks from street to street of trees, lawns and houses, once in a while coming to an avenue on which a street-car skates and gnaws, slowly progressing. The conductor, who has a handle-bar mustache, helps a young lady wearing a hat like a bowl with feathers on to the car. She lifts her long skirts slightly as she mounts the steps. He leisurely makes change and rings his bell. It is obviously Sunday, for everyone is wearing Sunday clothes, and the street-car's noises emphasize the quiet of the holiday. Is not Brooklyn the City of Churches? The shops are closed and their shades drawn, but for an occasional stationery store or drug-store with great green balls in the window.

My father has chosen to take this long walk because he likes to walk and think. He thinks about himself in the future and so arrives at the place he is to visit in a state of mild exaltation. He pays no attention to the houses he is passing, in which the Sunday dinner is being eaten, nor to the many trees which patrol each street, now coming to their full leafage and the time when they will room the whole street in cool shadow. An occasional carriage passes, the horse's hooves falling like stones in the quiet afternoon, and once in a while an automobile, looking like an enormous upholstered sofa, puffs and passes.

My father thinks of my mother, of how nice it will be to introduce her to his family. But he is not yet sure that he wants to marry her, and once in a while he becomes panicky about the bond already established. He reassures himself by thinking of the big men he admires who are married: William Randolph Hearst, and William Howard Taft, who has just become President of the United States.

My father arrives at my mother's house. He has come too early and so is suddenly embarrassed. My aunt, my mother's sister, answers the loud bell with her napkin in her hand, for the family is still at dinner. As my father enters, my grandfather rises from the table and shakes hands with him. My mother has run upstairs to tidy herself. My grandmother asks my father if he has had dinner, and tells him that Rose will be downstairs soon. My grandfather opens the conversation by remarking on the mild June weather. My father sits uncomfortably near the table, holding his hat in his hand. My grandmother tells my aunt to take my father's hat. My uncle, twelve years old, runs into the house, his hair tousled. He shouts a greeting to my father, who has often given him a nickel, and then runs upstairs. It is evident that the respect in which my father is held in the household is tempered by a good deal of mirth. He is impressive, yet he is very awkward.

II

Finally my mother comes downstairs, all dressed up, and my father being engaged in conversation with my grandfather becomes uneasy, not knowing whether to greet my mother or continue the conversation. He gets up from the chair clumsily and says "hello" gruffly. My grandfather watches, examining their congruence, such as it is, with a critical eye, and meanwhile rubbing his bearded cheek roughly, as he always does when he reflects. He is worried; he is afraid that my father will not make a good husband for his oldest daughter. At this point something happens to the film, just as my father is saying something funny to my mother; I am awakened to myself and my unhappiness just as my interest was rising. The audience begins to clap impatiently. Then the trouble is cared for but the film has been returned to a portion just shown, and once more I see my grandfather rubbing his bearded cheek and pondering my father's character. It is difficult to get back into the picture once more and forget myself, but as my mother giggles at my father's words, the darkness drowns me.

My father and mother depart from the house, my father shaking hands with my mother once more, out of some unknown uneasiness. I stir uneasily also, slouched in the hard chair of the theatre. Where is the older uncle, my mother's older brother? He is studying in his bedroom upstairs, studying for his final examination at the College of the City of New York, having been dead of rapid pneumonia for the last twenty-one years. My mother and father walk down the same quiet streets once more. My mother is holding my father's arm and telling him of the novel which she has been reading; and my father utters judgments of the characters as the plot is made clear to him. This is a habit which he very much enjoys, for he feels the utmost superiority and confidence when he approves and condemns the behavior of other people. At times he feels moved to utter a brief "Ugh"—whenever the story becomes what he would call sugary. This tribute is paid to his manliness. My mother feels satisfied by the interest which she has awakened; she is showing my father how intelligent she is, and how interesting.

They reach the avenue, and the street-car leisurely arrives. They are going to Coney Island this afternoon, although my mother considers that such pleasures are inferior. She has made up her mind to indulge only in a walk on the boardwalk and a pleasant dinner, avoiding the riotous amusements as being beneath the dignity of so dignified a couple.

My father tells my mother how much money he has made in the past week, exaggerating an amount which need not have been exaggerated. But my father has always felt that actualities somehow fall short. Suddenly I begin to weep. The determined old lady who sits next to me in the theatre is annoyed and looks at me with an angry face, and being intimidated, I stop. I drag out my handkerchief and dry my face, licking the drop which has fallen near my lips. Meanwhile I have missed something, for here are my mother and father alighting at the last stop, Coney Island.

III

They walk toward the boardwalk, and my father commands my mother to inhale the pungent air from the sea. They both breathe in deeply, both of them laughing as they do so. They have in common a great interest in health, although my father is strong and husky, my mother frail. Their minds are full of theories of what is good to eat and not good to eat, and sometimes they engage in heated discussions of the subject, the whole matter ending in my father's announcement, made with a scornful bluster, that you have to die sooner or later anyway. On the boardwalk's flagpole, the American flag is pulsing in an intermittent wind from the sea.

My father and mother go to the rail of the boardwalk and look down on the beach where a good many bathers are casually walking about. A few are in the surf. A peanut whistle pierces the air with its pleasant and active whine, and my father goes to buy peanuts. My mother remains at the rail and stares at the ocean. The ocean seems merry to her; it pointedly sparkles and again and again the pony waves are released. She notices the children digging in the wet sand, and the bathing costumes of the girls who are her own age. My father returns with the peanuts. Overhead the sun's lightning strikes and strikes, but neither of them are at all aware of it. The boardwalk is full of people dressed in their Sunday clothes and idly strolling. The tide does not reach as far as the boardwalk, and the strollers would feel no danger if it did. My mother and father lean on the rail of the boardwalk and absently stare at the ocean. The ocean is becoming rough; the waves come in slowly, tugging strength from far back. The moment before they somersault, the moment when they arch their backs so beautifully, showing green and white veins amid the black, that moment is intolerable. They finally crack, dashing fiercely upon the sand, actually driving, full force downward, against the sand, bouncing upward and forward, and at last petering out into a small stream which races up the beach and then is recalled. My parents gaze absentmindedly at the ocean, scarcely interested in its harshness. The sun overhead does not disturb them. But as I stare at the terrible sun which breaks up sight, and the fatal, merciless, passionate ocean, I forget my parents. I stare fascinated and finally, shocked by the indifference of my father and mother, I burst out weeping once more. The old lady next to me pats me on the shoulder and says "There, there, all of this is only a movie, young man, only a movie," but I look up once more at the terrifying sun and the terrifying ocean, and being unable to control my tears, I get up and go the men's room, stumbling over the feet of the other people seated in my row.

IV

When I return, feeling as if I had awakened in the morning sick for lack of sleep, several hours have apparently passed and my parents are riding on the merry-go-round. My father is on a black horse, my mother on a white one, and they seem to be making an eternal circuit for the single purpose of snatching the nickel rings which are attached to the arm of one of the posts. A hand-organ is playing; it is one with the ceaseless circling of the merry-go-round.

For a moment it seems that they will never get off the merry-go-round because it will never stop. I feel like one who looks down on the avenue from the 50th story of a building. But at length they do get off; even the music of the hand-organ has ceased for a moment. My father has acquired ten rings, my mother only two, although it was my mother who really wanted them.

They walk on along the boardwalk as the afternoon descends by imperceptible degrees into the incredible violet of dusk. Everything fades into a relaxed glow, even the ceaseless murmuring from the beach, and the revolutions of the merry-go-round. They look for a place to have dinner. My father suggests the best one on the boardwalk and my mother demurs, in accordance with her principles.

However they do go to the best place, asking for a table near the window, so that they can look out on the boardwalk and the mobile ocean. My father feels omnipotent as he places a quarter in the waiter's hand as he asks for a table. The place is crowded and here too there is music, this time from a kind of string trio. My father orders dinner with a fine confidence.

As the dinner is eaten, my father tells of his plans for the future, and my mother shows with expressive face how interested she is, and how impressed. My father becomes exultant. He is lifted up by the waltz that is being played, and his own future begins to intoxicate him. My father tells my mother that he is going to expand his business, for there is a great deal of money to be made. He wants to settle down. After all, he is twenty-nine, he has lived by himself since he was thirteen, he is making more and more money, and he is envious of his married friends when he visits them in the cozy security of their homes, surrounded, it seems, by the calm domestic pleasures, and by delightful children, and then, as the waltz reaches the moment when all the dancers swing madly, then, then with awful daring, then he asks my mother to marry him, although awkwardly enough and puzzled, even in his excitement, at how he had arrived at the proposal, and she, to make the whole business worse, begins to cry, and my father looks nervously about, not knowing at all what to do now, and my mother says: "It's all I've wanted from the moment I saw you," sobbing, and he finds all of this very difficult, scarcely to his taste, scarcely as he had thought it would be, on his long walks over the Brooklyn Bridge in the reverie of a fine cigar, and it was then that I stood up in the theatre and shouted: "Don't do it. It's not too late to change your minds, both of you. Nothing good will come of it, only remorse, hatred, scandal, and two children whose characters are monstrous." The whole audience turned to look at me, annoyed, the usher came hurrying down the aisle flashing his searchlight, and the old lady next to me tugged me down into my seat, saying: "Be quiet. You'll be put out, and you paid thirty-five cents to come in." And so I shut my eyes because I could not bear to see what was happening. I sat there quietly.

V

But after a while I begin to take brief glimpses, and at length I watch again with thirsty interest, like a child who wants to maintain his sulk although offered the bribe of candy. My parents are now having their picture taken in a photographer's booth along the boardwalk. The place is shadowed in the mauve light which is apparently necessary. The camera is set to the side on its tripod and looks like a Martian man. The photographer is instructing my parents in how to pose. My father has his arm over my mother's shoulder, and both of them smile emphatically. The photographer brings my mother a bouquet of flowers to hold in her hand but she holds it at the wrong angle. Then the photographer covers himself with the black cloth which drapes the camera and all that one sees of him is one protruding arm and his hand which clutches the rubber ball which he will squeeze when the picture is finally taken. But he is not satisfied with their appearance. He feels with certainty that somehow there is something wrong in their pose. Again and again he issues from his hidden place with new directions. Each suggestion merely makes matters worse. My father is becoming impatient. They try a seated pose. The photographer explains that he has pride, he is not interested in all of this for the money, he wants to make beautiful pictures. My father says: "Hurry up, will you? We haven't got all night." But the photographer only scurries about apologetically, and issues new directions. The photographer charms me. I approve of him with all my heart, for I know just how he feels, and as he criticizes each revised pose according to some unknown idea of rightness, I become quite hopeful. But then my father says angrily: "Come on, you've had enough time, we're not going to wait any longer." And the photographer, sighing unhappily, goes back under his black covering, holds out his hand, says: "One, two, three, Now!", and the picture is taken, with my father's smile turned to a grimace and my mother's, bright and false. It takes a few minutes for the picture to be developed and as my parents sit in the curious light they become quite depressed.

VI

They have passed a fortune-teller's booth, and my mother wishes to go in, but my father does not. They begin to argue about it. My mother becomes stubborn, my father once more impatient, and then they begin to quarrel, and what my father would like to do is walk off and leave my mother there, but he knows that that would never do. My mother refuses to budge. She is near to tears, but she feels an uncontrollable desire to hear what the palm-reader will say. My father consents angrily, and they both go into a booth which is in a way like the photographer's, since it is draped in black cloth and its light is shadowed. The place is too warm, and my father keeps saying this is all nonsense, pointing to the crystal ball on the table. The fortune-teller, a fat, short woman, garbed in what is supposed to be Oriental robes, comes into the room from the back and greets them, speaking with an accent. But suddenly my father feels that the whole thing is intolerable; he tugs at my mother's arm, but my mother refuses to budge. And then, in terrible anger, my father lets go of my mother's arm and strides out, leaving my mother stunned. She moves to go after my father, but the fortune-teller holds her arm tightly and begs her not to do so, and I in my seat am shocked more than can ever be said, for I feel as if I were walking a tight-rope a hundred feet over a circus-audience and suddenly the rope is showing signs of breaking, and I get up from my seat and begin to shout once more the first words I can think of to communicate my terrible fear and once more the usher comes hurrying down the aisle flashing his search-light, and the old lady pleads with me, and the shocked audience has turned to stare at me, and I keep shouting: "What are they doing? Don't they know what they are doing? Why doesn't my mother go after my father? If she does not do that, what will she do? Doesn't my father know what he is doing?"—But the usher has seized my arm and is dragging me away, and as he does so, he says: "What are *you* doing? Don't you know that you can't do whatever you want to do? Why should a young man like you, with your whole life before you, get hysterical like this? Why don't you *think* of what you're doing? You can't act like this even if other people aren't around! You will be sorry if you do not do what you should do, you can't carry on like this, it is not right, you will find that out soon enough, everything you do matters too much," and he said that dragging me through the lobby of the theatre into the cold light, and I woke up into the bleak winter morning of my 21st birthday, the windowsill shining with its lip of snow, and the morning already begun.

Ruth Prawer Jhabvala

My First Marriage

Last week Rahul went on a hunger strike. He didn't have to suffer long —his family got very frightened (he is the only son) and by the second day they were ready to do anything he wanted, even to let him marry me. So he had a big meal, and then he came to tell me of his achievement. He was so proud and happy that I too pretended to be happy. Now his father and Daddy are friends again, and they sit downstairs in the study and talk together about their university days in England. His mother too comes to the house, and yesterday his married sister Kamla paid me a visit. The last time I had met Kamla was when she told me all those things on their veranda, but neither of us seemed to have any recollection of that. Instead we had a very nice conversation about her husband's promotion and the annual flower show for which she had been asked to organize a raffle. Mama walks around the house looking pleased with herself and humming snatches of the national anthem (out of tune —she is completely unmusical). No one ever mentions M. any more.

It is two years now since he went away. I don't know where he is or what he is doing. Perhaps he is meditating somewhere in the

Himalayas, or wandering by the banks of the Ganges with an orange robe and a begging bowl; or perhaps he is just living in another town, trying to start a newspaper or a school. Sometimes I ask myself: can there really have been such a man? But it is not a question to which I require any answer. The first time I saw M., I was just going out to tennis with Rahul. I hardly glanced at him—he was just one of the people who came to see Daddy. But he returned many times, and I heard Daddy say: "That young man is a nuisance." "Of course," said Mama in a sarcastic way, "you can never say no to anyone." Daddy looked shy: it was true, he found it difficult to refuse people. He is the Director of Education, and because it is an important position, people are always coming, both to the house and to his office, to ask him to do something for them. Mostly there is nothing he can do, but because he is so nice and polite to them, they keep coming again. Then often Mama steps in.

One day, just as I was going out to Rahul's house, I heard her shouting outside the door of the study. "The Director is a busy man!" she was shouting. She had her back against the door and held her arms stretched out; M. stood in front of her, and his head was lowered. "Day after day you come and eat his life up!" she said.

I feel very embarrassed when I hear Mama shouting at people, so I went away quickly. But when I was walking down the road, he suddenly came behind me. He said, "Why are you walking so fast?"

I said nothing. I thought it was very rude of him to speak to me at all.

"You are running away," he said.

Then in spite of myself I had to laugh: "From what?"

"From the Real," he said, and he spoke so seriously that I was impressed and stood still in the middle of the road and looked at him.

He was not really young—not young like I am, or like Rahul. His hair was already going gray and he had lines around his eyes. But what eyes they were, how full of wisdom and experience! And he was looking at me with them. I can't describe how I felt suddenly.

He said he wanted Daddy to open a new department in the university. A department for moral training. He explained the scheme to me and we both stood still in the road. His eyes glowed. I understood at once; of course, not everything—I am not a brilliant person such as he—but I understood it was important and even grand. Here were many new ideas, which made life seem quite different. I began to see that I had been living wrongly because I had been brought up to think wrongly.

Everything I thought important, and Daddy and Mama and Rahul and everyone, was not important: these were the frivolities of life we were caught up in. For the first time someone was explaining to me the nature of reality. I promised to help him and to speak to Daddy. I was excited and couldn't stop thinking of everything he had said and the way he had said it. He often telephoned. I waited for his calls and was impatient and restless till they came. But I was also a little ashamed to talk to him because I could not tell him that I had succeeded. I spoke to Daddy many times. I said, "Education is no use without a firm moral basis."

"How philosophical my little girl is getting," Daddy said and smiled and was pleased that I was taking an interest in higher things.

Mama said, "Don't talk so much; it's not nice in a young girl."

When M. telephoned I could only say, "I'm trying."

"You are not trying!" he said; he spoke sternly to me. "You are thinking of your own pleasures only, of your tennis and games."

He was right—I often played tennis, and now that my examinations were finished, I spent a lot of time at the Club and went to the cinema and read novels. When he spoke to me, I realized all that was wrong; so that every time he telephoned I was thoughtful for many hours afterward and when Rahul came to fetch me for tennis, I said I had a headache.

But I tried to explain to Rahul. He listened carefully; Rahul listens carefully to everything I say. He becomes very serious, and his eyes, which are very large, become even larger. He looks so sweet then, just as he did when he was a little boy. I remember Rahul as a little boy, for we always played together. His father and Daddy were great friends, almost like brothers. So Rahul and I grew up together, and later it was decided we would be married. Everyone was happy: I also, and Rahul. We were to be married quite soon, for we had both finished our college and Rahul's father had already got him a good job in a business firm, with very fine prospects.

"You see, Rahul, we live in nice houses and have nice clothes and good education and everything, and all the time we don't know what reality is."

Rahul frowned a bit, the way he used to do over his sums when they were difficult; but he nodded and looked at me with his big sweet eyes and was ready to listen to everything else I would tell him. Rahul has very smooth cheeks and they are a little bit pink because he is so healthy.

One day when M. telephoned he asked me to go and meet him. At first I tried to say no, but I knew I really wanted to go. He called me to a coffeehouse I had never been to before, and I felt shy when going in—there were many men and no girls at all. Everyone looked at me; some of them may have been students from the university and perhaps they knew me. It was noisy in there and full of smoke and smelled of fritters and chutney. The tablecloths were dirty and so were the bearers' uniforms. But he was there, waiting for me. I had often tried to recall his face but I never could: now I saw it and—of course, of course, I cried to myself, that was how it was, how could I forget.

Then I began to meet him every day. Sometimes we met in that coffeehouse, at other times in a little park where there was a broken swing and an old tomb and clerks came to eat their lunch out of tiffin carriers. It was the end of winter and the sky was pale blue with little white lines on it and the sun was just beginning to get hot again and there were scarlet creepers all over the tomb and green parrots flew about. When I went home, I would lie on the bed in my room and think. Rahul came and I said I had a headache. I hardly knew anything anyone was saying. I ate very little. Mama often came into my room and asked, "Where did you go today?" She was very sweet and gentle, the way she always is when she wants to find out something from you. I would tell her anything that came into my head—an old college friend had come from Poona, we had been to the cinema together—"Which cinema?" Mama said, still sweet and gentle and tidying the handkerchiefs in my drawer. I would even tell her the story of the film I had not seen. "Tomorrow I'm meeting her again." "No, tomorrow I want you to come with me to Meena auntie—"

It began to be difficult to get out of the house. Mama watched me every minute, and when she saw me ready to leave, she stood in the doorway: "Today you are coming with me."

"I told you, I have to meet—"

"You are coming with me!"

We were both angry and shouted. Daddy came out of the study. He told Mama, "She is not a child . . ."

Then Mama started to shout at him and I ran out of the house and did not look back, though I could hear her calling me.

When I told M., he said, "You had better come with me." I also saw there was no other way. On Friday afternoons Mama goes to a committee meeting of the All-India Ladies' Council, so that was the best time.

I bundled up all my clothes and jewels in a sheet and I walked out of the house. Faqir Chand, our butler, saw me, but he said nothing—probably he thought I was sending my clothes to the washerman. M. was waiting for me in a tonga by the post office and he helped me climb up and sit beside him; the tonga was a very old and shaky one, and the driver was also old and so was the horse. We went very slowly, first by the river, past the Fort and through all the bazaars, he and I sitting side by side at the back of the tonga with my bundle between us.

We had such a strange wedding. I laugh even now when I think of it. He had a friend who was a sign painter and had a workshop on the other side of the river. The workshop was really only a shed, but they made it very nice—they turned all the signboards to the wall and they hung my saris over them and over the saris they hung flower garlands. It looked really artistic. They also bought sweetmeats and nuts and put them on a long table that they had borrowed from a carpenter. Several friends of his came and quite a lot of people who lived in sheds and huts nearby. There was a priest and a fire was lit and we sat in front of it and the priest chanted the holy verses. I was feeling very hot because of the fire and of course my face was completely covered by the sari. It wasn't a proper wedding sari, but my own old red sari that I had last worn when Mama gave a tea party for the professors' wives in our drawing room, with cakes from Wenger's.

M. got very impatient, he kept telling the priest, "Now hurry hurry, we have heard all that before."

The priest was offended and said, "These are all holy words."

I couldn't help laughing under my sari, even though I was crying at the same time because I was thinking of Daddy and Rahul and Mama.

There was a quarrel—his friends also told him to keep quiet and let the priest say his verses in the proper manner, and he got angry and shouted, "Is it my marriage or yours?"

At last it was finished and we were married and everyone ate sweetmeats and nuts, even people who just wandered in from the road and whom no one knew.

We stayed a few days with his friend. There was a little room built out of planks just off the workshop and in that we all slept at night, rolled up in blankets. In the day, when the friend painted signs, we stayed in the room by ourselves, M. and I, and no one came in to disturb us. When he slept, I would look at him and look; I studied all the lines on his face.

After I had looked my fill, I would shut my eyes and try to see his face in my mind, and when I opened them again, there he was really, his real face, and I cried out loud with joy.

After some days we went on a bus to Niripat. The journey was four hours long and the bus was crowded with farmers and laborers and many old women carrying little bundles. There was a strong smell of poor people who can't afford to change their clothes very often and of the food that the old women ate out of their bundles and the petrol from the bus. I began to feel a little sick. I often get carsick: when we used to drive up to Naini Tal for the summer holidays, Daddy always had to stop the car several times so that I could go out and take fresh air; and Mama would give me lemon drops to suck and rub my temples with eau de cologne.

In Niripat we stayed with M.'s cousin, who had a little brick house just outside the town. They were a big family, and the women lived in one side of the house, in a little set of dark rooms with only metal trunks and beds in them, and the men on the other side. But I ran all over the house; I was singing and laughing all the time. In the evenings I sat with the men and listened to them talking about religion and philosophy and their business (they had a grinding mill); and during the day I helped the women with their household work. M. and I went out for walks and sometimes we went swimming in a pond. The women of the house teased me a lot because I liked M. so much. "But look at him," they said, "he is so dark; and see! His hair is going gray like an old man's." Or, "He is just a loafer—it is only talking with him and never any work." I pretended to be annoyed with them (of course, I knew they were only joking) and that made them laugh more than ever. One of them said, "Now it is very fine, but just wait, in the end her fate will be the same as Savitri's."

"Savitri?" I said.

So that was how I first heard about Savitri and the children. At first I was unhappy, but M. explained everything. He had been married very young and to a simple girl from a village. After some years he had left her. She understood it was necessary for him to leave her because he had a task to fulfill in the world in which she could not help him. She went back to her parents, with the children. She was happy now, because she saw it was her duty to stay at home and look after the children and lead the good, simple, self-sacrificing life of a mother. He talked of her with affection: she was patient and good. I too learned to love her. I thought of her in the village, with the children, quietly doing her household tasks; early in the mornings and in the evenings she said her prayers. So her life passed. He had gone to see her a few times and she had welcomed him and been glad; but when he went away again, she never tried to keep him. I thought how it would be if he went away from me, but I could not even bear the idea. My heart hurt terribly and I stifled a cry. From that I saw how much nobler and more advanced Savitri was than I; and I hoped that, if the time ever came, I too could be strong like her. But not yet. Not yet. We sold my pearl brooch and sent money to her; he always sent money to her when he had it. Once he said of her: "She is a candle burning in a window of the world," and that was how I always thought of her—as a candle burning for him with a humble flame.

I had not yet written to Daddy and Mama, but I wrote to Rahul. I wrote, "Everything is for the best, Rahul. I often think about you. Please tell everyone that I am all right and happy." M. and I went to the post office together to buy a stamp and post the letter. On the way back he said, "You must write to your father also. He must listen to our ideas." How proud I was when he said *our* ideas.

Daddy and Mama came to Niripat. Daddy sent me a letter in which it said they were waiting for me at the Victoria Hotel. M. took me there, and then went away; he said I must talk to them and explain everything. The Victoria Hotel is the only hotel in Niripat and it is not very grand—it is certainly not the sort of hotel in which Mama is used to staying. In front there is the Victoria Restaurant, where meals can be had at a reduced rate on a monthly basis; there is an open passage at the side that leads to the hotel rooms. Some of the guests had pulled their beds out into the passage and were sitting on them: I noticed a very fat man in a dhoti and an undervest saying his prayers. But Daddy and Mama were inside their room.

It was a very small room with two big beds in it and a table with a blue cotton tablecloth in the middle. Mama was lying on one of the beds; she was crying, and when I came in, she cried more. Daddy and I embraced each other, but Mama turned her face away and pressed her eyes with her handkerchief and the tears rolled right down into her blouse. It made me impatient to see her like that: every mother must part with her daughter sometime, so what was there to cry about? I squeezed Daddy's hands, to show him how happy I was, but then he too turned his face away from me and he coughed. Here we were meeting after so many days, and they were both behaving in a ridiculous manner. I spoke to them quite sharply: "Every individual being must choose his own life and I have chosen mine."

"Don't, darling," Daddy said as if something were hurting him.

Mama suddenly shouted, "You are my shame and disgrace!"

"Quietly, quietly," Daddy said.

I felt like shouting back at her, but I controlled myself; I had not come there to quarrel with her, even if she had come to quarrel with me. I was a wiser person now than I had been. So I only said: "There are aspects of life which you will never grasp." A little servant boy came in with tea on a tray. Mama sat up on the bed—she is always very keen on her tea—but after a while she sank back again and said in a fainting sort of voice, "There is something dirty in the milk." I had a look and there were only bits of straw, from the cowshed, which I fished out easily with a teaspoon.

Daddy gave a big sigh and said, "You had better let me speak with the young man."

So then I was happy again: I knew that when Daddy really spoke to him and got to know him, he would soon realize what sort of a person M. was and everything would be all right.

And everything was all right. It was true, Daddy couldn't start the department of moral training for him, as we had hoped, because the university didn't have enough funds for a new department; and also, Daddy said, he couldn't get him an academic post because M. didn't have the necessary qualifications. (How stupid are these rules and regulations! Here was a wonderful gifted person like M., with great ideas and wide experience of life, who had so much to pass on; yet he had to take a backward place to some poor little M.A. or Ph.D. who knows nothing of life at all except what he has read in other people's books.) So all Daddy could do was get him a post as secretary to one of the college principals; and I think it was very nice of M. to accept it, because it was not the sort of post a person such as he had a right to expect. But he was always like that: he knew nothing of petty pride and never stood on his dignity, unlike many other people who have really no dignity at all to stand on.

I was sorry to leave Niripat, where I had been so happy with everyone, and to go home again. But of course it was different now, because M. was with me. We had the big guest room at the back of the house and at night we made our beds out on the lawn. Sometimes I thought how funny it was—only a few weeks ago Mama had tried to turn him out of the house and here he was back in the best guest room. It is true that the wheel of fate has many unexpected revolutions. I think he quite liked living in the house, though I was afraid at first he would feel stifled with so many servants and all that furniture and the carpets and clocks and Mama's china dinner-services. But he was too great in soul to be bothered by these trivial things; he transcended them and led his life and thought his thoughts in the same way as he would have done if he had been living in some little hut in the jungle.

If only Mama had had a different character. But she is too sunk in her own social station and habits to be able to look out and appreciate anything higher. She thinks if a person has not been abroad and doesn't wear suits and open doors for ladies, he is an inferior type of person. If M. had tried, I know he could have used a knife and fork quite as well as Mama or anyone, but why should he have tried? And there were other things like not making a noise when you drink your tea, which are just trivial little conventions we should all rise above. I often tried to explain this to Mama but I could never make her understand. So it became often quite embarrassing at meal times, with Mama looking at M., and pretending she couldn't eat her own food on account of the way he was eating his. M. of course never noticed, and I felt so ashamed of Mama that in the end I also refused to use any cutlery and ate with my hands. Daddy never said anything—in fact, Daddy said very little at all nowadays, and spent long hours in his office and went to a lot of meetings and, when he came home, he only sat in his study and did not come out to talk to us.

I often thought about Rahul. He had never answered my letter and when I tried to telephone, they said he was not at home. But I wanted very much to see him; there were so many things I had to tell him about. So one day I went to his house. The servants made me wait on the veranda and then Rahul's married sister Kamla came out. Kamla is a very ambitious person and she is always scheming for her husband's promotion (he is in the Ministry of Defense) so that she can take precedence over the other wives in his department. I was not surprised at the way she talked to me. I know a person like Kamla will always think only petty thoughts and doesn't understand that there is anything transcending the everyday life in which she is sunk up to her ears. So I let her say what she wanted and when she told me to go away, I went. When Mama found out that I had been to Rahul's house, she was furious. "All right, so you have lost all pride for yourself, but for your family—at least think of us!" At the word pride I laughed out loud: Mama's ideas of pride were so different from mine and M.'s. But I was sorry that they wouldn't let me see Rahul.

M. went out every day, and I thought he went to his job in the university. But one day Daddy called me into his study and he said that M. had lost his job because he hadn't been going there for weeks. I had a little shock at first, but then I thought it is all right, whatever he wants to do is all right; and anyway, it hadn't been a suitable post for him in the first place. I told Daddy so.

Daddy played with his silver paper-knife and he didn't look at me at all; then he said, "You know he has been married before?" and still he didn't look at me. I don't know how Daddy found out—I suppose he must have been making inquiries, it is the sort of thing people in our station of life always do about other people, we are so mistrustful—but I answered him quite calmly. I tried to explain to him about Savitri. After a while Daddy said, "I only wanted you to know that your marriage is not legal and can be dissolved any time you want."

Then I told him that marriages are not made in the sight of the law but in the sight of God, and that in the sight of God both Savitri and I were married to M., she there and I here. Daddy turned his head away and looked out of the window.

M. told me that he wanted to start a school and that he could do so if Daddy got him a grant from the Ministry. I thought it was a very exciting idea and we talked a lot about it that night, as we lay together on our beds. He had many wonderful ideas about how a school should be run and said that the children should be taught to follow only their instincts, which would lead them to the highest Good. He talked so beautifully like a prophet, a saint. I could hardly sleep all night, and first thing in the morning I talked to Daddy. Unfortunately Mama was listening at the door—she has a bad habit of doing that—and suddenly she came bursting in. "Why don't you leave your father alone?" she cried. "Isn't it enough that we give you both food and shelter?"

I said, "Mama please, I'm talking important business with Daddy."

She began to say all sorts of things about M. and why he had married me. Daddy tried to keep her quiet but she was beyond herself by that time, so I just covered my ears with my hands and ran out. She came after me, still shouting these horrible things.

There in the hall was M., and when I tried to run past him, he stopped me and took my hands from my ears and made me listen to everything Mama was saying. She got more and more furious, and then she went into one of her hysterical fits, in which she throws herself down and beats her head on the floor and tears at her clothes. Daddy tried to lift her up, but of course she is too heavy for him. She went on screaming and shouting at M. M. said, "Go and get your things," so I went and wrapped everything up in the sheet again, his things and mine, and he slung the bundle over his shoulder and went out of the house, with me walking behind him.

I hoped we would go back to Niripat, but he wanted to stay in the city because he had several schemes in mind—there was the school, and he also had hopes of starting a newspaper in which he could print all his ideas. So he had to go around and see a lot of people, in ministries and so on. Sometimes he got quite discouraged because it was so difficult to make people understand. Then he looked tired and the lines on his face became very deep and I felt such love and pity for him. But he had great inner strength, and next day he always started on his rounds again, as fresh and hopeful as before.

We had no proper home at that time, but lived in several places. There was the sign painter, and another friend had a bookshop in one of the government markets with a little room at the back where we could stay with him; and once we found a model house that was left over from a low-cost housing exhibition, and we lived in that till workmen came to tear it down. There were plenty of places where we could stay for a few days or even weeks. In the evenings there were always many friends and all sat and discussed their ideas, and some of them recited poetry or played the flute, so that sometimes we didn't go to sleep at all. We never had any worries about money—M. said if one doesn't think about money, one doesn't need it, and how true that is. Daddy sent me a check every month, care of the friends who kept the bookshop, and we still had some of my jewelry, which we could sell whenever we wanted; so there was even money to send to Savitri and the children.

Once I met Rahul, quite by chance. That was at the time when we had just moved out of the exhibition house. M. had to go to one of the ministries to see an under-secretary, and I was taking our bundle to an orphanage, run by a friend of M.'s, where we were going to stay. I was waiting for a bus, holding the bundle; it wasn't heavy at all anymore, so there was no need to take a tonga. Rahul came out of a music shop with some records that he had just bought (he is very fond of dance records—

how often we have danced together to his gramophone!). I called to him and when he didn't hear me, I went up to him. He lowered his eyes and wouldn't look at me and hardly greeted me. "Rahul," I said in the stern voice I always use with him when I think he is misbehaving. "Why did you do it?" he said. "My family are very angry with you and I'm also angry." He sulked, but he looked so sweet; he still had his pink cheeks.

"If you have your car, you can give me a lift," I said. Rahul is always a gentleman, and he even carried my bundle for me to his car.

It took us a long time to find the orphanage—it was right at the back of the Fatehpuri mosque somewhere—so there was plenty of time for me to talk to him. He listened quite quietly, driving the car through all that traffic. When at last we found the orphanage and I was ready to get out, he said. "Don't go yet." I stayed with him for a while, even though the car was parked very awkwardly in that crowded alleyway, and men with barrows swore at us because they could not get past.

Soon afterward a friend of M.'s who was in the railways got transferred, and as he lived in a house with a very low rent, it was a good opportunity for us and we took it over from him. There were two rooms and a little yard at the back, and upstairs two families were living. Daddy would send a check for the rent. I cooked for us and cleaned the house and talked with the families upstairs, while M. went out to see people about his ideas. But after a time he began to go out less and less, and he became depressed; he said the world had rejected him because he was not strong enough yet. Now it was his task to purify himself and make himself stronger. He stayed at home and meditated. A strange change came over him. Most of the time he sat in one of our rooms, in a corner of the floor by himself, and he wouldn't let me come in. Sometimes I heard him singing to himself and shouting—he made such strange noises, almost like an animal. For days he ate nothing at all and, when I tried to coax him, he upset the food I had brought and threw it on the floor. I tried to be patient and bear and understand everything.

His friends stopped coming and he hardly ever left that little room for two months. Then he started going out by himself—I never knew where and could not ask him. He had an expression on his face as if he were listening for something, so that one felt one couldn't disturb him. When he talked to me, he talked as if he were someone else and I were someone else. At night I slept in the yard at the back with the families from upstairs, who were always kind to me.

Then visitors began to come for him—not his old friends, but quite new people whom I had never seen before. They sat with him in the little room and I could hear him talking to them. At first only a few men used to come, but then more and more came, and women too. I also sat in the room sometimes and listened to him talk; he told strange stories about parrots and princes and tigers in the jungle, all of which had some deep meaning. When the people understood the deep meaning, they all exclaimed with pleasure and said God was speaking through his mouth.

Now they began to bring us gifts of food and money and clothes and even jewelry. M. never took any notice, and I just piled the things in the other room, which was soon very crowded. We ate the food and I also gave it to the families upstairs, but there was still plenty left over, and at night someone used to come from the beggars' home to take it away. I sent a lot of money to Savitri. The house was always full of people now, and they spilled over into the yard and out into the street. More and more women came —most of them were old but there were some young ones too, and the young ones were even more fervent and religious than the old ones. There was one plump and pretty young widow, who was always dressed very nicely and came every day. She said she was going mad with love of God and needed words of solace and comfort from M. She touched his feet and implored him to relieve her, and when he took no notice of her, she shook him and tugged at his clothes, so that he became quite angry.

Mama often came to see me. In the beginning she was very disgusted with the house and the way we lived and everything, but afterward, when she saw how many people came and all the things they brought and how they respected M., she kept quiet on that subject. Now she only said, "Who knows what is to become of it all?" Mama is not really a religious person, but she has a lot of superstitions. When holy men come begging to her house, she always gives them something—not because of their holiness, but because she is afraid they will curse her and bring the evil eye on us all. She no longer said anything bad about M., and when she talked about him, she didn't say, "that one" as she used to, but always "He." Once or twice she went and sat with the other people in the little room in which he was, and when she came out, she looked so grave and thoughtful that I had to laugh.

Rahul also visited me. At first he was stiff and sulky, as if he were doing me a favor by coming; but then he began to talk, all about how lonely he was and how his family were trying to persuade him to marry girls he didn't like. I felt sorry for him—I knew it is always difficult for him to make friends and he has never really had anyone except me. I let him talk, and he kept coming again and again. There was a little space with a roof of asbestos sheet over it in the yard where I did my cooking, and it was here that Rahul and I sat. It was not a very private place because of all the people in the yard, waiting to see M., but Rahul soon got used to it and talked just as he would have done if we had been sitting in Mama's drawing room. He was very melancholy, and when he had finished telling me about how lonely he was, he only sat and looked at me with big sad eyes. So I let him help me with the cooking—at first he only sifted the rice and lentils, but after a time I let him do some real cooking and he enjoyed it terribly. He would make all sorts of things—fritters and potato cakes and horseradish pancakes—and they were really delicious. We ate some ourselves and the rest we sent to the beggars' home.

There were always a few young men who stayed at night and slept outside the door of the room where M. was. I often heard him get up in the night and walk up and down; and sometimes he shouted at the young men sleeping outside his door, "Go home!" and he kicked them with his foot, he was so impatient and angry with them. He was often angry nowadays. I heard him shouting at people and scolding them for coming to pester him. When he scolded them, they said he was right to do so, because they were bad, sinful people; but they did not go away and, on the contrary, even more came.

One night I felt someone shaking me to wake up. I opened my eyes and it was M. I jumped up at once and we went out into the street together and sat on a doorstep. Here and there people were sleeping on the sidewalk or on the platforms of shuttered shops. It was very dark and quiet. Only sometimes someone coughed in his sleep or there was a watchman's cry and the tap of his stick. M. said, "Soon I shall have to go away."

Then I knew that the time I had always feared was near.

He said, "It will be best for you to go home again." He spoke very practically, and with gentleness and great concern for me.

But I didn't want to think about what I was going to do. For the moment I wanted it to be only now—always night and people always sleeping and he and I sitting together like this on the doorstep for ever and ever.

The plump young widow still came every day and every day in a different sari, and she made such scenes that in the end M. forbade her to come any more. So she hung about outside in the yard for a few days, and then she started peeping into his room and after that she crept in behind the others and sat quietly at the back; till finally she showed herself to him quite openly and even began to make scenes again. "Have pity!" she cried. "God is eating me up!" At last he quite lost his temper with her. He took off his slipper and began to beat her with it and when she ran away, screaming and clutching her sari about her, he ran after her, brandishing his slipper. They were a funny sight. He pursued her right out into the street, and then he turned back and began to chase all the other people out of the house. He scattered them right and left, beating at them with his slipper, and cursing and scolding. Everyone ran away very fast—even Rahul, who had been cooking potato cakes, made off in a great fright. When they had all gone, M. returned to his room and locked the door behind him. He looked hot and angry. And next day he was gone. People came as usual that day but when they realized he was no longer there, they went away again and also took their gifts back with them. That night the men from the beggars' home were disappointed. I stayed on by myself, it didn't matter to me where I was. Sometimes I sat in one of the rooms, sometimes I walked up and down. The families from upstairs tried to make me eat and sleep, but I heard nothing of what they said. I don't remember much about that time. Later Daddy came to take me away. For the last time I tied my things up in a sheet and I went with him.

I think sometimes of Savitri, and I wonder whether I too am like her now—a candle burning for him in a window of the world. I am patient and inwardly calm and lead the life that has been appointed for me. I play tennis again and I go out to tea and garden parties with Mama, and Rahul and I often dance to the gramophone. Probably I shall marry Rahul quite soon. I laugh and talk just as much as I used to and Mama says I am too frivolous, but Daddy smiles and encourages me. Mama has had a lot of new pieces of jewelry made for me to replace the ones I sold; she and I keep on quarreling as before.

I still try and see his face in my mind, and I never succeed. But I know—and that is how I can go on living the way I do, and even enjoy my life and be glad—that one day I shall succeed and I shall see that face as it really is. But whose face it is I shall see in that hour of happiness—and indeed, whose face it is I look for with such longing—is not quite clear to me.

Flannery O'Connor

Good Country People

Besides the neutral expression that she wore when she was alone, Mrs. Freeman had two others, forward and reverse, that she used for all her human dealings. Her forward expression was steady and driving like the advance of a heavy truck. Her eyes never swerved to left or right but turned as the story turned as if they followed a yellow line down the center of it. She seldom used the other expression because it was not often necessary for her to retract a statement, but when she did, her face came to a complete stop, there was an almost imperceptible movement of her black eyes, during which they seemed to be receding, and then the observer would see that Mrs. Freeman, though she might stand there as real as several grain sacks thrown on top of each other, was no longer there in spirit. As for getting anything across to her when this was the case, Mrs. Hopewell had given it up. She might talk her head off. Mrs. Freeman could never be brought to admit herself wrong to any point. She would stand there and if she could be brought to say anything, it was something like, "Well, I wouldn't of said it was and I wouldn't of said it wasn't" or letting her gaze range over the top kitchen shelf where there was an assortment of dusty bottles, she might remark, "I see you ain't ate many of them figs you put up last summer."

They carried on their most important business in the kitchen at breakfast. Every morning Mrs. Hopewell got up at seven o'clock and lit her gas heater and Joy's. Joy was her daughter, a large blonde girl who had an artificial leg. Mrs. Hopewell thought of her as a child though she was thirty-two years old and highly educated. Joy would get up while her mother was eating and lumber into the bathroom and slam the door, and before long, Mrs. Freeman would arrive at the back door. Joy would hear her mother call, "Come on in," and then they would talk for a while in low voices that were indistinguishable in the bathroom. By the time Joy came in, they had usually finished the weather report and were on one or the other of Mrs. Freeman's daughters, Glynese or Carramae. Joy called them Glycerin and Caramel. Glynese, a redhead, was eighteen and had many admirers; Carramae, a blonde, was only fifteen but already married and pregnant. She could not keep anything on her stomach. Every morning Mrs. Freeman told Mrs. Hopewell how many times she had vomited since the last report.

Mrs. Hopewell liked to tell people that Glynese and Carramae were two of the finest girls she knew and that Mrs. Freeman was a *lady* and that she was never ashamed to take her anywhere or introduce her to anybody they might meet. Then she would tell how she had happened to hire the Freemans in the first place and how they were a godsend to her and how she had had them four years. The reason for her keeping them so long was that they were not trash. They were good country people. She had telephoned the man whose name they had given as reference and he had told her that Mr. Freeman was a good farmer but that his wife was the nosiest woman ever to walk the earth. "She's got to be into everything," the man said. "If she don't get there before the dust settles, you can bet she's dead, that's all. She'll want to know all your business. I can stand him real good," he had said, "but me nor my wife neither could have stood that woman one more minute on this place." That had put Mrs. Hopewell off for a few days. She had hired them in the end because there were no other applicants but she had made up her mind beforehand exactly how she would handle the woman. Since she was the type who had to be into everything, then, Mrs. Hopewell had decided, she would not only let her be into everything, she would *see to it* that she was into everything—she would give her the responsibility of everything, she would put her in charge. Mrs. Hopewell had no bad qualities of her own but she was able to use other people's in such a constructive way that she had kept them four years.

Nothing is perfect. This was one of Mrs. Hopewell's favorite sayings. Another was: that is life! And still another, the most important, was: well, other people have their opinions too. She would make these statements, usually at the table, in a tone of gentle insistence as if no one held them but her, and the large hulking Joy, whose constant outrage had obliterated every expression from her face, would stare just a little to the side of her, her eyes icy blue, with the look of someone who had achieved blindness by an act of will and means to keep it.

When Mrs. Hopewell said to Mrs. Freeman that life was like that, Mrs. Freeman would say, "I always said so myself." Nothing had been arrived at by anyone that had not first been arrived at by her. She was quicker than Mr. Freeman. When Mrs. Hopewell said to her after they had been on the place for a while, "You know, you're the wheel behind the wheel," and winked, Mrs. Freeman had said, "I know it. I've always been quick. It's some that are quicker than others."

"Everybody is different," Mrs. Hopewell said.

"Yes, most people is," Mrs. Freeman said.

"It takes all kinds to make the world."

"I always said it did myself."

The girl was used to this kind of dialogue for breakfast and more of it for dinner; sometimes they had it for supper too. When they had no guest they ate in the kitchen because that was easier. Mrs. Freeman always managed to arrive at some point during the meal and to watch them finish it. She would stand in the doorway if it were summer but in the winter she would stand with one elbow on top of the refrigerator and look down at them, or she would stand by the gas heater, lifting the back of her skirt slightly. Occasionally she would stand against the wall and roll her head from side to side. At no time was she in any hurry to leave. All this was very trying on Mrs. Hopewell but she was a woman of great patience. She realized that nothing is perfect and that in the Freemans she had good country people and that if, in this day and age, you get good country people, you had better hang onto them.

She had had plenty of experience with trash. Before the Freemans she had averaged one tenant family a year. The wives of these farmers were not the kind you would want to be around you for very long. Mrs. Hopewell, who had divorced her husband long ago, needed someone to walk over the fields with her; and when Joy had to be impressed for these services, her remarks were usually so ugly and her face so glum that Mrs. Hopewell would say, "If you can't come pleasantly, I don't want you at all," to which the girl, standing square and rigid-shouldered with her neck thrust slightly forward, would reply, "If you want me, here I am—LIKE I AM."

Mrs. Hopewell excused this attitude because of the leg (which had been shot off in a hunting accident when Joy was ten). It was hard for Mrs. Hopewell to realize that her child was thirty-two now and that for more than twenty years she had had only one leg. She thought of her still as a child because it tore her heart to think instead of the poor stout girl in her thirties who had never danced a step or had any *normal* good times. Her name was really Joy but as soon as she was twenty-one and away from home, she had had it legally changed. Mrs. Hopewell was certain that she had thought and thought until she had hit upon the ugliest name in any language. Then she had gone and had the beautiful name, Joy, changed without telling her mother until after she had done it. Her legal name was Hulga.

When Mrs. Hopewell thought the name, Hulga, she thought of the broad blank hull of a battleship. She would not use it. She continued to call her Joy to which the girl responded but in a purely mechanical way.

Hulga had learned to tolerate Mrs. Freeman who saved her from taking walks with her mother. Even Glynese and Carramae were useful when they occupied attention that might otherwise have been directed at her. At first she had thought she could not stand Mrs. Freeman for she had found it was not possible to be rude to her. Mrs. Freeman would take on strange resentments and for days together she would be sullen but the source of her displeasure was always obscure; a direct attack, a positive leer, blatant ugliness to her face—these never touched her. And without warning one day, she began calling her Hulga.

She did not call her that in front of Mrs. Hopewell who would have been incensed but when she and the girl happened to be out of the house together, she would say something and add the name Hulga to the end of it, and the big spectacled Joy-Hulga would scowl and redden as if her privacy had been intruded upon. She considered the name her personal affair. She had arrived at it first purely on the basis of its ugly sound and then the full genius of its fitness had struck her. She had a vision of the name working like the ugly sweating Vulcan who stayed in the furnace and to whom, presumably, the goddess had to come when called. She saw it as the name of her highest creative act. One of her major triumphs was that her mother had not been able to turn her dust into Joy, but the greater one was that she had been able to turn it herself into Hulga. However, Mrs. Freeman's relish for using the name only irritated her. It was as if Mrs. Freeman's beady steel-pointed eyes had penetrated far enough behind her face to reach some secret fact. Something about her seemed to fascinate Mrs. Freeman and then one day Hulga realized that it was the artificial leg. Mrs. Freeman had a special fondness for the details of secret infections, hidden deformities, assaults upon children. Of diseases, she preferred the lingering or incurable. Hulga had heard Mrs. Hopewell give her the details of the hunting accident, how the leg had been literally blasted off, how she had never lost consciousness. Mrs. Freeman could listen to it any time as if it had happened an hour ago.

When Hulga stumped into the kitchen in the morning (she could walk without making the awful noise but she made it—Mrs. Hopewell was certain—because it was ugly-sounding), she glanced at them and did not speak. Mrs. Hopewell would be in her red kimono with her hair tied around her head in rags. She would be sitting at the table, finishing her breakfast and Mrs. Freeman would be hanging by her elbow outward from the refrigerator, looking down at the table. Hulga always put her eggs on the stove to boil and then stood over them with her arms folded, and Mrs. Hopewell would look at her—a kind of indirect gaze divided between her and Mrs. Freeman—and would think that if she would only keep herself up a little, she wouldn't be so bad looking. There was nothing wrong with her face that a pleasant expression wouldn't help. Mrs. Hopewell said that people who looked on the bright side of things would be beautiful even if they were not.

Whenever she looked at Joy this way, she could not help but feel that it would have been better if the child had not taken the Ph.D. It had certainly not brought her out any and now that she had it, there was no more excuse for her to go to school again. Mrs. Hopewell thought it was nice for girls to go to school to have a good time but Joy had "gone through." Anyhow, she would not have been strong enough to go again. The doctors had told Mrs. Hopewell that with the best of care, Joy might see forty-five. She had a weak heart. Joy had made it plain that if it had not been for this condition, she would be far from these red hills and good country people. She would be in a university lecturing to people who knew what she was talking about. And Mrs. Hopewell could very well picture her there, looking like a scarecrow and lecturing to more of the same. Here she went about all day in a six-year-old skirt and a yellow sweat shirt with a faded cowboy on a horse embossed on it. She thought this was funny; Mrs. Hopewell thought it was idiotic and showed simply that she was still a child. She was brilliant but she didn't have a grain of sense. It seemed to Mrs. Hopewell that every year she grew less like other people and more like herself—bloated, rude, and squint-eyed. And she said such strange things! To her own mother she had said—without warning, without excuse, standing up in the middle of a meal with her face purple and her mouth half full—"Woman! Do you ever look inside? Do you ever look inside and see what you are *not*? God!" she had cried sinking down again and staring at her plate, "Malebranche was right: we are not our own light. We are not our own light!" Mrs. Hopewell had no idea to this day what brought that on. She had only made the remark, hoping Joy would take it in, that a smile never hurt anyone.

The girl had taken the Ph.D. in philosophy and this left Mrs. Hopewell at a complete loss. You could say, "My daughter is a nurse," or "My daughter is a school teacher," or even, "My daughter is a chemical engineer." You could not say, "My daughter is a philosopher." That was something that had ended with the Greeks and Romans. All day Joy sat on her neck in a deep chair, reading. Sometimes she went for walks but she didn't like dogs or cats or birds or flowers or nature or nice young men. She looked at nice young men as if she could smell their stupidity.

One day Mrs. Hopewell had picked up one of the books the girl had just put down and opening it at random, she read, "Science, on the other hand, has to assert its soberness and seriousness afresh and declare that it is concerned solely with what-is. Nothing—how can it be for science anything but a horror and a phantasm? If science is right, then one thing stands firm: science wishes to know nothing of Nothing. Such is after all the strictly scientific approach to Nothing. We know it by wishing to know nothing of Nothing." These words had been underlined with a blue pencil and they worked on Mrs. Hopewell like some evil incantation in gibberish. She shut the book quickly and went out of the room as if she were having a chill.

This morning when the girl came in, Mrs. Freeman was on Carramae. "She thrown up four times after supper," she said, "and was up twict in the night after three o'clock. Yesterday she didn't do nothing but ramble in the bureau drawer. All she did. Stand up there and see what she could run up on."

"She's got to eat," Mrs. Hopewell muttered, sipping her coffee, while she watched Joy's back at the stove. She was wondering what the child had said to the Bible salesman. She could not imagine what kind of a conversation she could possibly have had with him.

He was a tall gaunt hatless youth who had called yesterday to sell them a Bible. He had appeared at the door, carrying a large black suitcase that weighted him so heavily on one side that he had to brace himself against the door facing. He seemed on the point of collapse but he said in a cheerful voice, "Good morning, Mrs. Cedars!" and set the suitcase down on the mat. He was not a bad-looking young man though he had on a bright blue suit and yellow socks that were not pulled up far enough. He had prominent face bones and a streak of sticky-looking brown hair falling across his forehead.

"I'm Mrs. Hopewell," she said.

"Oh!" he said, pretending to look puzzled but with his eyes sparkling, "I saw it said 'The Cedars' on the mailbox so I thought you was Mrs. Cedars!" and he burst out in a pleasant laugh. He picked up the satchel and under cover of a pant, he fell forward into her hall. It was rather as if the suitcase had moved first, jerking him after it. "Mrs. Hopewell!" he said and grabbed her hand. "I hope you are well!" and he laughed again and then all at once his face sobered completely. He paused and gave her a straight earnest look and said, "Lady, I've come to speak of serious things."

"Well, come in," she muttered, none too pleased because her dinner was almost ready. He came into the parlor and sat down on the edge of a straight chair and put the suitcase between his feet and glanced around the room as if he were sizing her up by it. Her silver gleamed on the two sideboards; she decided he had never been in a room as elegant as this.

"Mrs. Hopewell," he began, using her name in a way that sounded almost intimate, "I know you believe in Chrustian service."

"Well, yes," she murmured.

"I know," he said and paused, looking very wise with his head cocked on one side, "that you're a good woman. Friends have told me."

Mrs. Hopewell never liked to be taken for a fool. "What are you selling?" she asked.

"Bibles," the young man said and his eye raced around the room before he added, "I see you have no family Bible in your parlor, I see that is the one lack you got!"

Mrs. Hopewell could not say, "My daughter is an atheist and won't let me keep the Bible in the parlor." She said, stiffening slightly, "I keep my Bible by my bedside." This was not the truth. It was in the attic somewhere.

"Lady," he said, "the word of God ought to be in the parlor."

"Well, I think that's a matter of taste," she began, "I think . . ."

"Lady," he said, "for a Chrustian, the word of God ought to be in every room in the house besides in his heart. I know you're a Chrustian because I can see it in every line of your face."

She stood up and said, "Well, young man, I don't want to buy a Bible and I smell my dinner burning."

He didn't get up. He began to twist his hands and looking down at them, he said softly, "Well lady, I'll tell you the truth— not many people want to buy one nowadays and besides, I know I'm real simple. I don't know how to say a thing but to say it. I'm just a country boy." He glanced up into her unfriendly face. "People like you don't like to fool with country people like me!"

"Why!" she cried, "good country people are the salt of the earth! Besides, we all have different ways of doing, it takes all kinds to make the world go 'round. That's life!"

"You said a mouthful," he said.

"Why, I think there aren't enough good country people in the world!" she said, stirred. "I think that's what's wrong with it!"

His face had brightened. "I didn't intraduce myself," he said. "I'm Manley Pointer from out in the country around Willohobie, not even from a place, just from near a place."

"You wait a minute," she said. "I have to see about my dinner." She went out to the kitchen and found Joy standing near the door where she had been listening.

"Get rid of the salt of the earth," she said, "and let's eat."

Mrs. Hopewell gave her a pained look and turned the heat down under the vegetables. "*I* can't be rude to anybody," she murmured and went back into the parlor.

He had opened the suitcase and was sitting with a Bible on each knee.

"I appreciate your honesty," he said. "You don't see any more real honest people unless you go way out in the country."

"I know," she said, "real genuine folks!" Through the crack in the door she heard a groan.

"I guess a lot of boys come telling you they're working their way through college," he said, "but I'm not going to tell you that. Somehow," he said, "I don't want to go to college. I want to devote my life to Chrustian service. See," he said, lowering his voice, "I got this heart condition. I may not live long. When you know it's something wrong with you and you may not live long, well then, lady . . ." He paused, with his mouth open, and stared at her.

He and Joy had the same condition! She knew that her eyes were filling with tears but she collected herself quickly and murmured, "Won't you stay for dinner? We'd love to have you!" and was sorry the instant she heard herself say it.

"Yes mam," he said in an abashed voice. "I would sher love to do that!"

Joy had given him one look on being introduced to him and then throughout the meal had not glanced at him again. He had addressed several remarks to her, which she had pretended not to hear. Mrs. Hopewell could not understand deliberate rudeness, although she lived with it, and she felt she had always to overflow with hospitality to make up for Joy's lack of courtesy. She urged him to talk about himself and he did. He said he was the seventh child of twelve and that his father had been crushed under a tree when he himself was eight years old. He had been crushed very badly, in fact, almost cut in two and was practically not recognizable. His mother had got along the best she could by hard working and she had always seen that her children went to Sunday School and that they read the Bible every evening. He was now nineteen years old and he had been selling Bibles for four months. In that time he had sold seventy-seven Bibles and had the promise of two more sales. He wanted to become a missionary because he thought that was the way you could do most for people. "He who losest his life shall find it," he said simply and he was so sincere, so genuine and earnest that Mrs. Hopewell would not for the world have smiled. He prevented his peas from sliding onto the table by blocking them with a piece of bread which he later cleaned his plate with. She could see Joy observing sidewise how he handled his knife and fork and she saw too that every few minutes, the boy would dart a keen appraising glance at the girl as if he were trying to attract her attention.

After dinner Joy cleared the dishes off the table and disappeared and Mrs. Hopewell was left to talk with him. He told her again about his childhood and his father's accident and about various things that had happened to him. Every five minutes or so she would stifle a yawn. He sat for two hours until finally she told him she must go because she had an appointment in town. He packed his Bibles and thanked her and prepared to leave, but in the doorway he stopped and wrung her hand and said that not on any of his trips had he met a lady as nice as her and he asked if he could come again. She had said she would always be happy to see him.

Joy had been standing in the road, apparently looking at something in the distance, when he came down the steps toward her, bent to the side with his heavy valise. He stopped where she was standing and confronted her directly. Mrs. Hopewell could not hear what he said but she trembled to think what Joy would say to him. She could see that after a minute Joy said something and that then the boy began to speak again, making an excited gesture with his free hand. After a minute Joy said something else at which the boy began to speak once more. Then to her amazement, Mrs. Hopewell saw the two of them walk off together, toward the gate. Joy had walked all the way to the gate with him and Mrs. Hopewell could not imagine what they had said to each other, and she had not yet dared to ask.

Mrs. Freeman was insisting upon her attention. She had moved from the refrigerator to the heater so that Mrs. Hopewell had to turn and face her in order to seem to be listening. "Glynese gone out with Harvey Hill again last night," she said. "She had this sty."

"Hill," Mrs. Hopewell said absently, "is that the one who works in the garage?"

"Nome, he's the one that goes to chiropractor school," Mrs. Freeman said. "She had this sty. Been had it two days. So she says when he brought her in the other night he says, 'Lemme get rid of that sty for you,' and she says, 'How?' and he says, 'You just lay yourself down acrost the seat of that car and I'll show you.' So she done it and he popped her neck. Kept on a-popping it several times until she made him quit. This morning," Mrs. Freeman said, "she ain't got no sty. She ain't got no traces of a sty."

"I never heard of that before," Mrs. Hopewell said.

"He ast her to marry him before the Ordinary," Mrs. Freeman went on, "and she told him she wasn't going to be married in no office."

"Well, Glynese is a fine girl," Mrs. Hopewell said. "Glynese and Carramae are both fine girls."

"Carramae said when her and Lyman was married Lyman said it sure felt sacred to him. She said he said he wouldn't take five hundred dollars for being married by a preacher."

"How much would he take?" the girl asked from the stove.

"He said he wouldn't take five hundred dollars," Mrs. Freeman repeated.

"Well we all have work to do," Mrs. Hopewell said.

"Lyman said it just felt more sacred to him," Mrs. Freeman said. "The doctor wants Carramae to eat prunes. Says instead of medicine. Says them cramps is coming from pressure. You know where I think it is?"

"She'll be better in a few weeks," Mrs. Hopewell said.

"In the tube," Mrs. Freeman said. "Else she wouldn't be as sick as she is."

Hulga had cracked her two eggs into a saucer and was bringing them to the table along with a cup of coffee that she had filled too full. She sat down carefully and began to eat, meaning to keep Mrs. Freeman there by questions if for any reason she showed an inclination to leave. She could perceive her mother's eye on her. The first round-about question would be about the Bible salesman and she did not wish to bring it on. "How did he pop her neck?" she asked.

Mrs. Freeman went into a description of how he had popped her neck. She said he owned a '55 Mercury but that Glynese said she would rather marry a man with only a '36 Plymouth who would be married by a preacher. The girl asked what if he had a '32 Plymouth and Mrs. Freeman said what Glynese had said was a '36 Plymouth.

Mrs. Hopewell said there were not many girls with Glynese's common sense. She said what she admired in those girls was their common sense. She said that reminded her that they had had a nice visitor yesterday, a young man selling Bibles. "Lord," she said, "he bored me to death but he was so sincere and genuine I couldn't be rude to him. He was just good country people, you know," she said, "—just the salt of the earth."

"I seen him walk up," Mrs. Freeman said, "and then later—I seen him walk off," and Hulga could feel the slight shift in her voice, the slight insinuation, that he had not walked off alone, had he? Her face remained expressionless but the color rose into her neck and she seemed to swallow it down with the next spoonful of egg. Mrs. Freeman was looking at her as if they had a secret together.

"Well, it takes all kinds of people to make the world go 'round," Mrs. Hopewell said. "It's very good we aren't all alike."

"Some people are more alike than others," Mrs. Freeman said.

Hulga got up and stumped, with about twice the noise that was necessary, into her room and locked the door. She was to meet the Bible salesman at ten o'clock at the gate. She had thought about it half the night. She had started thinking of it as a great joke and then she had begun to see profound implications in it. She had lain in bed imagining dialogues for them that were insane on the surface but that reached below the depths that no Bible salesman would be aware of. Their conversation yesterday had been of this kind.

He had stopped in front of her and had simply stood there. His face was bony and sweaty and bright, with a little pointed nose in the center of it, and his look was different from what it had been at the dinner table. He was gazing at her with open curiosity, with fascination, like a child watching a new fantastic animal at the zoo, and he was breathing as if he had run a great distance to reach her. His gaze seemed somehow familiar but she could not think where she had been regarded with it before. For almost a minute he didn't say anything. Then on what seemed an insuck of breath, he whispered, "You ever ate a chicken that was two days old?"

The girl looked at him stonily. He might have just put this question up for consideration at the meeting of a philosophical association. "Yes," she presently replied as if she had considered it from all angles.

"It must have been mighty small!" he said triumphantly and shook all over with little nervous giggles, getting very red in the face, and subsiding finally into his gaze of complete admiration, while the girl's expression remained exactly the same.

"How old are you?" he asked softly.

She waited some time before she answered. Then in a flat voice she said, "Seventeen."

His smiles came in succession like waves breaking on the surface of a little lake. "I see you got a wooden leg," he said. "I think you're real brave. I think you're real sweet."

The girl stood blank and solid and silent.

"Walk to the gate with me," he said. "You're a brave sweet little thing and I liked you the minute I seen you walk in the door."

Hulga began to move forward.

"What's your name?" he asked, smiling down on the top of her head.

"Hulga," she said.

"Hulga," he murmured, "Hulga. Hulga. I never heard of anybody name Hulga before. You're shy, aren't you, Hulga?" he asked.

She nodded, watching his large red hand on the handle of the giant valise.

"I like girls that wear glasses," he said. "I think a lot. I'm not like these people that a serious thought don't ever enter their heads. It's because I may die."

"I may die too," she said suddenly and looked up at him. His eyes were very small and brown, glittering feverishly.

"Listen," he said, "don't you think some people was meant to meet on account of what all they got in common and all? Like they both think serious thoughts and all?" He shifted the valise to his other hand so that the hand nearest her was free. He caught hold of her elbow and shook it a little. "I don't work on Saturday," he said. "I like to walk in the woods and see what Mother Nature is wearing. O'er the hills and far away. Picnics and things. Couldn't we go on a picnic tomorrow? Say yes, Hulga," he said and gave her a dying look as if he felt his insides about to drop out of him. He had even seemed to sway slightly toward her.

During the night she had imagined that she seduced him. She imagined that the two of them walked on the place until they came to the storage barn beyond the two back fields and there, she imagined, that things came to such a pass that she very easily seduced him and that then, of course, she had to reckon with his remorse. True genius can get an idea across even to an inferior mind. She imagined that she took his remorse in hand and changed it into a deeper understanding of life. She took all his shame away and turned it into something useful.

She set off for the gate at exactly ten o'clock, escaping without drawing Mrs. Hopewell's attention. She didn't take anything to eat, forgetting that food is usually taken on a picnic. She wore a pair of slacks and a dirty white shirt, and as an afterthought, she had put some Vapex on the collar of it since she did not own any perfume. When she reached the gate no one was there.

She looked up and down the empty highway and had the furious feeling that she had been tricked, that he only meant to make her walk to the gate after the idea of him. Then suddenly he stood up, very tall, from behind a bush on the opposite embankment. Smiling, he lifted his hat which was new and wide-brimmed. He had not worn it yesterday and she wondered if he had bought it for the occasion. It was toast-colored with a red and white band around it and was slightly too large for him. He stepped from behind the bush still carrying the black valise. He had on the same suit and the same yellow socks sucked down in his shoes from walking. He crossed the highway and said, "I knew you'd come!"

The girl wondered acidly how he had known this. She pointed to the valise and asked, "Why did you bring your Bibles?"

He took her elbow, smiling down on her as if he could not stop. "You can never tell when you'll need the word of God, Hulga," he said. She had a moment in which she doubted that this was actually happening and then they began to climb the embankment. They went down into the pasture toward the woods. The boy walked lightly by her side, bouncing on his toes. The valise did not seem to be heavy today; he even swung it. They crossed half the pasture without saying anything and then, putting his hand easily on the small of her back, he asked softly, "Where does your wooden leg join on?"

She turned an ugly red and glared at him and for an instant the boy looked abashed. "I didn't mean you no harm," he said. "I only meant you're so brave and all. I guess God takes care of you."

"No," she said, looking forward and walking fast, "I don't even believe in God."

At this he stopped and whistled. "No!" he exclaimed as if he were too astonished to say anything else.

She walked on and in a second he was bouncing at her side, fanning with his hat. "That's very unusual for a girl," he remarked, watching her out of the corner of his eye. When they reached the edge of the wood, he put his hand on her back again and drew her against him without a word and kissed her heavily.

The kiss, which had more pressure than feeling behind it, produced that extra surge of adrenalin in the girl that enables one to carry a packed trunk out of a burning house, but in her, the power went at once to the brain. Even before he released her, her mind, clear and detached and ironic anyway, was regarding him from a great distance, with amusement but with pity. She had never been kissed before and she was pleased to discover that it was an unexceptional experience and all a matter of the mind's control. Some people might enjoy drain water if they were told it was vodka. When the boy, looking expectant but uncertain, pushed her gently away, she turned and walked on, saying nothing as if such business, for her, were common enough.

He came along panting at her side, trying to help her when he saw a root that she might trip over. He caught and held back the long swaying blades of thorn vine until she had passed beyond them. She led the way and he came breathing heavily behind her. Then they came out on a sunlit hillside, sloping softly into another one a little smaller. Beyond, they could see the rusted top of the old barn where the extra hay was stored.

The hill was sprinkled with small pink weeds. "Then you ain't saved?" he asked suddenly, stopping.

The girl smiled. It was the first time she had smiled at him at all. "In my economy," she said, "I'm saved and you are damned but I told you I didn't believe in God."

Nothing seemed to destroy the boy's look of admiration. He gazed at her now as if the fantastic animal at the zoo had put its paw through the bars and given him a loving poke. She thought he looked as if he wanted to kiss her again and she walked on before he had the chance.

"Ain't there somewheres we can sit down sometime?" he murmured, his voice softening toward the end of the sentence.

"In that barn," she said.

They made for it rapidly as if it might slide away like a train. It was a large two-story barn, cool and dark inside. The boy pointed up the ladder that led into the loft and said, "It's too bad we can't go up there."

"Why can't we?" she asked.

"Yer leg," he said reverently.

The girl gave him a contemptuous look and putting both hands on the ladder, she climbed it while he stood below, apparently awestruck. She pulled herself expertly through the opening and then looked down at him and said, "Well, come on if you're coming," and he began to climb the ladder, awkwardly bringing the suitcase with him.

"We won't need the Bible," she observed.

"You never can tell," he said, panting. After he had got into the loft, he was a few seconds catching his breath. She had sat down in a pile of straw. A wide sheath of sunlight, filled with dust particles, slanted over her. She lay back against a bale, her face turned away, looking out the front opening of the barn where hay was thrown from a wagon into the loft. The two pink-speckled hillsides lay back against a dark ridge of woods. The sky was cloudless and cold blue. The boy dropped down by her side and put one arm under her and the other over her and began methodically kissing her face, making little noises like a fish. He did not remove his hat but it was pushed far enough back not to interfere. When her glasses got in his way, he took them off of her and slipped them into his pocket.

The girl at first did not return any of the kisses but presently she began to and after she had put several on his cheek, she reached his lips and remained there, kissing him again and again as if she were trying to draw all the breath out of him. His breath was clear and sweet like a child's and the kisses were sticky like a child's. He mumbled about loving her and about knowing when he first seen her that he loved her, but the mumbling was like the sleepy fretting of a child being put to sleep by his mother. Her mind, throughout this, never stopped or lost itself for a second to her feelings. "You ain't said you loved me none," he whispered finally, pulling back from her. "You got to say that."

She looked away from him off into the hollow sky and then down at a black ridge and then down farther into what appeared to be two green swelling lakes. She didn't realize he had taken her glasses but this landscape could not seem exceptional to her for she seldom paid any close attention to her surroundings.

"You got to say it," he repeated. "You got to say you love me."

She was always careful how she committed herself. "In a sense," she began, "if you use the word loosely, you might say that. But it's not a word I use. I don't have illusions. I'm one of those people who see *through* to nothing."

The boy was frowning. "You got to say it. I said it and you got to say it," he said.

The girl looked at him almost tenderly. "You poor baby," she murmured. "It's just as well you don't understand," and she pulled him by the neck, face-down, against her. "We are all damned," she said, "but some of us have taken off our blindfolds and see that there's nothing to see. It's a kind of salvation."

The boy's astonished eyes looked blankly through the ends of her hair. "Okay," he almost whined, "but do you love me or don'tcher?"

"Yes," she said and added, "in a sense. But I must tell you something. There mustn't be anything dishonest between us." She lifted his head and looked him in the eye. "I am thirty years old," she said. "I have a number of degrees."

The boy's look was irritated but dogged. "I don't care," he said. "I don't care a thing about what all you done. I just want to know if you love me or don'tcher?" and he caught her to him and wildly planted her face with kisses until she said, "Yes, yes."

"Okay then," he said, letting her go. "Prove it."

She smiled, looking dreamily out on the shifty landscape. She had seduced him without even making up her mind to try. "How?" she asked, feeling that he should be delayed a little.

He leaned over and put his lips to her ear. "Show me where your wooden leg joins on," he whispered.

The girl uttered a sharp little cry and her face instantly drained of color. The obscenity of the suggestion was not what shocked her. As a child she had sometimes been subject to feelings of shame but education had removed the last traces of that as a good surgeon scrapes for cancer; she would no more have felt it over what he was asking than she would have believed in his Bible. But she was as sensitive about the artificial leg as a peacock about his tail. No one ever touched it but her. She took care of it as someone else would his soul, in private and almost with her own eyes turned away. "No," she said.

"I known it," he muttered, sitting up. "You're just playing me for a sucker."

"Oh no no!" she cried. "It joins on at the knee. Only at the knee. Why do you want to see it?"

The boy gave her a long penetrating look. "Because," he said, "it's what makes you different. You ain't like anybody else."

She sat staring at him. There was nothing about her face or her round freezing-blue eyes to indicate that this had moved her; but she felt as if her heart had stopped and left her mind to pump her blood. She decided that for the first time in her life she was face to face with real innocence. This boy, with an instinct that came from beyond wisdom, had touched the truth about her. When after a minute, she said in a hoarse high voice, "All right," it was like surrendering to him completely. It was like losing her own life and finding it again, miraculously, in his.

Very gently, he began to roll the slack leg up. The artificial limb, in a white sock and brown flat shoe, was bound in a heavy material like canvas and ended in an ugly jointure where it was attached to the stump. The boy's face and his voice were entirely reverent as he uncovered it and said, "Now show me how to take it off and on."

She took it off for him and put it back on again and then he took it off himself, handling it as tenderly as if it were a real one. "See!" he said with a delighted child's face. "Now I can do it myself!"

"Put it back on," she said. She was thinking that she would run away with him and that every night he would take the leg off and every morning put it back on again. "Put it back on," she said.

"Not yet," he murmured, setting it on its foot out of her reach. "Leave it off for awhile. You got me instead."

She gave a little cry of alarm but he pushed her down and began to kiss her again. Without the leg she felt entirely dependent on him. Her brain seemed to have stopped thinking altogether and to be about some other function that it was not very good at. Different expressions raced back and forth over her face. Every now and then the boy, his eyes like two steel spikes, would glance behind him where the leg stood. Finally she pushed him off and said, "Put it back on me now."

"Wait," he said. He leaned the other way and pulled the valise toward him and opened it. It had a pale blue spotted lining and there were only two Bibles in it. He took one of these out and opened the cover of it. It was hollow and contained a pocket flask of whiskey, a pack of cards, and a small blue box with printing on it. He laid these out in front of her one at a time in an evenly-spaced row, like one presenting offerings at the shrine of a goddess. He put the blue box in her hand. THIS PRODUCT TO BE USED ONLY FOR THE PREVENTION OF DISEASE, she read, and dropped it. The boy was unscrewing the top of the flask. He stopped and pointed, with a smile, to the deck of cards. It was not an ordinary deck but one with an obscene picture on the back of each card. "Take a swig," he said, offering her the bottle first. He held it in front of her, but like one mesmerized, she did not move.

Her voice when she spoke had an almost pleading sound. "Aren't you," she murmured, "aren't you just good country people?"

The boy cocked his head. He looked as if he were just beginning to understand that she might be trying to insult him. "Yeah," he said, curling his lip slightly, "but it ain't held me back none. I'm as good as you any day in the week."

"Give me my leg," she said.

He pushed it farther away with his foot. "Come on now, let's begin to have us a good time," he said coaxingly. "We ain't got to know one another good yet."

"Give me my leg!" she screamed and tried to lunge for it but he pushed her down easily.

"What's the matter with you all of a sudden?" he asked, frowning as he screwed the top on the flask and put it quickly back inside the Bible. "You just a while ago said you didn't believe in nothing. I thought you was some girl!"

Her face was almost purple. "You're a Christian!" she hissed. "You're a fine Christian! You're just like them all—say one thing and do another. You're a perfect Christian, you're . . ."

The boy's mouth was set angrily. "I hope you don't think," he said in a lofty indignant tone, "that I believe in that crap! I may sell Bibles but I know which end is up and I wasn't born yesterday and I know where I'm going!"

"Give me my leg!" she screeched. He jumped up so quickly that she barely saw him sweep the cards and the blue box back into the Bible and throw the Bible into the valise. She saw him grab the leg and then she saw it for an instant slanted forlornly across the inside of the suitcase with a Bible at either side of its opposite ends. He slammed the lid shut and snatched up the valise and swung it down the hole and then stepped through himself. When all of him had passed but his head, he turned and regarded her with a look that no longer had any admiration in it. "I've gotten a lot of interesting things," he said. "One time I got a woman's glass eye this way. And you needn't to think you'll catch me because Pointer ain't really my name. I use a different name at every house I call at and don't stay nowhere long. And I'll tell you another thing, Hulga," he said, using the name as if he didn't think much of it, "you ain't so smart. I been believing in nothing ever since I was born!" and then the toast-colored hat disappeared down the hole and the girl was left, sitting on the straw in the dusty sunlight. When she turned her churning face toward the opening, she saw his blue figure struggling successfully over the green speckled lake.

Mrs. Hopewell and Mrs. Freeman, who were in the back pasture, digging up onions, saw him emerge a little later from the woods and head across the meadow toward the highway. "Why, that looks like that nice dull young man that tried to sell me a Bible yesterday," Mrs. Hopewell said, squinting. "He must have been selling them to the Negroes back in there. He was so simple," she said, "but I guess the world would be better off if we were all that simple."

Mrs. Freeman's gaze drove forward and just touched him before he disappeared under the hill. Then she returned her attention to the evil-smelling onion shoot she was lifting from the ground. "Some can't be that simple," she said. "I know I never could."

James Joyce

THE DEAD

Lily, the caretaker's daughter, was literally run off her feet. Hardly had she brought one gentleman into the little pantry behind the office on the ground floor and helped him off with his overcoat than the wheezy hall-door bell clanged again and she had to scamper along the bare hallway to let in another guest. It was well for her she had not to attend to the ladies also. But Miss Kate and Miss Julia had thought of that and had converted the bathroom upstairs into a ladies' dressing-room. Miss Kate and Miss Julia were there, gossiping and laughing and fussing, walking after each other to the head of the stairs, peering down over the banisters and calling down to Lily to ask her who had come.

It was always a great affair, the Misses Morkan's annual dance. Everybody who knew them came to it, members of the family, old friends of the family, the members of Julia's choir, any of Kate's pupils that were grown up enough, and even some of Mary Jane's pupils too. Never once had it fallen flat. For years and years it had gone off in splendid style, as long as anyone could remember; ever since Kate and Julia, after the death of their brother Pat, had left the house in

Stoney Batter and taken Mary Jane, their only niece, to live with them in the dark, gaunt house on Usher's Island, the upper part of which they had rented from Mr. Fulham, the corn-factor on the ground floor. That was a good thirty years ago if it was a day. Mary Jane, who was then a little girl in short clothes, was now the main prop of the household, for she had the organ in Haddington Road. She had been through the Academy and gave a pupils' concert every year in the upper room of the Antient Concert Rooms. Many of her pupils belonged to the better-class families on the Kingstown and Dalkey line. Old as they were, her aunts also did their share. Julia, though she was quite grey, was still the leading soprano in Adam and Eve's, and Kate, being too feeble to go about much, gave music lessons to beginners on the old square piano in the back room. Lily, the caretaker's daughter, did housemaid's work for them. Though their life was modest, they believed in eating well; the best of everything: diamond-bone sirloins, three-shilling tea and the best bottled stout. But Lily seldom made a mistake in the orders, so that she got on well with her three mistresses. They were fussy, that was all. But the only thing they would not stand was back answers.

Of course, they had good reason to be fussy on such a night. And then it was long after ten o'clock and yet there was no sign of Gabriel and his wife. Besides they were dreadfully afraid that Freddy Malins might turn up screwed. They would not wish for worlds that any of Mary Jane's pupils should see him under the influence; and when he was like that it was sometimes very hard to manage him. Freddy Malins always came late, but they wondered what could be keeping Gabriel: and that was what brought them every two minutes to the banisters to ask Lily had Gabriel or Freddy come.

"O, Mr. Conroy," said Lily to Gabriel when she opened the door for him, "Miss Kate and Miss Julia thought you were never coming. Good-night, Mrs. Conroy."

"I'll engage they did," said Gabriel, "but they forget that my wife here takes three mortal hours to dress herself."

He stood on the mat, scraping the snow from his goloshes, while Lily led his wife to the foot of the stairs and called out:

"Miss Kate, here's Mrs. Conroy."

Kate and Julia came toddling down the dark stairs at once. Both of them kissed Gabriel's wife, said she must be perished alive, and asked was Gabriel with her.

"Here I am as right as the mail, Aunt Kate! Go on up. I'll follow," called out Gabriel from the dark.

He continued scraping his feet vigorously while the three women went upstairs, laughing, to the ladies' dressing-room. A light fringe of snow lay like a cape on the shoulders of his overcoat and like toecaps on the toes of his goloshes; and, as the buttons of his overcoat slipped with a squeaking noise through the snow-stiffened frieze, a cold, fragrant air from out-of-doors escaped from crevices and folds.

"Is it snowing again, Mr. Conroy?" asked Lily.

She had preceded him into the pantry to help him off with his overcoat. Gabriel smiled at the three syllables she had given his surname and glanced at her. She was a slim, growing girl, pale in complexion and with hay-coloured hair. The gas in the pantry made her look still paler. Gabriel had known her when she was a child and used to sit on the lowest step nursing a rag doll.

"Yes, Lily," he answered, "and I think we're in for a night of it."

He looked up at the pantry ceiling, which was shaking with the stamping and shuffling of feet on the floor above, listened for a moment to the piano and then glanced at the girl, who was folding his overcoat carefully at the end of a shelf.

"Tell me. Lily," he said in a friendly tone, "do you still go to school?"

"O no, sir," she answered. "I'm done schooling this year and more."

"O, then," said Gabriel gaily, "I suppose we'll be going to your wedding one of these fine days with your young man, eh?"

The girl glanced back at him over her shoulder and said with great bitterness:

"The men that is now is only all palaver and what they can get out of you."

Gabriel coloured, as if he felt he had made a mistake and, without looking at her, kicked off his goloshes and flicked actively with his muffler at his patent-leather shoes.

He was a stout, tallish young man. The high colour of his cheeks pushed upwards even to his forehead, where it scattered itself in a few formless patches of pale red; and on his hairless face there scintillated restlessly the polished lenses and the bright gilt rims of the glasses which screened his delicate and restless eyes. His glossy black hair was parted in the middle and brushed in a long curve behind his ears where it curled slightly beneath the groove left by his hat.

When he had flicked lustre into his shoes he stood up and pulled his waistcoat down more tightly on his plump body. Then he took a coin rapidly from his pocket.

"O Lily," he said, thrusting it into her hands, "it's Christmastime, isn't it? Just . . . here's a little . . ."

He walked rapidly towards the door.

"O no, sir!" cried the girl, following him. "Really, sir, I wouldn't take it."

"Christmas-time! Christmas-time!" said Gabriel, almost trotting to the stairs and waving his hand to her in deprecation.

The girl, seeing that he had gained the stairs, called out after him:

"Well, thank you, sir."

He waited outside the drawing-room door until the waltz should finish, listening to the skirts that swept against it and to the shuffling of feet. He was still discomposed by the girl's bitter and sudden retort. It had cast a gloom over him which he tried to dispel by arranging his cuffs and the bows of his tie. He then took from his waistcoat pocket a little paper and glanced at the headings he had made for his speech. He was undecided about the lines from Robert Browning, for he feared they would be above the heads of his hearers. Some quotation that they would recognise from Shakespeare or from the Melodies would be better. The indelicate clacking of the men's heels and the shuffling of their soles reminded him that their grade of culture differed from his. He would only make himself ridiculous by quoting poetry to them which they could not understand. They would think that he was airing his superior education. He would fail with them just as he had failed with the girl in the pantry. He had taken up a wrong tone. His whole speech was a mistake from first to last, an utter failure.

Just then his aunts and his wife came out of the ladies' dressing-room. His aunts were two small, plainly dressed old women. Aunt Julia was an inch or so the taller. Her hair, drawn low over the tops of her ears, was grey; and grey also, with darker shadows, was her large flaccid face. Though she was stout in build and stood erect, her slow eyes and parted lips gave her the appearance of a woman who did not know where she was or where she was going. Aunt Kate was more vivacious. Her face, healthier than her sister's, was all puckers and creases, like a shrivelled red apple, and her hair, braided in the same old-fashioned way, had not lost its ripe nut colour.

They both kissed Gabriel frankly. He was their favourite nephew, the son of their dead elder sister, Ellen, who had married T. J. Conroy of the Port and Docks.

"Gretta tells me you're not going to take a cab back to Monkstown tonight, Gabriel," said Aunt Kate.

"No," said Gabriel, turning to his wife, "we had quite enough of that last year, hadn't we? Don't you remember, Aunt Kate, what a cold Gretta got out of it? Cab windows rattling all the way, and the east wind blowing in after we passed Merrion. Very jolly it was. Gretta caught a dreadful cold."

Aunt Kate frowned severely and nodded her head at every word.

"Quite right, Gabriel, quite right," she said. "You can't be too careful."

"But as for Gretta there," said Gabriel, "she'd walk home in the snow if she were let."

Mrs. Conroy laughed.

"Don't mind him, Aunt Kate," she said. "He's really an awful bother, what with green shades for Tom's eyes at night and making him do the dumb-bells, and forcing Eva to eat the stirabout. The poor child! And she simply hates the sight of it! . . . O, but you'll never guess what he makes me wear now!"

She broke out into a peal of laughter and glanced at her husband, whose admiring and happy eyes had been wandering from her dress to her face and hair. The two aunts laughed heartily, too, for Gabriel's solicitude was a standing joke with them.

"Goloshes!" said Mrs. Conroy. "That's the latest. Whenever it's wet underfoot I must put on my goloshes. Tonight even, he wanted me to put them on, but I wouldn't. The next thing he'll buy me will be a diving suit."

Gabriel laughed nervously and patted his tie reassuringly, while Aunt Kate nearly doubled herself, so heartily did she enjoy the joke. The smile soon faded from Aunt Julia's face and her mirthless eyes were directed towards her nephew's face. After a pause she asked:

"And what are goloshes, Gabriel?"

"Goloshes, Julia!" exclaimed her sister "Goodness me, don't you know what goloshes are? You wear them over your . . . over your boots, Gretta, isn't it?"

"Yes," said Mrs. Conroy. "Guttapercha things. We both have a pair now. Gabriel says everyone wears them on the Continent."

"O, on the Continent," murmured Aunt Julia, nodding her head slowly.

Gabriel knitted his brows and said, as if he were slightly angered:

"It's nothing very wonderful, but Gretta thinks it very funny because she says the word reminds her of Christy Minstrels."

"But tell me, Gabriel," said Aunt Kate, with brisk tact. "Of course, you've seen about the room. Gretta was saying . . ."

"O, the room is all right," replied Gabriel. "I've taken one in the Gresham."

"To be sure," said Aunt Kate, "by far the best thing to do. And the children, Gretta, you're not anxious about them?"

"O, for one night," said Mrs. Conroy. "Besides, Bessie will look after them."

"To be sure," said Aunt Kate again. "What a comfort it is to have a girl like that, one you can depend on! There's that Lily, I'm sure I don't know what has come over her lately. She's not the girl she was at all."

Gabriel was about to ask his aunt some questions on this point, but she broke off suddenly to gaze after her sister, who had wandered down the stairs and was craning her neck over the banisters.

"Now, I ask you," she said almost testily, "where is Julia going? Julia! Julia! Where are you going?"

Julia, who had gone half way down one flight, came back and announced blandly:

"Here's Freddy."

At the same moment a clapping of hands and a final flourish of the pianist told that the waltz had ended. The drawing-room door was opened from within and some couples came out. Aunt Kate drew Gabriel aside hurriedly and whispered into his ear:

"Slip down, Gabriel, like a good fellow and see if he's all right, and don't let him up if he's screwed. I'm sure he's screwed. I'm sure he is."

Gabriel went to the stairs and listened over the banisters. He could hear two persons talking in the pantry. Then he recognised Freddy Malins' laugh. He went down the stairs noisily.

"It's such a relief," said Aunt Kate to Mrs. Conroy, "that Gabriel is here. I always feel easier in my mind when he's here. . . . Julia, there's Miss Daly and Miss Power will take some refreshment. Thanks for your beautiful waltz, Miss Daly. It made lovely time."

A tall wizen-faced man, with a stiff grizzled moustache and swarthy skin, who was passing out with his partner, said:

"And may we have some refreshment, too, Miss Morkan?"

"Julia," said Aunt Kate summarily, "and here's Mr. Browne and Miss Furlong. Take them in, Julia, with Miss Daly and Miss Power."

"I'm the man for the ladies," said Mr. Browne, pursing his lips until his moustache bristled and smiling in all his wrinkles. "You know, Miss Morkan, the reason they are so fond of me is—"

He did not finish his sentence, but, seeing that Aunt Kate was out of earshot, at once led the three young ladies into the back room. The middle of the room was occupied by two square tables placed end to end, and on these Aunt Julia and the caretaker were straightening and smoothing a large cloth. On the sideboard were arrayed dishes and plates, and glasses and bundles of knives and forks and spoons. The top of the closed square piano served also as a sideboard for viands and sweets. At a smaller sideboard in one corner two young men were standing, drinking hop-bitters.

Mr. Browne led his charges thither and invited them all, in jest, to some ladies' punch, hot, strong and sweet. As they said they never took anything strong, he opened three bottles of lemonade for them. Then he asked one of the young men to move aside, and, taking hold of the decanter, filled out for himself a goodly measure of whisky. The young men eyed him respectfully while he took a trial sip.

"God help me," he said, smiling, "it's the doctor's orders."

His wizened face broke into a broader smile, and the three young ladies laughed in musical echo to his pleasantry, swaying their bodies to and fro, with nervous jerks of their shoulders. The boldest said:

"O, now, Mr. Browne, I'm sure the doctor never ordered anything of the kind."

Mr. Browne took another sip of his whisky and said, with sidling mimicry:

"Well, you see, I'm like the famous Mrs. Cassidy, who is reported to have said: 'Now, Mary Grimes, if I don't take it, make me take it, for I feel I want it.'"

His hot face had leaned forward a little too confidentially and he had assumed a very low Dublin accent so that the young ladies, with one instinct, received his speech in silence. Miss Furlong, who was one of Mary Jane's pupils, asked Miss Daly what was the name of the pretty waltz she had played; and Mr. Browne, seeing that he was ignored, turned promptly to the two young men who were more appreciative.

A red-faced young woman, dressed in pansy, came into the room, excitedly clapping her hands and crying:

"Quadrilles! Quadrilles!"

Close on her heels came Aunt Kate, crying:

"Two gentlemen and three ladies, Mary Jane!"

"O, here's Mr. Bergin and Mr. Kerrigan," said Mary Jane. "Mr. Kerrigan, will you take Miss Power? Miss Furlong, may I get you a partner, Mr. Bergin. O, that'll just do now."

"Three ladies, Mary Jane," said Aunt Kate.

The two young gentlemen asked the ladies if they might have the pleasure, and Mary Jane turned to Miss Daly.

"O, Miss Daly, you're really awfully good, after playing for the last two dances, but really we're so short of ladies tonight."

"I don't mind in the least, Miss Morkan."

"But I've a nice partner for you, Mr. Bartell D'Arcy, the tenor. I'll get him to sing later on. All Dublin is raving about him."

"Lovely voice, lovely voice!" said Aunt Kate.

As the piano had twice begun the prelude to the first figure Mary Jane led her recruits quickly from the room. They had hardly gone when Aunt Julia wandered slowly into the room, looking behind her at something.

"What is the matter, Julia?" asked Aunt Kate anxiously. "Who is it?"

Julia, who was carrying in a column of table-napkins, turned to her sister and said, simply, as if the question had surprised her:

"It's only Freddy, Kate, and Gabriel with him."

In fact right behind her Gabriel could be seen piloting Freddy Malins across the landing. The latter, a young man of about forty, was of Gabriel's size and build, with very round shoulders. His face was fleshy and pallid, touched with colour only at the thick hanging lobes of his ears and at the wide wings of his nose. He had coarse features, a blunt nose, a convex and receding brow, tumid and protruded lips. His heavy-lidded eyes and the disorder of his scanty hair made him look sleepy. He was laughing heartily in a high key at a story which he had been telling Gabriel on the stairs and at the same time rubbing the knuckles of his left fist backwards and forwards into his left eye.

"Good-evening, Freddy," said Aunt Julia.

Freddy Malins bade the Misses Morkan good-evening in what seemed an offhand fashion by reason of the habitual catch in his voice and then, seeing that Mr. Browne was grinning at him from the sideboard, crossed the room on rather shaky legs and began to repeat in an undertone the story he had just told to Gabriel.

"He's not so bad, is he?" said Aunt Kate to Gabriel.

Gabriel's brows were dark but he raised them quickly and answered:

"O, no, hardly noticeable."

"Now, isn't he a terrible fellow!" she said. "And his poor mother made him take the pledge on New Year's Eve. But come on, Gabriel, into the drawing-room."

Before leaving the room with Gabriel she signalled to Mr. Browne by frowning and shaking her forefinger in warning to and fro. Mr. Browne nodded in answer and, when she had gone, said to Freddy Malins:

"Now, then, Teddy, I'm going to fill you out a good glass of lemonade just to buck you up."

Freddy Malins, who was nearing the climax of his story, waved the offer aside impatiently but Mr. Browne, having first called Freddy Malins' attention to a disarray in his dress, filled out and handed him a full glass of lemonade. Freddy Malins' left hand accepted the glass mechanically, his right hand being engaged in the mechanical readjustment of his dress. Mr. Browne, whose face was once more wrinkling with mirth, poured out for himself a glass of whisky while Freddy Malins exploded, before he had well reached the climax of his story, in a kink of high-pitched bronchitic laughter and, setting down his untasted and overflowing glass, began to rub the knuckles of his left fist backwards and forwards into his left eye, repeating words of his last phrase as well as his fit of laughter would allow him.

Gabriel could not listen while Mary Jane was playing her Academy piece, full of runs and difficult passages, to the hushed drawing-room. He liked music but the piece she was playing had no melody for him and he doubted whether it had any melody for the other listeners, though they had begged Mary Jane to play something. Four young men, who had come from the refreshment-room to stand in the doorway at the sound of the piano, had gone away quietly in couples after a few minutes. The only persons who seemed to follow the music were Mary Jane herself, her hands racing along the key-board or lifted from it at the pauses like those of a priestess in momentary imprecation, and Aunt Kate standing at her elbow to turn the page.

Gabriel's eyes, irritated by the floor, which glittered with beeswax under the heavy chandelier, wandered to the wall above the piano. A picture of the balcony scene in *Romeo and Juliet* hung there and beside it was a picture of the two murdered princes in the Tower which Aunt

Julia had worked in red, blue and brown wools when she was a girl. Probably in the school they had gone to as girls that kind of work had been taught for one year. His mother had worked for him as a birthday present a waistcoat of purple tabinet, with little foxes' heads upon it, lined with brown satin and having round mulberry buttons. It was strange that his mother had had no musical talent though Aunt Kate used to call her the brains carrier of the Morkan family. Both she and Julia had always seemed a little proud of their serious and matronly sister. Her photograph stood before the pierglass. She held an open book on her knees and was pointing out something in it to Constantine who, dressed in a man-o-war suit, lay at her feet. It was she who had chosen the name of her sons for she was very sensible of the dignity of family life. Thanks to her, Constantine was now senior curate in Balbrigan and, thanks to her, Gabriel himself had taken his degree in the Royal University. A shadow passed over his face as he remembered her sullen opposition to his marriage. Some slighting phrases she had used still rankled in his memory; she had once spoken of Gretta as being country cute and that was not true of Gretta at all. It was Gretta who had nursed her during all her last long illness in their house at Monkstown.

He knew that Mary Jane must be near the end of her piece for she was playing again the opening melody with runs of scales after every bar and while he waited for the end the resentment died down in his heart. The piece ended with a trill of octaves in the treble and a final deep octave in the bass. Great applause greeted Mary Jane as, blushing and rolling up her music nervously, she escaped from the room. The most vigorous clapping came from the four young men in the doorway who had gone away to the refreshment-room at the beginning of the piece but had come back when the piano had stopped.

Lancers were arranged. Gabriel found himself partnered with Miss Ivors. She was a frank-mannered talkative young lady, with a freckled face and prominent brown eyes. She did not wear a low-cut bodice and the large brooch which was fixed in the front of her collar bore on it an Irish device and motto.

When they had taken their places she said abruptly:

"I have a crow to pluck with you."

"With me?" said Gabriel.

She nodded her head gravely.

"What is it?" asked Gabriel, smiling at her solemn manner.

"Who is G. C.?" answered Miss Ivors, turning her eyes upon him.

Gabriel coloured and was about to knit his brows, as if he did not understand, when she said bluntly:

"O, innocent Amy! I have found out that you write for *The Daily Express*. Now, aren't you ashamed of yourself?"

"Why should I be ashamed of myself?" asked Gabriel, blinking his eyes and trying to smile.

"Well, I'm ashamed of you," said Miss Ivors frankly. "To say you'd write for a paper like that. I didn't think you were a West Briton."

A look of perplexity appeared on Gabriel's face. It was true that he wrote a literary column every Wednesday in *The Daily Express*, for which he was paid fifteen shillings. But that did not make him a West Briton surely. The books he received for review were almost more welcome than the paltry cheque. He loved to feel the covers and turn over the pages of newly printed books. Nearly every day when his teaching in the college was ended he used to wander down the quays to the second-hand booksellers, to Hickey's on Bachelor's Walk, to Web's or Massey's on Aston's Quay, or to O'Clohissey's in the bystreet. He did not know how to meet her charge. He wanted to say that literature was above politics. But they were friends of many years' standing and their careers had been parallel, first at the University and then as teachers: he could not risk a grandiose phrase with her. He continued blinking his eyes and trying to smile and murmured lamely that he saw nothing political in writing reviews of books.

When their turn to cross had come he was still perplexed and inattentive. Miss Ivors promptly took his hand in a warm grasp and said in a soft friendly tone:

"Of course, I was only joking. Come, we cross now."

When they were together again she spoke of the University question and Gabriel felt more at ease. A friend of hers had shown her his review of Browning's poems. That was how she had found out the secret: but she liked the review immensely. Then she said suddenly:

"O, Mr. Conroy, will you come for an excursion to the Aran Isles this summer? We're going to stay there a whole month. It will be splendid out in the Atlantic. You ought to come. Mr. Clancy is coming, and Mr. Kilkelly and Kathleen Kearney. It would be splendid for Gretta too if she'd come. She's from Connacht, isn't she?"

"Her people are," said Gabriel shortly.

"But you will come, won't you?" said Miss Ivors, laying her warm hand eagerly on his arm.

"The fact is," said Gabriel, "I have just arranged to go—"

"Go where?" asked Miss Ivors.

"Well, you know, every year I go for a cycling tour with some fellows and so—"

"But where?" asked Miss Ivors.

"Well, we usually go to France or Belgium or perhaps Germany," said Gabriel awkwardly.

"And why do you go to France and Belgium," said Miss Ivors, "instead of visiting your own land?"

"Well," said Gabriel, "it's partly to keep in touch with the languages and partly for a change."

"And haven't you your own language to keep in touch with—Irish?" asked Miss Ivors.

"Well," said Gabriel, "if it comes to that, you know, Irish is not my language."

Their neighbours had turned to listen to the cross-examination. Gabriel glanced right and left nervously and tried to keep his good humour under the ordeal which was making a blush invade his forehead.

"And haven't you your own land to visit," continued Miss Ivors, "that you know nothing of, your own people, and your own country?"

"O, to tell you the truth," retorted Gabriel suddenly, "I'm sick of my own country, sick of it!"

"Why?" asked Miss Ivors.

Gabriel did not answer for his retort had heated him.

"Why?" repeated Miss Ivors.

They had to go visiting together and, as he had not answered her, Miss Ivors said warmly:

"Of course, you've no answer."

Gabriel tried to cover his agitation by taking part in the dance with great energy. He avoided her eyes for he had seen a sour expression on her face. But when they met in the long chain he was surprised to feel his hand firmly pressed. She looked at him from under her brows for a moment quizzically until he smiled. Then, just as the chain was about to start again, she stood on tiptoe and whispered into his ear:

"West Briton!"

When the lancers were over Gabriel went away to a remote corner of the room where Freddy Malins' mother was sitting. She was a stout feeble old woman with white hair. Her voice had a catch in it like her son's and she stuttered slightly. She had been told that Freddy had come and that he was nearly all right. Gabriel asked her whether she had had a good crossing. She lived with her married daughter in Glasgow and came to Dublin on a visit once a year. She answered placidly that she had had a beautiful crossing and that the captain had been most attentive to her. She spoke also of the beautiful house her daughter kept in Glasgow, and of all the friends they had there. While her tongue rambled on Gabriel tried to banish from his mind all memory of the unpleasant incident with Miss Ivors. Of course the girl or woman, or whatever she was, was an enthusiast but there was a time for all things. Perhaps he ought not to have answered her like that. But she had no right to call him a West Briton before people, even in joke. She had tried to make him ridiculous before people, heckling him and staring at him with her rabbit's eyes.

He saw his wife making her way towards him through the waltzing couples. When she reached him she said into his ear:

"Gabriel. Aunt Kate wants to know won't you carve the goose as usual. Miss Daly will carve the ham and I'll do the pudding."

"All right," said Gabriel.

"She's sending in the younger ones first as soon as this waltz is over so that we'll have the table to ourselves."

"Were you dancing?" asked Gabriel.

"Of course I was. Didn't you see me? What row had you with Molly Ivors?"

"No row. Why? Did she say so?"

"Something like that. I'm trying to get that Mr. D'Arcy to sing. He's full of conceit, I think."

"There was no row," said Gabriel moodily, "only she wanted me to go for a trip to the west of Ireland and I said I wouldn't."

His wife clasped her hands excitedly and gave a little jump.

"O, do go, Gabriel," she cried. "I'd love to see Galway again."

"You can go if you like," said Gabriel coldly.

She looked at him for a moment, then turned to Mrs. Malins and said:

"There's a nice husband for you, Mrs. Malins."

While she was threading her way back across the room Mrs. Malins, without adverting to the interruption, went on to tell Gabriel what beautiful places there were in Scotland and beautiful scenery. Her son-in-law brought them every year to the lakes and they used to go fishing. Her son-in-law was a splendid fisher. One day he caught a beautiful big fish and the man in the hotel cooked it for their dinner.

Gabriel hardly heard what she said. Now that supper was coming near he began to think again about his speech and about the quotation. When he saw Freddy Malins coming across the room to visit his mother Gabriel left the chair free for him and retired into the embrasure of the window. The room had already cleared and from the back room came the clatter of plates and knives. Those who still remained in the drawing room seemed tired of dancing and were conversing quietly in little groups. Gabriel's warm trembling fingers tapped the cold pane of the window. How cool it must be outside! How pleasant it would be to walk out alone, first along by the river and then through the park! The snow would be lying on the branches of the trees and forming a bright cap on the top of the Wellington Monument. How much more pleasant it would be there than at the supper-table!

He ran over the headings of his speech: Irish hospitality, sad memories, the Three Graces, Paris, the quotation from Browning. He repeated to himself a phrase he had written in his review: "One feels that one is listening to a thought-tormented music." Miss Ivors had praised the review. Was she sincere? Had she really any life of her own behind all her propagandism? There had never been any ill-feeling between them until that night. It unnerved him to think that she would be at the supper-table, looking up at him while he spoke with her critical quizzing eyes. Perhaps she would not be sorry to see him fail in his speech. An idea came into his mind and gave him courage. He would say, alluding to Aunt Kate and Aunt Julia: "Ladies and Gentlemen, the generation which is now on the wane among us may have had its faults but for my part I think it had certain qualities of hospitality, of humour, of humanity, which the new and very serious and hypereducated generation that is growing up around us seems to me to lack." Very good: that was one for Miss Ivors. What did he care that his aunts were only two ignorant old women?

A murmur in the room attracted his attention. Mr. Browne was advancing from the door, gallantly escorting Aunt Julia, who leaned upon his arm, smiling and hanging her head. An irregular musketry of applause escorted her also as far as the piano and then, as Mary Jane seated herself on the stool, and Aunt Julia, no longer smiling, half turned so as to pitch her voice fairly into the room, gradually ceased. Gabriel recognised the prelude. It was that of an old song of Aunt Julia's—"Arrayed for the Bridal." Her voice, strong and clear in tone, attacked with great spirit the runs which embellish the air and though she sang very rapidly she did not miss even the smallest of the grace notes. To follow the voice, without looking at the singer's face, was to feel and share the excitement of swift and secure flight. Gabriel applauded loudly with all the others at the close of the song and loud applause was borne in from the invisible supper-table. It sounded so genuine that a little colour struggled into Aunt Julia's face as she bent to replace in the music-stand the old leather-bound songbook that had her initials on the cover. Freddy Malins, who had listened with his head perched sideways to hear her better, was still applauding when everyone else had ceased and talking animatedly to his mother who nodded her head gravely and slowly in acquiescence. At last, when he could clap no more, he stood up suddenly and hurried across the room to Aunt Julia whose hand he seized and held in both his hands, shaking it when words failed him or the catch in his voice proved too much for him.

"I was just telling my mother," he said, "I never heard you sing so well, never. No, I never heard your voice so good as it is tonight. Now! Would you believe that now? That's the truth. Upon my word and honour that's the truth. I never heard your voice sound so fresh and so . . . so clear and fresh, never."

Aunt Julia smiled broadly and murmured something about compliments as she released her hand from his grasp. Mr. Browne extended his open hand towards her and said to those who were near him in the manner of a showman introducing a prodigy to an audience:

"Miss Julia Morkan, my latest discovery!"

He was laughing very heartily at this himself when Freddy Malins turned to him and said:

"Well, Browne, if you're serious you might make a worse discovery. All I can say is I never heard her sing half so well as long as I am coming here. And that's the honest truth."

"Neither did I," said Mr. Browne. "I think her voice has greatly improved."

Aunt Julia shrugged her shoulders and said with meek pride:

"Thirty years ago I hadn't a bad voice as voices go."

"I often told Julia," said Aunt Kate emphatically, "that she was simply thrown away in that choir. But she never would be said by me."

She turned as if to appeal to the good sense of the others against a refractory child while Aunt Julia gazed in front of her, a vague smile of reminiscence playing on her face.

"No," continued Aunt Kate, "she wouldn't be said or led by anyone, slaving there in that choir night and day, night and day. Six o'clock on Christmas morning! And all for what?"

"Well, isn't it for the honour of God, Aunt Kate?" asked Mary Jane, twisting round on the piano-stool and smiling.

Aunt Kate turned fiercely on her niece and said:

"I know all about the honour of God, Mary Jane, but I think it's not at all honourable for the pope to turn out the women out of the choirs that have slaved there all their lives and put little whipper-snappers of boys over their heads. I suppose it is for the good of the Church if the pope does it. But it's not just, Mary Jane, and it's not right."

She had worked herself into a passion and would have continued in defence of her sister for it was a sore subject with her but Mary Jane, seeing that all the dancers had come back, intervened pacifically:

"Now, Aunt Kate, you're giving scandal to Mr. Browne who is of the other persuasion."

Aunt Kate turned to Mr. Browne, who was grinning at this allusion to his religion, and said hastily:

"O, I don't question the pope's being right. I'm only a stupid old woman and I wouldn't presume to do such a thing. But there's such a thing as common everyday politeness and gratitude. And if I were in Julia's place I'd tell that Father Healey straight up to his face . . ."

"And besides, Aunt Kate," said Mary Jane, "we really are all hungry and when we are hungry we are all very quarrelsome."

"And when we are thirsty we are also quarrelsome," added Mr. Browne.

"So that we had better go to supper," said Mary Jane, "and finish the discussion afterwards."

On the landing outside the drawing-room Gabriel found his wife and Mary Jane trying to persuade Miss Ivors to stay for supper. But Miss Ivors, who had put on her hat and was buttoning her cloak, would not stay. She did not feel in the least hungry and she had already overstayed her time.

"But only for ten minutes, Molly," said Mrs. Conroy. "That won't delay you."

"To take a pick itself," said Mary Jane, "after all your dancing."

"I really couldn't," said Miss Ivors.

"I am afraid you didn't enjoy yourself at all," said Mary Jane hopelessly.

"Ever so much, I assure you," said Miss Ivors, "but you really must let me run off now."

"But how can you get home?" asked Mrs. Conroy.

"O, it's only two steps up the quay."

Gabriel hesitated a moment and said:

"If you will allow me, Miss Ivors, I'll see you home if you are really obliged to go."

But Miss Ivors broke away from them.

"I won't hear of it," she cried. "For goodness' sake go in to your suppers and don't mind me. I'm quite well able to take care of myself."

"Well, you're the comical girl, Molly," said Mrs. Conroy frankly.

"Beannacht libh," cried Miss Ivors, with a laugh, as she ran down the staircase.

Mary Jane gazed after her, a moody puzzled expression on her face, while Mrs. Conroy leaned over the banisters to listen for the hall-door. Gabriel asked himself was he the cause of her abrupt departure. But she did not seem to be in ill humour: she had gone away laughing. He stared blankly down the staircase.

At the moment Aunt Kate came toddling out of the supper-room, almost wringing her hands in despair.

"Where is Gabriel?" she cried. "Where on earth is Gabriel? There's everyone waiting in there, stage to let, and nobody to carve the goose!"

"Here I am, Aunt Kate!" cried Gabriel, with sudden animation, "ready to carve a flock of geese, if necessary."

A fat brown goose lay at one end of the table and at the other end, on a bed of creased paper strewn with sprigs of parsley, lay a great ham, stripped of its outer skin and peppered over with crust crumbs, a neat paper frill round its shin and beside this was a round of spiced beef. Between these rival ends ran parallel lines of side-dishes: two little minsters of jelly, red and yellow; a shallow dish full of blocks of blancmange and red jam, a large green leaf-shaped dish with a stalk-shaped handle, on which lay bunches of purple raisins and peeled almonds, a companion dish on which lay a solid rectangle of Smyrna figs, a dish of custard topped with grated nutmeg, a small bowl full of chocolates and sweets wrapped in gold and silver papers and a glass vase in which stood some tall celery stalks. In the centre of the table there stood, as sentries to a fruit-stand which upheld a pyramid of oranges and American apples, two squat old-fashioned decanters of cut glass, one containing port and the other dark sherry. On the closed square piano a pudding in a huge yellow dish lay in waiting and behind it were three squads of bottles of stout and ale and minerals, drawn up according to the colours of their uniforms, the first two black, with brown and red labels, the third and smallest squad white, with transverse green sashes.

Gabriel took his seat boldly at the head of the table and, having looked to the edge of the carver, plunged his fork firmly into the goose. He felt quite at ease now for he was an expert carver and liked nothing better than to find himself at the head of a well-laden table.

"Miss Furlong, what shall I send you?" he asked. "A wing or a slice of the breast?"

"Just a small slice of the breast."

"Miss Higgins, what for you?"

"O, anything at all, Mr. Conroy."

While Gabriel and Miss Daly exchanged plates of goose and plates of ham and spiced beef Lily went from guest to guest with a dish of hot floury potatoes wrapped in a white napkin. This was Mary Jane's idea and she had also suggested apple sauce for the goose but Aunt Kate had said that plain roast goose without any apple sauce had always been good enough for her and she hoped she might never eat worse. Mary Jane waited on her pupils and saw that they got the best slices and Aunt Kate and Aunt Julia opened and carried across from the piano bottles of stout and ale for the gentlemen and bottles of minerals for the ladies. There was a great deal of confusion and laughter and noise, the noise of orders and counter-orders, of knives and forks, of corks and glass-stoppers. Gabriel began to carve second helpings as soon as he had finished the first round without serving himself. Everyone protested loudly so that he compromised by taking a long draught of stout for he had found the carving hot work. Mary Jane settled down quietly to her supper but Aunt Kate and Aunt Julia were still toddling round the table, walking on each other's heels, getting in each other's way and giving each other unheeded orders. Mr. Browne begged of them to sit down and eat their suppers and so did Gabriel but they said there was time enough, so that, at last, Freddy Malins stood up and, capturing Aunt Kate, plumped her down on her chair amid general laughter.

When everyone had been well served Gabriel said, smiling:

"Now, if anyone wants a little more of what vulgar people call stuffing let him or her speak."

A chorus of voices invited him to begin his own supper and Lily came forward with three potatoes which she had reserved for him.

"Very well," said Gabriel amiably, as he took another preparatory draught, "kindly forget my existence, ladies and gentlemen, for a few minutes."

He set to his supper and took no part in the conversation with which the table covered Lily's removal of the plates. The subject of talk was the opera company which was then at the Theatre Royal. Mr. Bartell D'Arcy, the tenor, a dark-complexioned young man with a smart moustache, praised very highly the leading contralto of the company but Miss Furlong thought she had a rather vulgar style of production. Freddy Malins said there was a Negro chieftain singing in the second part of the Gaiety pantomime who had one of the finest tenor voices he had ever heard.

"Have you heard him?" he asked Mr. Bartell D'Arcy across the table.

"No," answered Mr. Bartell D'Arcy carelessly.

"Because," Freddy Malins explained, "now I'd be curious to hear your opinion of him. I think he has a grand voice."

"It takes Teddy to find out the really good things," said Mr. Browne familiarly to the table.

"And why couldn't he have a voice too?" asked Freddy Malins sharply. "Is it because he's only a black?"

Nobody answered this question and Mary Jane led the table back to the legitimate opera. One of her pupils had given her a pass for *Mignon*. Of course it was very fine, she said, but it made her think of poor Georgina Burns. Mr. Browne could go back farther still, to the old Italian companies that used to come to Dublin—Tietjens, Ilma de Murzka, Campanini, the great Trebelli, Giuglini, Ravelli, Aramburo. Those were the days, he said, when there was something like singing to be heard in Dublin. He told too of how the top gallery of the old Royal used to be packed night after night, of how one night an Italian tenor had sung five encores to "Let Me Like a Soldier Fall," introducing a high C every time, and of how the gallery boys would sometimes in their enthusiasm unyoke the horses from the carriage of some great prima donna and pull her themselves through the streets to her hotel. Why did they never play the grand old operas now, he asked, *Dinorah, Lucrezia Borgia*? Because they could not get the voices to sing them: that was why.

"Oh, well," said Mr. Bartell D'Arcy, "I presume there are as good singers today as there were then."

"Where are they?" asked Mr. Browne defiantly.

"In London, Paris, Milan," said Mr. Bartell D'Arcy warmly. "I suppose Caruso, for example, is quite as good, if not better than any of the men you have mentioned."

"Maybe so," said Mr. Browne. "But I may tell you I doubt it strongly."

"O, I'd give anything to hear Caruso sing," said Mary Jane.

"For me," said Aunt Kate, who had been picking a bone, "there was only one tenor. To please me, I mean. But I suppose none of you ever heard of him."

"Who was he, Miss Morkan?" asked Mr. Bartell D'Arcy politely.

"His name," said Aunt Kate, "was Parkinson. I heard him when he was in his prime and I think he had then the purest tenor voice that was ever put into a man's throat."

"Strange," said Mr. Bartell D'Arcy. "I never even heard of him."

"Yes, yes, Miss Morkan is right," said Mr. Browne. "I remember hearing of old Parkinson but he's too far back for me."

"A beautiful, pure, sweet, mellow English tenor," said Aunt Kate with enthusiasm.

Gabriel having finished, the huge pudding was transferred to the table. The clatter of forks and spoons began again. Gabriel's wife served out spoonfuls of the pudding and passed the plates down the table. Midway down they were held up by Mary Jane, who replenished them with raspberry or orange jelly or with blancmange and jam. The pudding was of Aunt Julia's making and she received praises for it from all quarters. She herself said that it was not quite brown enough.

"Well, I hope, Miss Morkan," said Mr. Browne, "that I'm brown enough for you because, you know, I'm all brown."

All the gentlemen, except Gabriel, ate some of the pudding out of compliment to Aunt Julia. As Gabriel never ate sweets the celery had been left for him. Freddy Malins also took a stalk of celery and ate it with his pudding. He had been told that celery was a capital thing for the blood and he was just then under doctor's care. Mrs. Malins, who had been silent all through the supper, said that her son was going down to Mount Melleray in a week or so. The table then spoke of Mount Melleray, how bracing the air was down there, how hospitable the monks were and how they never asked for a penny-piece from their guests.

"And do you mean to say," asked Mr. Browne incredulously, "that a chap can go down there and put up there as if it were a hotel and live on the fat of the land and then come away without paying anything?"

"O, most people give some donation to the monastery when they leave," said Mary Jane.

"I wish we had an institution like that in our Church," said Mr. Browne candidly.

He was astonished to hear that the monks never spoke, got up at two in the morning and slept in their coffins. He asked what they did it for.

"That's the rule of the order," said Aunt Kate firmly.

"Yes, but why?" asked Mr. Browne.

Aunt Kate repeated that it was the rule, that was all. Mr. Browne still seemed not to understand. Freddy Malins explained to him, as best he could, that the monks were trying to make up for the sins committed by all the sinners in the outside world. The explanation was not very clear for Mr. Browne grinned and said:

"I like that idea very much but wouldn't a comfortable spring bed do them as well as a coffin?"

"The coffin," said Mary Jane, "is to remind them of their last end."

As the subject had grown lugubrious it was buried in a silence of the table during which Mrs. Malins could be heard saying to her neighbour in an indistinct undertone:

"They are very good men, the monks, very pious men."

The raisins and almonds and figs and apples and oranges and chocolates and sweets were now passed about the table and Aunt Julia invited all the guests to have either port or sherry. At first Mr. Bartell D'Arcy refused to take either but one of his neighbours nudged him and whispered something to him upon which he allowed his glass to be filled. Gradually as the last glasses were being filled the conversation ceased. A pause followed, broken only by the noise of the wine and by unsettlings of chairs. The Misses Morkan, all three, looked down at the tablecloth. Someone coughed once or twice and then a few gentlemen patted the table gently as a signal for silence. The silence came and Gabriel pushed back his chair.

The patting at once grew louder in encouragement and then ceased altogether. Gabriel leaned his ten trembling fingers on the tablecloth and smiled nervously at the company. Meeting a row of upturned faces he raised his eyes to the chandelier. The piano was playing a waltz tune and he could hear the skirts sweeping against the drawing-room door. People, perhaps, were standing in the snow on the quay outside, gazing up at the lighted windows and listening to the waltz music. The air was pure there. In the distance lay the park where the trees were weighted with snow. The Wellington Monument wore a gleaming cap of snow that flashed westward over the white field of Fifteen Acres.

He began:

"Ladies and Gentlemen, it has fallen to my lot this evening, as in years past, to perform a very pleasing task but a task for which I am afraid my poor powers as a speaker are all too inadequate."

"No, no!" said Mr. Browne.

"But, however that may be, I can only ask you tonight to take the will for the deed and to lend me your attention for a few moments while I endeavour to express to you in words what my feelings are on this occasion.

"Ladies and Gentlemen, it is not the first time that we have gathered together under this hospitable roof, around this hospitable board. It is not the first time that we have been the recipients—or perhaps, I had better say, the victims—of the hospitality of certain good ladies."

He made a circle in the air with his arm and paused. Everyone laughed or smiled at Aunt Kate and Aunt Julia and Mary Jane who all turned crimson with pleasure. Gabriel went on more boldly:

"I feel more strongly with every recurring year that our country has no tradition which does it so much honour and which it should guard so jealously as that of its hospitality. It is a tradition that is unique as far as my experience goes (and I have visited not a few places abroad) among the modern nations. Some would say, perhaps, that with us it is rather a failing than anything to be boasted of. But granted even that, it is, to my mind, a princely failing, and one that I trust will long be cultivated among us. Of one thing, at least, I am sure. As long as this one roof shelters the good ladies aforesaid—and I wish from my heart it may do so for many and many a long year to come—the tradition of genuine warm-hearted courteous Irish hospitality, which our forefathers have handed down to us and which we in turn must hand down to our descendants, is still alive among us."

A hearty murmur of assent ran round the table. It shot through Gabriel's mind that Miss Ivors was not there and that she had gone away discourteously: and he said with confidence in himself:

"Ladies and Gentlemen, a new generation is growing up in our midst, a generation actuated by new ideas and new principles. It is serious and enthusiastic for these new ideas and its enthusiasm, even when it is misdirected, is, I believe, in the main sincere. But we are living in a sceptical and, if I may use the phrase, a thought-tormented age: and sometimes I fear that this new generation, educated or hypereducated as it is, will lack those qualities of humanity, of hospitality, of kindly humour which belonged to an older day. Listening tonight to the names of all those great singers of the past it seemed to me, I must confess, that we were living in a less spacious age. Those days might, without exaggeration, be called spacious days: and if they are gone beyond recall let us hope, at least, that in gatherings such as this we shall still speak of them with pride and affection, still cherish in our hearts the memory of those dead and gone great ones whose fame the world will not willingly let die."

"Hear, hear!" said Mr. Browne loudly.

"But yet," continued Gabriel, his voice falling into a softer inflection, "there are always in gatherings such as this sadder thoughts that will recur to our minds: thoughts of the past, of youth, of changes, of absent faces that we miss here tonight. Our path through life is strewn with many such sad memories: and were we to brood upon them always we could not find the heart to go on bravely with our work among the living. We have all of us living duties and living affections which claim, and rightly claim, our strenuous endeavours.

"Therefore, I will not linger on the past. I will not let any gloomy moralising intrude upon us here tonight. Here we are gathered together for a brief moment from the bustle and rush of our everyday routine. We are met here as friends, in the spirit of good-fellowship, as colleagues, also to a certain extent, in the true spirit of camaraderie, and as the guests of—what shall I call them?—the Three Graces of the Dublin musical world."

The table burst into applause and laughter at this allusion. Aunt Julia vainly asked each of her neighbours in turn to tell her what Gabriel had said.

"He says we are the Three Graces, Aunt Julia," said Mary Jane.

Aunt Julia did not understand but she looked up, smiling, at Gabriel, who continued in the same vein:

"Ladies and Gentlemen,

"I will not attempt to play tonight the part that Paris played on another occasion. I will not attempt to choose between them. The task would be an invidious one and one beyond my poor powers. For when I view them in turn, whether it be our chief hostess herself, whose good heart, whose too good heart, has become a byword with all who know her, or her sister, who seems to be gifted with perennial youth and whose singing must have been a surprise and a revelation to us all tonight, or, last but not least, when I consider our youngest hostess, talented, cheerful, hard-working and the best of nieces, I confess, Ladies and Gentlemen, that I do not know to which of them I should award the prize."

Gabriel glanced down at his aunts and, seeing the large smile on Aunt Julia's face and the tears which had risen to Aunt Kate's eyes, hastened to his close. He raised his glass of port gallantly, while every member of the company fingered a glass expectantly, and said loudly:

"Let us toast them all three together. Let us drink to their health, wealth, long life, happiness and prosperity and may they long continue to hold the proud and self-won position which they hold in their profession and the position of honour and affection which they hold in our hearts."

All the guests stood up, glass in hand, and turning towards the three seated ladies, sang in unison, with Mr. Browne as leader:

For they are jolly gay fellows,
For they are jolly gay fellows,
For they are jolly gay fellows,
Which nobody can deny.

Aunt Kate was making frank use of her handkerchief and even Aunt Julia seemed moved. Freddy Malins beat time with his pudding-fork and the singers turned towards one another, as if in melodious conference, while they sang with emphasis:

Unless he tells a lie,
Unless he tells a lie,

Then, turning once more towards their hostesses, they sang:

For they are jolly gay fellows,
For they are jolly gay fellows,
For they are jolly gay fellows,
Which nobody can deny.

The acclamation which followed was taken up beyond the door of the supper-room by many of the other guests and renewed time after time, Freddy Malins acting as officer with his fork on high.

The piercing morning air came into the hall where they were standing so that Aunt Kate said:

"Close the door, somebody. Mrs. Malins will get her death of cold."

"Browne is out there, Aunt Kate," said Mary Jane.

"Browne is everywhere," said Aunt Kate, lowering her voice.

Mary Jane laughed at her tone.

"Really," she said archly, "he is very attentive."

"He has been laid on here like the gas," said Aunt Kate in the same tone, "all during the Christmas."

She laughed herself this time good-humouredly and then added quickly:

"But tell him to come in, Mary Jane, and close the door. I hope to goodness he didn't hear me."

At that moment the hall-door was opened and Mr. Browne came in from the doorstep, laughing as if his heart would break. He was dressed in a long green overcoat with mock astrakhan cuffs and collar and wore on his head an oval fur cap. He pointed down the snow-covered quay from where the sound of shrill prolonged whistling was borne in.

"Teddy will have all the cabs in Dublin out," he said.

Gabriel advanced from the little pantry behind the office, struggling into his overcoat and, looking round the hall, said:

"Gretta not down yet?"

"She's getting on her things, Gabriel," said Aunt Kate.

"Who's playing up there?" asked Gabriel.

"Nobody. They're all gone."

"O no, Aunt Kate," said Mary Jane. "Bartell D'Arcy and Miss O'Callaghan aren't gone yet."

"Someone is fooling at the piano anyhow," said Gabriel.

Mary Jane glanced at Gabriel and Mr. Browne and said with a shiver:

"It makes me feel cold to look at you two gentlemen muffled up like that. I wouldn't like to face your journey home at this hour."

"I'd like nothing better this minute," said Mr. Browne stoutly, "than a rattling fine walk in the country or a fast drive with a good spanking goer between the shafts."

"We used to have a very good horse and trap at home," said Aunt Julia sadly.

"The never-to-be-forgotten Johnny," said Mary Jane, laughing.

Aunt Kate and Gabriel laughed too.

"Why, what was wonderful about Johnny?" asked Mr. Browne.

"The late lamented Patrick Morkan, our grandfather, that is," explained Gabriel, "commonly known in his later years as the old gentleman, was a glue-boiler."

"O, now, Gabriel," said Aunt Kate, laughing, "he had a starch mill."

"Well, glue or starch," said Gabriel, "the old gentleman had a horse by the name of Johnny. And Johnny used to work in the old gentleman's mill, walking round and round in order to drive the mill. That was all very well; but now comes the tragic part about Johnny. One fine day the old gentleman thought he'd like to drive out with the quality to a military review in the park."

"The Lord have mercy on his soul," said Aunt Kate compassionately.

"Amen," said Gabriel. "So the old gentleman, as I said, harnessed Johnny and put on his very best tall hat and his very best stock collar and drove out in grand style from his ancestral mansion somewhere near Back Lane, I think."

Everyone laughed, even Mrs. Malins, at Gabriel's manner and Aunt Kate said:

"O, now, Gabriel, he didn't live in Back Lane, really. Only the mill was there."

"Out from the mansion of his forefathers," continued Gabriel, "he drove with Johnny. And everything went on beautifully until Johnny came in sight of King Billy's statue: and whether he fell in love with the horse King Billy sits on or whether he thought he was back again in the mill, anyhow he began to walk round the statue."

Gabriel paced in a circle round the hall in his goloshes amid the laughter of the others.

"Round and round he went," said Gabriel, "and the old gentleman, who was a very pompous old gentleman, was highly indignant. 'Go on, sir! What do you mean, sir? Johnny! Johnny! Most extraordinary conduct! Can't understand the horse!'"

The peal of laughter which followed Gabriel's imitation of the incident was interrupted by a resounding knock at the hall door. Mary Jane ran to open it and let in Freddy Malins. Freddy Malins, with his hat well back on his head and his shoulders humped with cold, was puffing and steaming after his exertions.

"I could only get one cab," he said.

"O, we'll find another along the quay," said Gabriel.

"Yes," said Aunt Kate. "Better not keep Mrs. Malins standing in the draught."

Mrs. Malins was helped down the front steps by her son and Mr. Browne and, after many manoeuvres, hoisted into the cab. Freddy Malins clambered in after her and spent a long time settling her on the seat, Mr. Browne helping him with advice. At last she was settled comfortably and Freddy Malins invited Mr. Browne into the cab. There was a good deal of confused talk, and then Mr. Browne got into the cab. The cabman settled his rug over his knees, and bent down for the address. The confusion grew greater and the cabman was directed differently by Freddy Malins and Mr. Browne, each of whom had his head out through a window of the cab. The difficulty was to know where to drop Mr. Browne along the route, and Aunt Kate, Aunt Julia and Mary Jane helped the discussion from the doorstep with cross-directions and contradictions and abundance of laughter. As for Freddy Malins he was speechless with laughter. He popped his head in and out of the window every moment to the great danger of his hat, and told his mother how the discussion was progressing, till at last Mr. Browne shouted to the bewildered cabman above the din of everybody's laughter:

"Do you know Trinity College?"

"Yes, sir," said the cabman.

"Well, drive bang up against Trinity College gates," said Mr. Browne, "and then we'll tell you where to go. You understand now?"

"Yes, sir," said the cabman.

"Make like a bird for Trinity College."

"Right, sir," said the cabman.

The horse was whipped up and the cab rattled off along the quay amid a chorus of laughter and adieus.

Gabriel had not gone to the door with the others. He was in a dark part of the hall gazing up the staircase. A woman was standing near the top of the first flight, in the shadow also. He could not see her face but he could see the terra-cotta and salmon-pink panels of her skirt which the shadow made appear black and white. It was his wife. She was leaning on the banisters, listening to something. Gabriel was surprised at her stillness and strained his ear to listen also. But he could hear little save the noise of laughter and dispute on the front steps, a few chords struck on the piano and a few notes of a man's voice singing.

He stood still in the gloom of the hall, trying to catch the air that the voice was singing and gazing up at his wife. There was grace and mystery in her attitude as if she were a symbol of something. He asked himself what is a woman standing on the stairs in the shadow, listening to distant music, a symbol of. If he were a painter he would paint her in that attitude. Her blue felt hat would show off the bronze of her hair against the darkness and the dark panels of her skirt would show off the light ones. *Distant Music* he would call the picture if he were a painter.

The hall-door was closed; and Aunt Kate, Aunt Julia and Mary Jane came down the hall, still laughing.

"Well, isn't Freddy terrible?" said Mary Jane. "He's really terrible."

Gabriel said nothing but pointed up the stairs towards where his wife was standing. Now that the hall-door was closed the voice and the piano could be heard more clearly. Gabriel held up his hand for them to be silent. The song seemed to be in the old Irish tonality and the singer seemed uncertain both of his words and of his voice. The voice, made plaintive by distance and by the singer's hoarseness, faintly illuminated the cadence of the air with words expressing grief:

O, the rain falls on my heavy locks
And the dew wets my skin,
My babe lies cold . . .

"O," exclaimed Mary Jane. "It's Bartell D'Arcy singing and he wouldn't sing all the night. O, I'll get him to sing a song before he goes."

"O, do, Mary Jane," said Aunt Kate.

Mary Jane brushed past the others and ran to the staircase, but before she reached it the singing stopped and the piano was closed abruptly.

"O, what a pity!" she cried. "Is he coming down, Gretta?"

Gabriel heard his wife answer yes and saw her come down towards them. A few steps behind her were Mr. Bartell D'Arcy and Miss O'Callaghan.

"O, Mr. D'Arcy," cried Mary Jane, "it's downright mean of you to break off like that when we were all in raptures listening to you."

"I have been at him all the evening," said Miss O'Callaghan, "and Mrs. Conroy, too, and he told us he had a dreadful cold and couldn't sing."

"O, Mr. D'Arcy," said Aunt Kate, "now that was a great fib to tell."

"Can't you see that I'm as hoarse as a crow?" said Mr. D'Arcy roughly.

He went into the pantry hastily and put on his overcoat. The others, taken aback by his rude speech, could find nothing to say. Aunt Kate wrinkled her brows and made signs to the others to drop the subject. Mr. D'Arcy stood swathing his neck carefully and frowning.

"It's the weather," said Aunt Julia, after a pause.

"Yes, everybody has colds," said Aunt Kate readily, "everybody."

"They say," said Mary Jane, "we haven't had snow like it for thirty years; and I read this morning in the newspapers that the snow is general all over Ireland."

"I love the look of snow," said Aunt Julia sadly.

"So do I," said Miss O'Callaghan. "I think Christmas is never really Christmas unless we have the snow on the ground."

"But poor Mr. D'Arcy doesn't like the snow," said Aunt Kate, smiling.

Mr. D'Arcy came from the pantry, fully swathed and buttoned, and in a repentant tone told them the history of his cold. Everyone gave him advice and said it was a great pity and urged him to be very careful of his throat in the night air. Gabriel watched his wife, who did not join in the conversation. She was standing right under the dusty fanlight and the flame of the gas lit up the rich bronze of her hair, which he had seen her drying at the fire a few days before. She was in the same attitude and seemed unaware of the talk about her. At last she turned towards them and Gabriel saw that there was colour on her cheeks and that her eyes were shining. A sudden tide of joy went leaping out of his heart.

"Mr. D'Arcy," she said, "what is the name of that song you were singing?"

"It's called 'The Lass of Aughrim,'" said Mr. D'Arcy, "but I couldn't remember it properly. Why? Do you know it?"

"'The Lass of Aughrim,'" she repeated. "I couldn't think of the name."

"It's a very nice air," said Mary Jane. "I'm sorry you were not in voice tonight."

"Now, Mary Jane," said Aunt Kate, "don't annoy Mr. D'Arcy. I won't have him annoyed."

Seeing that all were ready to start she shepherded them to the door, where good-night was said:

"Well, good-night, Aunt Kate, and thanks for the pleasant evening."

"Good-night, Gabriel. Good-night, Gretta!"

"Good-night, Aunt Kate, and thanks ever so much. Goodnight, Aunt Julia."

"O, good-night, Gretta, I didn't see you."

"Good-night, Mr. D'Arcy. Good-night, Miss O'Callaghan."

"Good-night, Miss Morkan."

"Good-night, again."

"Good-night, all. Safe home."

"Good-night. Good-night."

The morning was still dark. A dull, yellow light brooded over the houses and the river; and the sky seemed to be descending. It was slushy underfoot; and only streaks and patches of snow lay on the roofs, on the parapets of the quay and on the area railings. The lamps were still burning redly in the murky air and, across the river, the palace of the Four Courts stood out menacingly against the heavy sky.

She was walking on before him with Mr. Bartell D'Arcy, her shoes in a brown parcel tucked under one arm and her hands holding her skirt up from the slush. She had no longer any grace of attitude, but Gabriel's eyes were still bright with happiness. The blood went bounding along his veins; and the thoughts went rioting through his brain, proud, joyful, tender, valorous.

She was walking on before him so lightly and so erect that he longed to run after her noiselessly, catch her by the shoulders and say something foolish and affectionate into her ear. She seemed to him so frail that he longed to defend her against something and then to be alone with her. Moments of their secret life together burst like stars upon his memory. A heliotrope envelope was lying beside his breakfast-cup and he was caressing it with his hand. Birds were twittering in the ivy and the sunny web of the curtain was shimmering along the floor: he could not eat for happiness. They were standing on the crowded platform and he was placing a ticket inside the warm palm of her glove. He was standing with her in the cold, looking in through a grated window at a man making bottles in a roaring furnace. It was very cold. Her face, fragrant in the cold air, was quite close to his; and suddenly he called out to the man at the furnace:

"Is the fire hot, sir?"

But the man could not hear with the noise of the furnace. It was just as well. He might have answered rudely.

A wave of yet more tender joy escaped from his heart and went coursing in warm flood along his arteries. Like the tender fire of stars moments of their life together, that no one knew of or would ever know of, broke upon and illumined his memory. He longed to recall to her those moments, to make her forget the years of their dull existence together and remember only their moments of ecstasy. For the years, he felt, had not quenched his soul or hers. Their children, his writing, her household cares had not quenched all their souls' tender fire. In one letter that he had written to her then he had said: "Why is it that words like these seem to me so dull and cold? Is it because there is no word tender enough to be your name?"

Like distant music these words that he had written years before were borne towards him from the past. He longed to be alone with her. When the others had gone away, when he and she were in the room in the hotel, then they would be alone together. He would call her softly:

"Gretta!"

Perhaps she would not hear at once: she would be undressing. Then something in his voice would strike her. She would turn and look at him. . . .

At the corner of Winetavern Street they met a cab. He was glad of its rattling noise as it saved him from conversation. She was looking out of the window and seemed tired. The others spoke only a few words, pointing out some building or street. The horse galloped along wearily under the murky morning sky, dragging his old rattling box after his heels, and Gabriel was again in a cab with her, galloping to catch the boat, galloping to their honeymoon.

As the cab drove across O'Connell Bridge Miss O'Callaghan said:

"They say you never cross O'Connell Bridge without seeing a white horse."

"I see a white man this time," said Gabriel.

"Where?" asked Mr. Bartell D'Arcy.

Gabriel pointed to the statue, on which lay patches of snow. Then he nodded familiarly to it and waved his hand.

"Good-night, Dan," he said gaily.

When the cab drew up before the hotel, Gabriel jumped out and, in spite of Mr. Bartell D'Arcy's protest, paid the driver. He gave the man a shilling over his fare. The man saluted and said:

"A prosperous New Year to you, sir."

"The same to you," said Gabriel cordially.

She leaned for a moment on his arm in getting out of the cab and while standing at the curbstone, bidding the others good- night. She leaned lightly on his arm, as lightly as when she had danced with him a few hours before. He had felt proud and happy then, happy that she was his, proud of her grace and wifely carriage. But now, after the kindling again of so many memories, the first touch of her body, musical and strange and perfumed, sent through him a keen pang of lust. Under cover of her silence he pressed her arm closely to his side; and, as they stood at the hotel door, he felt that they had escaped from their lives and duties, escaped from home and friends and run away together with wild and radiant hearts to a new adventure.

An old man was dozing in a great hooded chair in the hall. He lit a candle in the office and went before them to the stairs. They followed him in silence, their feet falling in soft thuds on the thickly carpeted stairs. She mounted the stairs behind the porter, her head bowed in the ascent, her frail shoulders curved as with a burden, her skirt girt tightly about her. He could have flung his arms about her hips and held her still, for his arms were trembling with desire to seize her and only the stress of his nails against the palms of his hands held the wild impulse of his body in check. The porter halted on the stairs to settle his guttering candle. They halted, too, on the steps below him. In the silence Gabriel could hear the falling of the molten wax into the tray and the thumping of his own heart against his ribs.

The porter led them along a corridor and opened a door. Then he set his unstable candle down on a toilet-table and asked at what hour they were to be called in the morning.

"Eight," said Gabriel.

The porter pointed to the tap of the electric-light and began a muttered apology, but Gabriel cut him short.

"We don't want any light. We have light enough from the street. And I say," he added, pointing to the candle, "you might remove that handsome article, like a good man."

The porter took up his candle again, but slowly, for he was surprised by such a novel idea. Then he mumbled good-night and went out. Gabriel shot the lock to.

A ghostly light from the street lamp lay in a long shaft from one window to the door. Gabriel threw his overcoat and hat on a couch and crossed the room towards the window. He looked down into the street in order that his emotion might calm a little. Then he turned and leaned against a chest of drawers with his back to the light. She had taken off her hat and cloak and was standing before a large swinging mirror, unhooking her waist. Gabriel paused for a few moments, watching her, and then said:

"Gretta!"

She turned away from the mirror slowly and walked along the shaft of light towards him. Her face looked so serious and weary that the words would not pass Gabriel's lips. No, it was not the moment yet.

"You looked tired," he said.

"I am a little," she answered.

"You don't feel ill or weak?"

"No, tired: that's all."

She went on to the window and stood there, looking out. Gabriel waited again and then, fearing that diffidence was about to conquer him, he said abruptly:

"By the way, Gretta!"

"What is it?"

"You know that poor fellow Malins?" he said quickly.

"Yes. What about him?"

"Well, poor fellow, he's a decent sort of chap, after all," continued Gabriel in a false voice. "He gave me back that sovereign I lent him, and I didn't expect it, really. It's a pity he wouldn't keep away from that Browne, because he's not a bad fellow, really."

He was trembling now with annoyance. Why did she seem so abstracted? He did not know how he could begin. Was she annoyed, too, about something? If she would only turn to him or come to him of her own accord! To take her as she was would be brutal. No, he must see some ardour in her eyes first. He longed to be master of her strange mood.

"When did you lend him the pound?" she asked, after a pause.

Gabriel strove to restrain himself from breaking out into brutal language about the sottish Malins and his pound. He longed to cry to her from his soul, to crush her body against his, to overmaster her. But he said:

"O, at Christmas, when he opened that little Christmas-card shop in Henry Street."

He was in such a fever of rage and desire that he did not hear her come from the window. She stood before him for an instant, looking at him strangely. Then, suddenly raising herself on tiptoe and resting her hands lightly on his shoulders, she kissed him.

"You are a very generous person, Gabriel," she said.

Gabriel, trembling with delight at her sudden kiss and at the quaintness of her phrase, put his hands on her hair and began smoothing it back, scarcely touching it with his fingers. The washing had made it fine and brilliant. His heart was brimming over with happiness. Just when he was wishing for it she had come to him of her own accord. Perhaps her thoughts had been running with his. Perhaps she had felt the impetuous desire that was in him, and then the yielding mood had come upon her. Now that she had fallen to him so easily, he wondered why he had been so diffident.

He stood, holding her head between his hands. Then, slipping one arm swiftly about her body and drawing her towards him, he said softly:

"Gretta, dear, what are you thinking about?"

She did not answer nor yield wholly to his arm. He said again, softly:

"Tell me what it is, Gretta. I think I know what is the matter. Do I know?"

She did not answer at once. Then she said in an outburst of tears:

"O, I am thinking about that song, 'The Lass of Aughrim.'"

She broke loose from him and ran to the bed and, throwing her arms across the bed-rail, hid her face. Gabriel stood stockstill for a moment in astonishment and then followed her. As he passed in the way of the cheval-glass he caught sight of himself in full length, his broad, well-filled shirt-front, the face whose expression always puzzled him when he saw it in a mirror, and his glimmering gilt-rimmed eyeglasses. He halted a few paces from her and said:

"What about the song? Why does that make you cry?"

She raised her head from her arms and dried her eyes with the back of her hand like a child. A kinder note than he had intended went into his voice.

"Why, Gretta?" he asked.

"I am thinking about a person long ago who used to sing that song."

"And who was the person long ago?" asked Gabriel, smiling.

"It was a person I used to know in Galway when I was living with my grandmother," she said.

The smile passed away from Gabriel's face. A dull anger began to gather again at the back of his mind and the dull fires of his lust began to glow angrily in his veins.

"Someone you were in love with?" he asked ironically.

"It was a young boy I used to know," she answered, "named Michael Furey. He used to sing that song, 'The Lass of Aughrim.' He was very delicate."

Gabriel was silent. He did not wish her to think that he was interested in this delicate boy.

"I can see him so plainly," she said, after a moment. "Such eyes as he had: big, dark eyes! And such an expression in them—an expression!"

"O, then, you are in love with him?" said Gabriel.

"I used to go out walking with him," she said, "when I was in Galway."

A thought flew across Gabriel's mind.

"Perhaps that was why you wanted to go to Galway with that Ivors girl?" he said coldly.

She looked at him and asked in surprise:

"What for?"

Her eyes made Gabriel feel awkward. He shrugged his shoulders and said:

"How do I know? To see him, perhaps."

She looked away from him along the shaft of light towards the window in silence.

"He is dead," she said at length. "He died when he was only seventeen. Isn't it a terrible thing to die so young as that?"

"What was he?" asked Gabriel, still ironically.

"He was in the gasworks," she said.

Gabriel felt humiliated by the failure of his irony and by the evocation of this figure from the dead, a boy in the gasworks. While he had been full of memories of their secret life together, full of tenderness and joy and desire, she had been comparing him in her mind with another. A shameful consciousness of his own person assailed him. He saw himself as a ludicrous figure, acting as a pennyboy for his aunts, a nervous, well-meaning sentimentalist, orating to vulgarians and idealising his own clownish lusts, the pitiable fatuous fellow he had caught a glimpse of in the mirror. Instinctively he turned his back more to the light lest she might see the shame that burned upon his forehead.

He tried to keep up his tone of cold interrogation, but his voice when he spoke was humble and indifferent.

"I suppose you were in love with this Michael Furey, Gretta," he said.

"I was great with him at that time," she said.

Her voice was veiled and sad. Gabriel, feeling now how vain it would be to try to lead her whither he had purposed, caressed one of her hands and said, also sadly:

"And what did he die of so young, Gretta? Consumption, was it?"

"I think he died for me," she answered.

A vague terror seized Gabriel at this answer, as if, at that hour when he had hoped to triumph, some impalpable and vindictive being was coming against him, gathering forces against him in its vague world. But he shook himself free of it with an effort of reason and continued to caress her hand. He did not question her again, for he felt that she would tell him of herself. Her hand was warm and moist: it did not respond to his touch, but he continued to caress it just as he had caressed her first letter to him that spring morning.

"It was in the winter," she said, "about the beginning of the winter when I was going to leave my grandmother's and come up here to the convent. And he was ill at the time in his lodgings in Galway and wouldn't be let out, and his people in Oughterard were written to. He was in decline, they said, or something like that. I never knew rightly."

She paused for a moment and sighed.

"Poor fellow," she said. "He was very fond of me and he was such a gentle boy. We used to go out together, walking, you know, Gabriel, like the way they do in the country. He was going to study singing only for his health. He had a very good voice, poor Michael Furey."

"Well; and then?" asked Gabriel.

"And then when it came to the time for me to leave Galway and come up to the convent he was much worse and I wouldn't be let see him so I wrote him a letter saying I was going up to Dublin and would be back in the summer, and hoping he would be better then."

She paused for a moment to get her voice under control, and then went on:

"Then the night before I left, I was in my grandmother's house in Nuns' Island, packing up, and I heard gravel thrown up against the window. The window was so wet I couldn't see, so I ran downstairs as I was and slipped out the back into the garden and there was the poor fellow at the end of the garden, shivering."

"And did you not tell him to go back?" asked Gabriel.

"I implored of him to go home at once and told him he would get his death in the rain. But he said he did not want to live. I can see his eyes as well! He was standing at the end of the wall where there was a tree."

"And did he go home?" asked Gabriel.

"Yes, he went home. And when I was only a week in the convent he died and he was buried in Oughterard, where his people came from. O, the day I heard that, that he was dead!"

She stopped, choking with sobs, and, overcome by emotion, flung herself face downward on the bed, sobbing in the quilt. Gabriel held her hand for a moment longer, irresolutely, and then, shy of intruding on her grief, let it fall gently and walked quietly to the window.

She was fast asleep.

Gabriel, leaning on his elbow, looked for a few moments unresentfully on her tangled hair and half-open mouth, listening to her deep-drawn breath. So she had had that romance in her life: a man had died for her sake. It hardly pained him now to think how poor a part he, her husband, had played in her life. He watched her while she slept, as though he and she had never lived together as man and wife. His curious eyes rested long upon her face and on her hair: and, as he thought of what she must have been then, in that time of her first girlish beauty, a strange, friendly pity for her entered his soul. He did not like to say even to himself that her face was no longer beautiful, but he knew that it was no longer the face for which Michael Furey had braved death.

Perhaps she had not told him all the story. His eyes moved to the chair over which she had thrown some of her clothes. A petticoat string dangled to the floor. One boot stood upright, its limp upper fallen down: the fellow of it lay upon its side. He wondered at his riot of emotions of an hour before. From what had it proceeded? From his aunt's supper, from his own foolish speech, from the wine and dancing, the merry-making when saying good-night in the hall, the pleasure of the walk along the river in the snow. Poor Aunt Julia! She, too, would soon be a shade with the shade of Patrick Morkan and his horse. He had caught that haggard look upon her face for a moment when she was singing "Arrayed for the Bridal." Soon, perhaps, he would be sitting in that same drawing-room, dressed in black, his silk hat on his knees. The blinds would be drawn down and Aunt Kate would be sitting beside him, crying and blowing her nose and telling him how Julia had died. He would cast about in his mind for some words that might console her, and would find only lame and useless ones. Yes, yes: that would happen very soon.

The air of the room chilled his shoulders. He stretched himself cautiously along under the sheets and lay down beside his wife. One by one, they were all becoming shades. Better pass boldly into that other world, in the full glory of some passion, than fade and wither dismally with age. He thought of how she who lay beside him had locked in her heart for so many years that image of her lover's eyes when he had told her that he did not wish to live.

Generous tears filled Gabriel's eyes. He had never felt like that himself towards any woman, but he knew that such a feeling must be love. The tears gathered more thickly in his eyes and in the partial darkness he imagined he saw the form of a young man standing under a dripping tree. Other forms were near. His soul had approached that region where dwell the vast hosts of the dead. He was conscious of, but could not apprehend, their wayward and flickering existence. His own identity was fading out into a grey impalpable world: the solid world itself, which these dead had one time reared and lived in, was dissolving and dwindling.

A few light taps upon the pane made him turn to the window. It had begun to snow again. He watched sleepily the flakes, silver and dark, falling obliquely against the lamplight. The time had come for him to set out on his journey westward. Yes, the newspapers were right: snow was general all over Ireland. It was falling on every part of the dark central plain, on the treeless hills, falling softly upon the Bog of Allen and, farther westward, softly falling into the dark mutinous Shannon waves. It was falling, too, upon every part of the lonely churchyard on the hill where Michael Furey lay buried. It lay thickly drifted on the crooked crosses and headstones, on the spears of the little gate, on the barren thorns. His soul swooned slowly as he heard the snow falling faintly through the universe and faintly falling, like the descent of their last end, upon all the living and the dead.

Albert Camus

THE ADULTEROUS WOMAN

A housefly had been circling for the last few minutes in the bus, though the windows were closed. An odd sight here, it had been silently flying back and forth on tired wings. Janine had lost track of it, then saw it light on her husband's motionless hand. The weather was cold. The fly shuddered with each gust of sandy wind that scratched against the windows. In the meager light of the winter morning, with great fracas of sheet metal and axles, the vehicle was rolling, pitching, and making hardly any progress. Janine looked at her husband. With wisps of graying hair growing low on a narrow forehead, a broad nose, a flabby mouth, Marcel looked like a pouting faun. At each hollow in the pavement she felt him jostle against her. Then his heavy torso would slump back on his widespread legs and he would become inert again and absent, with vacant stare. Nothing about him seemed active but his thick hairless hands, made even shorter by the flannel underwear extending below his cuffs and covering his wrists. His hands were holding so tight to a little canvas suitcase set between his knees that they appeared not to feel the fly's halting progress.

Suddenly the wind was distinctly heard to howl and the gritty fog surrounding the bus became even thicker. The sand now struck the windows in packets as if hurled by invisible hands. The fly shook a chilled wing, flexed its legs, and took flight. The bus slowed and seemed on the point of stopping. But the wind apparently died down, the fog lifted slightly, and the vehicle resumed speed. Gaps of light opened up in the dust-drowned landscape. Two or three frail, whitened palm trees which seemed cut out of metal flashed into sight in the window only to disappear the next moment.

"What a country!" Marcel said.

The bus was full of Arabs pretending to sleep, shrouded in their burnooses. Some had folded their legs on the seat and swayed more than the others in the car's motion. Their silence and impassivity began to weigh upon Janine; it seemed to her as if she had been traveling for days with that mute escort. Yet the bus had left only at dawn from the end of the rail line and for two hours in the cold morning it had been advancing on a stony, desolate plateau which, in the beginning at least, extended its straight lines all the way to reddish horizons. But the wind had risen and gradually swallowed up the vast expanse. From that moment on, the passengers had seen nothing more; one after another, they had ceased talking and were silently progressing in a sort of sleepless night, occasionally wiping their lips and eyes irritated by the sand that filtered into the car.

"Janine!" She gave a start at her husband's call. Once again she thought how ridiculous that name was for someone tall and sturdy like her. Marcel wanted to know where his sample case was. With her foot she explored the empty space under the seat and encountered an object which she decided must be it. She could not stoop over without gasping somewhat. Yet in school she had won the first prize in gymnastics and hadn't known what it was to be winded. Was that so long ago? Twenty-five years. Twenty-five years were nothing, for it seemed to her only yesterday when she was hesitating between an independent life and marriage, just yesterday when she was thinking anxiously of the time she might be growing old alone. She was not alone and that law student who always wanted to be with her was now at her side. She had eventually accepted him although he was a little shorter than she and she didn't much like his eager, sharp laugh or his black, protruding eyes. But she liked his courage in facing up to life, which he shared with all the French of this country. She also liked his crestfallen look when events or men failed to live up to his expectations. Above all, she liked being loved, and he had showered her with attentions. By so often making her aware that she existed for him he made her exist in reality. No, she was not alone . . .

The bus, with many loud honks, was plowing its way through invisible obstacles. Inside the car, however, no one stirred. Janine suddenly felt someone staring at her and turned toward the seat across the aisle. He was not an Arab, and she was surprised not to have noticed him from the beginning. He was wearing the uniform of the French regiments of the Sahara and an unbleached linen cap above his tanned face, long and pointed like a jackal's. His gray eyes were examining her with a sort of glum disapproval, in a fixed stare. She suddenly blushed and turned back to her husband, who was still looking straight ahead in the fog and wind. She snuggled down in her coat. But she could still see the French soldier, long and thin, so thin in his fitted tunic that he seemed constructed of a dry, friable material, a mixture of sand and bone. Then it was that she saw the thin hands and burned faces of the Arabs in front of her and noticed that they seemed to have plenty of room, despite their ample garments, on the seat where she and her husband felt wedged in. She pulled her coat around her knees. Yet she wasn't so fat—tall and well rounded rather, plump and still desirable, as she was well aware when men looked at her, with her rather childish face, her bright, naïve eyes contrasting with this big body she knew to be warm and inviting.

No, nothing had happened as she had expected. When Marcel had wanted to take her along on his trip she had protested. For some time he had been thinking of this trip—since the end of the war, to be precise, when business had returned to normal. Before the war the small dry-goods business he had taken over from his parents on giving up his study of law had provided a fairly good living. On the coast the years of youth can be happy ones. But he didn't much like physical effort and very soon had given up taking her to the beaches. The little car took them out of town solely for the Sunday afternoon ride. The rest of the time he preferred his shop full of multi-colored piece-goods shaded by the arcades of this half-native, half-European quarter. Above the shop they lived in three rooms furnished with Arab hangings and furniture from the Galerie Barbes. They had not had children. The years had passed in the semi-darkness behind the half-closed shutters. Summer, the beaches, excursions, the mere sight of the sky were things of the past. Nothing seemed to interest Marcel but business. She felt she had discovered his true passion to be money, and, without really knowing why, she didn't like that. After all, it was to her advantage. Far from being miserly, he was generous, especially where she was concerned. "If something happened to me," he used to say, "you'd be provided for." And, in fact, it is essential to provide for one's needs. But for all the rest, for what is not the most elementary need, how to provide? This is what she felt vaguely, at infrequent intervals. Meanwhile she helped Marcel keep his books and occasionally substituted for him in the shop. Summer was always the hardest, when the heat stifled even the sweet sensation of boredom.

Suddenly, in summer as it happened, the war, Marcel called up then rejected on grounds of health, the scarcity of piece-goods, business at a standstill, the streets empty and hot. If something happened now, she would no longer be provided for. This is why, as soon as piece-goods came back on the market, Marcel had thought of covering the villages of the Upper Plateaus and of the South himself in order to do without a middleman and sell directly to the Arab merchants. He had wanted to take her along. She knew that travel was difficult, she had trouble breathing, and she would have preferred staying at home. But he was obstinate and she had accepted because it would have taken too much energy to refuse. Here they were and, truly, nothing was like what she had imagined. She had feared the heat, the swarms of flies, the filthy hotels reeking of aniseed. She had not thought of the cold, of the biting wind, of these semi-polar plateaus cluttered with moraines. She had dreamed too of palm trees and soft sand. Now she saw that the desert was not that at all, but merely stone, stone everywhere, in the sky full of nothing but stone-dust, rasping and cold, as on the ground, where nothing grew among the stones except dry grasses.

The bus stopped abruptly. The driver shouted a few words in that language she had heard all her life without ever understanding it. "What's the matter?" Marcel asked. The driver, in French this time, said that the sand must have clogged the carburetor, and again Marcel cursed this country. The driver laughed hilariously and asserted that it was nothing, that he would clean the carburetor and they'd be off again. He opened the door and the cold wind blew into the bus, lashing their faces with myriad grains of sand. All the Arabs silently plunged their noses into their burnooses and huddled up. "Shut the door," Marcel shouted. The driver laughed as he came back to the door. Without hurrying, he took some tools from under the dashboard, then, tiny in the fog, again disappeared ahead without closing the door. Marcel sighed. "You may be sure he's never seen a motor in his life." "Oh, be quiet! said Janine. Suddenly she gave a start. On the shoulder of the road close to the bus, draped forms were standing still. Under the burnoose's hood and behind a rampart of veils, only their eyes were visible. Mute, come from nowhere, they were staring at the travelers. "Shepherds," Marcel said.

Inside the car there was total silence. All the passengers, heads lowered, seemed to be listening to the voice of the wind loosed across these endless plateaus. Janine was all of a sudden struck by the almost complete absence of luggage. At the end of the railroad line the driver had hoisted their trunk and a few bundles onto the roof. In the racks inside the bus could be seen nothing but gnarled sticks and shopping-baskets. All these people of the South apparently were traveling empty-handed.

But the driver was coming back, still brisk. His eyes alone were laughing above the veils with which he too had masked his face. He announced that they would soon be under way. He closed the door, the wind became silent, and the rain of sand on the windows could be heard better. The motor coughed and died. After having been urged at great length by the starter, it finally sparked and the driver raced it by pressing on the gas. With a big hiccough the bus started off. From the ragged clump of shepherds, still motionless, a hand rose and then faded into the fog behind them. Almost at once the vehicle began to bounce on the road, which had become worse. Shaken up, the Arabs constantly swayed. Nonetheless, Janine was feeling overcome with sleep when there suddenly appeared in front of her a little yellow box filled with lozenges. The jackal-soldier was smiling at her. She hesitated, took one, and thanked him. The jackal pocketed the box and simultaneously swallowed his smile. Now he was staring at the road, straight in front of him. Janine turned toward Marcel and saw only the solid back of his neck. Through the window he was watching a denser fog rising from the crumbly embankment.

They had been traveling for hours and fatigue had extinguished all life in the car when shouts burst forth outside. Children wearing burnooses, whirling like tops, leaping, clapping their hands, were running around the bus. It was now going down a long street lined with low houses; they were entering the oasis. The wind was still blowing, but the walls intercepted the grains of sand which had previously cut off the light. Yet the sky was still cloudy. Amidst shouts, in a great screeching of brakes, the bus stopped in front of the adobe arcades of a hotel with dirty windows. Janine got out and, once on the pavement, staggered. Above the houses she could see a slim yellow minaret. On her left rose the first palm trees of the oasis, and she would have liked to go toward them. But although it was close to noon, the cold was bitter; the wind made her shiver. She turned toward Marcel and saw the soldier coming toward her. She was expecting him to smile or salute. He passed without looking at her and disappeared. Marcel was busy getting down the trunk of piece-goods, a black foot-locker perched on the bus's roof. It would not be easy. The driver was the only one to take care of the luggage and he had already stopped, standing on the roof, to hold forth to the circle of burnooses gathered around the bus. Janine, surrounded with faces that seemed cut out of bone and leather, besieged by guttural shouts, suddenly became aware of her fatigue. "I'm going in," she said to Marcel, who was shouting impatiently at the driver.

She entered the hotel. The manager, a thin, laconic Frenchman, came to meet her. He led her to a second-floor balcony overlooking the street and into a room which seemed to have but an iron bed, a white-enameled chair, an uncurtained wardrobe, and, behind a rush screen, a washbasin covered with fine sand-dust. When the manager had closed the door, Janine felt the cold coming from the bare, whitewashed walls. She didn't know where to put her bag, where to put herself. She had either to lie down or to remain standing, and to shiver in either case. She remained standing, holding her bag and staring at a sort of window-slit that opened onto the sky near the ceiling. She was waiting, but she didn't know for what. She was aware only of her solitude, and of the penetrating cold, and of a greater weight in the region of her heart. She was in fact dreaming, almost deaf to the sounds rising from the street along with Marcel's vocal outbursts, more aware on the other hand of that sound of a river coming from the window-slit and caused by the wind in the palm trees, so close now, it seemed to her. Then the wind seemed to increase and the gentle ripple of waters became a hissing of waves. She imagined, beyond the walls, a sea of erect, flexible palm trees unfurling in the storm. Nothing was like what she had expected, but those invisible waves refreshed her tired eyes. She was standing, heavy, with dangling arms, slightly stooped, as the cold climbed her thick legs. She was dreaming of the erect and flexible palm trees and of the girl she had once been.

After having washed, they went down to the dining-room. On the bare walls had been painted camels and palm trees drowned in a sticky background of pink and lavender. The arcaded windows let in a meager light. Marcel questioned the hotel manager about the merchants. Then an elderly Arab wearing a military decoration on his tunic served them. Marcel, preoccupied, tore his bread into little pieces. He kept his wife from drinking water. "It hasn't been boiled. Take wine." She didn't like that, for wine made her sleepy. Besides, there was pork on the menu. "They don't eat it because of the Koran. But the Koran didn't know that well-done pork doesn't cause illness. We French know how to cook. What are you thinking about?" Janine was not thinking of anything, or perhaps of that victory of the cooks over the prophets. But she had to hurry. They were to leave the next morning for still farther south; that afternoon they had to see all the important merchants. Marcel urged the elderly Arab to hurry the coffee. He nodded without smiling and pattered out. "Slowly in the morning, not too fast in the afternoon," Marcel said, laughing. Yet eventually the coffee came. They barely took time to swallow it and went out into the dusty, cold street. Marcel called a young Arab to help him carry the trunk, but as a matter of principle quibbled about the payment. His opinion, which he once more expressed to Janine, was in fact based on the vague principle that they always asked for twice as much in the hope of settling for a quarter of the amount. Janine, ill at ease, followed the two trunk-bearers. She had put on a wool dress under her heavy coat and would have liked to take up less space. The pork, although well done, and the small quantity of wine she had drunk also bothered her somewhat.

They walked along a diminutive public garden planted with dusty trees. They encountered Arabs who stepped out of their way without seeming to see them, wrapping themselves in their burnooses. Even when they were wearing rags, she felt they had a look of dignity unknown to the Arabs of her town. Janine followed the trunk, which made a way for her through the crowd. They went through the gate in an earthen rampart and emerged on a little square planted with the same mineral trees and bordered on the far side, where it was widest, with arcades and shops. But they stopped on the square itself in front of a small construction shaped like an artillery shell and painted chalky blue. Inside, in the single room lighted solely by the entrance, an old Arab with white mustaches stood behind a shiny plank. He was serving tea, raising and lowering the teapot over three tiny multicolored glasses. Before they could make out anything else in the darkness, the cool scent of mint tea greeted Marcel and Janine at the door. Marcel had barely crossed the threshold and dodged the garlands of pewter teapots, cups and trays, and the postcard displays when he was up against the counter. Janine stayed at the door. She stepped a little aside so as not to cut off the light. At that moment she perceived in the darkness behind the old merchant two Arabs smiling at them, seated on the bulging sacks that filled the back of the shop. Red-and-black rugs and embroidered scarves hung on the walls; the floor was cluttered with sacks and little boxes filled with aromatic seeds. On the counter, beside a sparkling pair of brass scales and an old yardstick with figures effaced, stood a row of loaves of sugar. One of them had been unwrapped from its coarse blue paper and cut into on top. The smell of wool and spices in the room became apparent behind the scent of tea when the old merchant set down the teapot and said good-day.

Marcel talked rapidly in the low voice he assumed when talking business. Then he opened the trunk, exhibited the wools and silks, pushed back the scale and yardstick to spread out his merchandise in front of the old merchant. He got excited, raised his voice, laughed nervously, like a woman who wants to make an impression and is not sure of herself. Now, with hands spread wide, he was going though the gestures of selling and buying. The old man shook his head, passed the tea tray to the two Arabs behind him, and said just a few words that seemed to discourage Marcel. He picked up his goods, piled them back into the trunk, then wiped an imaginary sweat from his forehead. He called the little porter and they started off toward the arcades. In the first shop, although the merchant began by exhibiting the same Olympian manner, they were a little luckier. "They think they're God almighty," Marcel said, "but they're in business too! Life is hard for everyone."

Janine followed without answering. The wind had almost ceased. The sky was clearing in spots. A cold, harsh light came from the deep holes that opened up in the thickness of the clouds. They had now left the square. They were walking in narrow streets along earthen walls over which hung rotted December roses or, from time to time, a pomegranate, dried and wormy. An odor of dust and coffee, the smoke of a wood fire, the smell of stone and of sheep permeated this quarter. The shops, hollowed out of the walls, were far from one another; Janine felt her feet getting heavier. But her husband was gradually becoming more cheerful. He was beginning to sell and was feeling more kindly; he called Janine "Baby"; the trip would not be wasted. "Of course," Janine said mechanically, "it's better to deal directly with them."

They came back by another street, toward the center. It was late in the afternoon; the sky was now almost completely clear. They stopped in the square. Marcel rubbed his hands and looked affectionately at the trunk in front of them. "Look," said Janine. From the other end of the square was coming a tall Arab, thin, vigorous, wearing a sky-blue burnoose, soft brown boots and gloves, and bearing his bronzed aquiline face loftily. Nothing but the *chèche* that he was wearing swathed as a turban distinguished him from those French officers in charge of native affairs whom Janine had occasionally admired. He was advancing steadily toward them, but seemed to be looking beyond their group as he slowly removed the glove from one hand. "Well," said Marcel as he shrugged his shoulders, "there's one who thinks he's a general." Yes, all of them here had that look of pride; but this one, really, was going too far. Although they were surrounded by the empty space of the square, he was walking straight toward the trunk without seeing it, without seeing them. Then the distance separating them decreased rapidly and the Arab was upon them when Marcel suddenly seized the handle of the foot-locker and pulled it out of the way. The Arab passed without seeming to notice anything and headed with the same regular step toward the ramparts. Janine looked at her husband; he had his crestfallen look. "They think they can get away with anything now," he said. Janine did not reply. She loathed that Arab's stupid arrogance and suddenly felt unhappy. She wanted to leave and thought of her little apartment. The idea of going back to the hotel, to that icy room, discouraged her. It suddenly occurred to her that the manager had advised her to climb up to the terrace around the fort to see the desert. She said this to Marcel and that he could leave the trunk at the hotel. But he was tired and wanted to sleep a little before dinner. "Please," said Janine. He looked at her, suddenly attentive. "Of course, my dear," he said.

She waited for him in the street in front of the hotel. The white-robed crowd was becoming larger and larger. Not a single woman could be seen, and it seemed to Janine that she had never seen so many men. Yet none of them looked at her. Some of them, without appearing to see her, slowly turned toward her that thin, tanned face that made them all look alike to her, the face of the French soldier in the bus and that of the gloved Arab, a face both shrewd and proud. They turned that face toward the foreign woman, they didn't see her, and then, light and silent, they walked around her as she stood there with swelling ankles.

And her discomfort, her need of getting away increased. "Why did I come?" But already Marcel was coming back.

When they climbed the stairs to the fort, it was five o'clock. The wind had died down altogether. The sky, completely clear, was now periwinkle blue. The cold, now drier, made their cheeks smart. Halfway up the stairs an old Arab, stretched out against the wall, asked them if they wanted a guide, but didn't budge, as if he had been sure of their refusal in advance. The stairs were long and steep despite several landings of packed earth. As they climbed, the space widened and they rose into an ever broader light, cold and dry, in which every sound from the oasis reached them pure and distinct. The bright air seemed to vibrate around them with a vibration increasing in length as they advanced, as if their progress struck from the crystal of light a sound wave that kept spreading out. And as soon as they reached the terrace and their gaze was lost in the vast horizon beyond the palm grove, it seemed to Janine that the whole sky rang with a single short and piercing note, whose echoes gradually filled the space above her, then suddenly died and left her silently facing the limitless expanse.

From east to west, in fact, her gaze swept slowly, without encountering a single obstacle, along a perfect curve. Beneath her, the blue-and-white terraces of the Arab town overlapped one another, splattered with the dark-red spots of peppers drying in the sun. Not a soul could be seen, but from the inner courts, together with the aroma of roasting coffee, there rose laughing voices or incomprehensible stamping of feet. Farther off, the palm grove, divided into uneven squares by clay walls, rustled its upper foliage in a wind that could not be felt up on the terrace. Still farther off and all the way to the horizon extended the ocher-and-gray realm of stones, in which no life was visible. At some distance from the oasis, however, near the wadi that bordered the palm grove on the west could be seen broad black tents. All around them a flock of motionless dromedaries, tiny at that distance, formed against the gray ground the black signs of a strange handwriting, the meaning of which had to be deciphered. Above the desert, the silence was as vast as the space.

Janine, leaning her whole body against the parapet, was speechless, unable to tear herself away from the void opening before her. Beside her, Marcel was getting restless. He was cold; he wanted to go back down. What was there to see here, after all? But she could not take her gaze from the horizon. Over yonder, still farther south, at that point where sky and earth met in a pure line—over yonder it suddenly seemed there was awaiting her something of which, though it had always been lacking, she had never been aware until now. In the advancing afternoon the light relaxed and softened; it was passing from the crystalline to the liquid. Simultaneously, in the heart of a woman brought there by pure chance a knot tightened by the years, habit, and boredom was slowly loosening. She was looking at the nomads' encampment. She had not even seen the men living in it; nothing was stirring among the black tents, and yet she could think only of them whose existence she had barely known until this day. Homeless, cut off from the world, they were a handful wandering over the vast territory she could see, which however was but a paltry part of an even greater expanse whose dizzying course stopped only thousands of miles farther south, where the first river finally waters the forest. Since the beginning of time, on the dry earth of this limitless land scraped to the bone, a few men had been ceaselessly trudging, possessing nothing but serving no one, poverty-stricken but free lords of a strange kingdom. Janine did not know why this thought filled her with such a sweet, vast melancholy that it closed her eyes. She knew that this kingdom had been eternally promised her and yet that it would never be hers, never again, except in this fleeting moment perhaps when she opened her eyes again on the suddenly motionless sky and on its waves of steady light, while the voices rising from the Arab town suddenly fell silent. It seemed to her that the world's course had just stopped and that, from that moment on, no one would ever age any more or die. Everywhere, henceforth, life was suspended—except in her heart, where, at the same moment, someone was weeping with affliction and wonder.

But the light began to move; the sun, clear and devoid of warmth, went down toward the west, which became slightly pink, while a gray wave took shape in the east ready to roll slowly over the vast expanse. A first dog barked and its distant bark rose in the now even colder air. Janine noticed that her teeth were chattering. "We are catching our death of cold," Marcel said. "You're a fool. Let's go back." But he took her hand awkwardly. Docile now, she turned away from the parapet and followed him. Without moving, the old Arab on the stairs watched them go down toward the town. She walked along without seeing anyone, bent under a tremendous and sudden fatigue, dragging her body, whose weight now seemed to her unbearable. Her exaltation had left her. Now she felt too tall, too thick, too white too for this world she had just entered. A child, the girl, the dry man, the furtive jackal were the only creatures who could silently walk that earth. What would she do there henceforth except to drag herself toward sleep, toward death?

She dragged herself, in fact, toward the restaurant with a husband suddenly taciturn unless he was telling how tired he was, while she was struggling weakly against a cold, aware of a fever rising within her. Then she dragged herself toward her bed, where Marcel came to join her and put the light out at once without asking anything of her. The room was frigid. Janine felt the cold creeping up while the fever was increasing. She breathed with difficulty, her blood pumped without warming her; a sort of fear grew within her. She turned over and the old iron bedstead groaned under her weight. No, she didn't want to fall ill. Her husband was already asleep; it was essential. The muffled sounds of the town reached her through the window-slit. With a nasal twang old phonographs in the Moorish cafes ground out tunes she recognized vaguely; they reached her borne on the sound of a slow-moving crowd. She must sleep. But she was counting black tents; behind her eyelids motionless camels were grazing; immense solitudes were whirling within her. Yes, why had she come? She fell asleep on that question.

She awoke a little later. The silence around her was absolute. But, on the edges of town, hoarse dogs were howling in the soundless night. Janine shivered. She turned over, felt her husband's hard shoulder against hers, and suddenly, half asleep, huddled against him. She was drifting on the surface of sleep without sinking in and she clung to that shoulder with unconscious eagerness as her safest haven. She was talking, but no sound issued from her mouth. She was talking, but she herself hardly heard what she was saying. She could feel only Marcel's warmth. For more than twenty years every night thus, in his warmth, just the two of them, even when ill, even when traveling, as at present . . . Besides, what would she have done alone at home? No child! Wasn't that what she lacked? She didn't know. She simply followed Marcel, pleased to know that someone needed her. The only joy he gave her was the knowledge that she was necessary. Probably he didn't love her. Love, even, when filled with hate, doesn't have that sullen face. But what is his face like? They made love in the dark by feel, without seeing each other. Is there another love than that of darkness, a love that would cry aloud in daylight? She didn't know, but she did know that Marcel needed her and that she needed that need, that she lived on it night and day, at night especially—every night, when he didn't want to be alone, or to age to die, with that set expression he assumed which she occasionally recognized on other men's faces, the only common expression of those madmen hiding under an appearance of wisdom until the madness seizes them and hurls them desperately toward a woman's body to bury in it, without desire, everything terrifying that solitude and night reveals to them.

Marcel stirred as if to move away from her. No, he didn't love her; he was merely afraid of what was not she, and she and he should long ago have separated and slept alone until the end. But who can always sleep alone? Some men do, cut off from others by a vocation or misfortune, who go to bed every night in the same bed as death. Marcel never could do so—he above all, a weak and disarmed child always frightened by suffering, her own child indeed who needed her and who, just at that moment, let out a sort of whimper. She cuddled a little closer and put her hand on his chest. And to herself she called him with the little love-name she had once given him, which they still used from time to time without even thinking of what they were saying.

She called him with all her heart. After all, she too needed him, his strength, his little eccentricities, and she too was afraid of death. "If I could overcome that fear, I'd be happy . . ." Immediately, a nameless anguish seized her. She drew back from Marcel. No, she was overcoming nothing, she was not happy, she was going to die, in truth, without having been liberated. Her heart pained her; she was stifling under a huge weight that she suddenly discovered she had been dragging around for twenty years. Now she was struggling under it with all her strength. She wanted to be liberated even if Marcel, even if the others, never were! Fully awake, she sat up in bed and listened to a call that seemed very close. But from the edges of night the exhausted and yet indefatigable voices of the dogs of the oasis were all that reached her ears. A slight wind had risen and she heard its light waters flow in the palm grove. It came from the south, where desert and night mingled now under the again unchanging sky, where life stopped, where no one would ever age or die any more. Then the waters of the wind dried up and she was not even sure of having heard anything except a mute call that she could, after all, silence or notice. But never again would she know its meaning unless she responded to it at once. At once—yes, that much was certain at least!

She got up gently and stood motionless beside the bed, listening to her husband's breathing. Marcel was asleep. The next moment, the bed's warmth left her and the cold gripped her. She dressed slowly, feeling for her clothes in the faint light coming though the blinds from the street-lamps. Her shoes in her hand, she reached the door. She waited a moment more in the darkness, then gently opened the door. The knob squeaked and she stood still. Her heart was beating madly. She listened with her body tense and, reassured by the silence, turned her hand a little more. The knob's turning seemed to her interminable. At last she opened the door, slipped outside, and closed the door with the same stealth. Then, with her cheek against the wood, she waited. After a moment she made out, in the distance, Marcel's breathing. She faced about, felt the icy night air against her cheek, and ran the length of the balcony. The outer door was closed. While she was slipping the bolt, the night watchman appeared at the top of the stairs, his face blurred with sleep, and spoke to her in Arabic. "I'll be back," said Janine as she stepped out into the night.

Garlands of stars hung down from the black sky over the palm trees and houses. She ran along the short avenue, now empty, that led to the fort. The cold, no longer having to struggle against the sun, had invaded the night; the icy air burned her lungs. But she ran, half blind, in the darkness. At the top of the avenue, however, lights appeared, then descended toward her, zigzagging. She stopped, caught the whir of turning sprockets and, behind the enlarging lights, soon saw vast burnooses surmounting fragile bicycle wheels. The burnooses flapped against her; then three red lights sprang out of the black behind her and disappeared at once. She continued running toward the fort. Halfway up the stairs, the air burned her lungs with such cutting effect that she wanted to stop. A final burst of energy hurled her despite herself onto the terrace, against the parapet, which was now pressing her belly. She was panting and everything was hazy before her eyes. Her running had not warmed her and she was still trembling all over. But the cold air she was gulping down soon flowed evenly inside her and a spark of warmth began to glow amidst her shivers. Her eyes opened at last on the expanse of night.

Not a breath, not a sound—except at intervals the muffled crackling of stones that the cold was reducing to sand—disturbed the solitude and silence surrounding Janine. After a moment, however, it seemed to her that the sky above her was moving in a sort of slow gyration. In the vast reaches of the dry, cold night, thousands of stars were constantly appearing, and their sparkling icicles, loosened at once, began to slip gradually toward the horizon. Janine could not tear herself away from contemplating those drifting flares. She was turning with them, and the apparently stationary progress little by little identified her with the core of her being, where cold and desire were now vying with each other. Before her the stars were falling one by one and being snuffed out among the stones of the desert, and each time Janine opened a little more to the night. Breathing deeply, she forgot the cold, the dead weight of others, the craziness or stuffiness of life, the long anguish of living and dying. After so many years of mad, aimless fleeing from fear, she had come to a stop at last. At the same time, she seemed to recover her roots and the sap again rose in her body, which had ceased trembling. Her whole belly pressed against the parapet as she strained toward the moving sky; she was merely waiting for her fluttering heart to calm down and establish silence within her. The last stars of the constellations dropped their clusters a little lower on the desert horizon and became still. Then, with unbearable gentleness, the water of night began to fill Janine, drowned the cold, rose gradually from the hidden core of her being and overflowed in wave after wave, rising up even to her mouth full of moans. The next moment, the whole sky stretched out over her, fallen on her back on the cold earth.

When Janine returned to the room, with the same precautions, Marcel was not awake. But he whimpered as she got back in bed and a few seconds later sat up suddenly. He spoke and she didn't understand what he was saying. He got up, turned on the light, which blinded her. He staggered toward the washbasin and drank a long draught from the bottle of mineral water. He was about to slip between the sheets when, one knee on the bed, he looked at her without understanding. She was weeping copiously, unable to restrain herself. "It's nothing, dear," she said, "it's nothing."

Katherine Anne Porter

He

Life was very hard for the Whipples. It was hard to feed all the hungry mouths, it was hard to keep the children in flannels during the winter, short as it was. "God knows what would become of us if we lived north," they would say; keeping them decently clean was hard. "It looks like our luck won't never let up on us," said Mr. Whipple, but Mrs. Whipple was all for taking what was sent and calling it good, anyhow when the neighbors were in earshot. "Don't ever let a soul hear us complain," she kept saying to her husband. She couldn't stand to be pitied. "No, not if it comes to it that we have to live in a wagon and pick cotton around the country," she said, "nobody's going to get a chance to look down on us."

Mrs. Whipple loved her second son, the simple-minded one, better than she loved the other two children put together. She was forever saying so, and when she talked with certain of her neighbors, she would even throw in her husband and her mother for good measure.

"You needn't keep on saying that," said Mr. Whipple, "you'll make people think nobody else has any feelings about Him but . . ."

"It's natural for a mother," Mrs. Whipple would remind him. "You know yourself it's more natural for a mother to be that way. People don't expect so much of fathers, some way."

This didn't keep the neighbors from talking plainly among themselves. "A Lord's pure mercy if He should die," they said. "It's the sins of the fathers," they agreed among themselves. "There's bad blood and bad doings somewhere, you can bet on that." This behind the Whipples' back. To their faces everybody said, "He's not so bad off. He'll be all right yet. Look how He grows!"

Mrs. Whipple hated to talk about it, she tried to keep her mind off it, but every time anybody set foot in the house, the subject always came up, and she had to talk about Him first, before she could get on to anything else. It seemed to ease her mind. "I wouldn't have anything happen to Him for all the world, but it just looks like I can't keep Him out of mischief. He's so strong and active, He's always into everything; He was like that since He could walk. It's actually funny sometimes, the way He can do anything; it's laughable to see Him up to His tricks. Emly has more accidents; I'm forever tying up her bruises, and Adna can't fall a foot without cracking a bone. But He can do anything and not get a scratch. The preacher said such a nice thing once when he was here. He said, and I'll remember it to my dying day, "The innocent walk with God—that's why He don't get hurt." Whenever Mrs. Whipple repeated these words, she always felt a warm pool spread in her breast, and the tears would fill her eyes, and then she could talk about something else.

He did grow and He never got hurt. A plank blew off the chicken house and struck Him on the head and He never seemed to know it. He had learned a few words, and after this He forgot them. He didn't whine for food as the other children did, but waited until it was given Him; He ate squatting in the corner, smacking and mumbling. Rolls of fat covered Him like an overcoat, and He could carry twice as much wood and water as Adna. Emly had a cold in the head most of the time—"she takes that after me," said Mrs. Whipple—so in bad weather they gave her the extra blanket off His cot. He never seemed to mind the cold.

Just the same, Mrs. Whipple's life was a torment for fear something might happen to Him. He climbed the peach trees much better than Adna and went skittering along the branches like a monkey, just a regular monkey.

"Oh, Mrs. Whipple, you hadn't ought to let Him do that. He'll lose His balance sometime. He can't rightly know what He's doing."

Mrs. Whipple almost screamed out at the neighbor. "He does know what He's doing! He's as able as any other child! Come down out of there, you!" When He finally reached the ground she could hardly keep her hands off Him for acting like that before people, a grin all over His face and her worried sick about Him all the time.

"It's the neighbors," said Mrs. Whipple to her husband. "Oh, I do mortally wish they would keep out of our business. I can't afford to let Him do anything for fear they'll come nosing around about it. Look at the bees, now. Adna can't handle them, they sting him up so; I haven't got time to do everything, and now I don't dare let Him. But if He gets a sting He don't really mind."

"It's just because He ain't got sense enough to be scared of anything," said Mr. Whipple.

"You ought to be ashamed of yourself," said Mrs. Whipple, "talking that way about your own child. Who's to take up for Him if we don't, I'd like to know? He sees a lot that goes on, He listens to things all the time. And anything I tell Him to do He does it. Don't never let anybody hear you say such things. They'd think you favored the other children over Him."

"Well, now I don't, and you know it, and what's the use of getting all worked up about it? You always think the worst of everything. Just let Him alone, He'll get along somehow. He gets plenty to eat and wear, don't He?" Mr. Whipple suddenly felt tired out. "Anyhow, it can't be helped now."

Mrs. Whipple felt tired too, she complained in a tired voice. "What's done can't never be undone, I know that as good as anybody; but He is my child, and I'm not going to have people say anything. I get sick of people coming around saying things all the time."

In the early fall Mrs. Whipple got a letter from her brother saying he and his wife and two children were coming over for a little visit next Sunday week. "Put the big pot in the little one," he wrote at the end. Mrs. Whipple read this part out loud twice, she was so pleased. Her brother was a great one for saying funny things. "We'll just show him that's no joke," she said, "we'll just butcher one of the suckling pigs."

"It's a waste and I don't hold with waste the way we are now," said Mr. Whipple. "That pig'll be worth money by Christmas."

"It's a shame and a pity we can't have a decent meal's vittles once in a while when my own family comes to see us," said Mrs. Whipple. "I'd hate for his wife to go back and say there wasn't a thing in the house to eat. My God, it's better than buying up a great chance of meat in town. There's where you'd spend the money!"

"All right, do it yourself then," said Mr. Whipple. "Christamighty, no wonder we can't get ahead!"

The question was how to get the little pig away from his ma, a great fighter, worse than a Jersey cow. Adna wouldn't try it: "That sow'd rip my insides out all over the pen." "All right, old fraidy," said Mrs. Whipple, "He's not scared. Watch Him do it." And she laughed as though it was all a good joke and gave Him a little push towards the pen. He sneaked up and snatched the pig right away from the teat and galloped back and was over the fence with the sow raging at His heels. The little black squirming thing was screeching like a baby in a tantrum, stiffening its back and stretching its mouth to the ears. Mrs. Whipple took the pig with her face stiff and sliced its throat with one stroke. When He saw the blood He gave a great jolting breath and ran away. "But He'll forget and eat plenty, just the same," thought Mrs. Whipple. Whenever she was thinking, her lips moved making words. "He'd eat it all if I didn't stop Him. He'd eat up every mouthful from the other two if I'd let Him."

She felt badly about it. He was ten years old now and a third again as large as Adna, who was going on fourteen. "It's a shame, a shame," she kept saying under her breath, "and Adna with so much brains!"

She kept on feeling badly about all sorts of things. In the first place it was the man's work to butcher; the sight of the pig scraped pink and naked made her sick. He was too fat and soft and pitiful-looking. It was simply a shame the way things had to happen. By the time she had finished it up, she almost wished her brother would stay at home.

Early Sunday morning Mrs. Whipple dropped everything to get Him all cleaned up. In an hour He was dirty again, with crawling under fences after a possum, and straddling along the rafters of the barn looking for eggs in the hayloft. "My Lord, look at you now after all my trying! And here's Adna and Emly staying so quiet. I get tired trying to keep you decent. Get off that shirt and put on another, people will say I don't half dress you!" And she boxed Him on the ears, hard. He blinked and blinked and rubbed His head, and His face hurt Mrs. Whipple's feelings. Her knees began to tremble, she had to sit down while she buttoned His shirt. "I'm just all gone before the day starts."

The brother came with his plump healthy wife and two great roaring-hungry boys. They had a grand dinner, with the pig roasted to a crackling in the middle of the table, full of dressing, a pickled peach in his mouth and plenty of gravy for the sweet potatoes.

"This looks like prosperity all right," said the brother; "you're going to have to roll me home like I was a barrel when I'm done."

Everybody laughed out loud; it was fine to hear them laughing all at once around the table. Mrs. Whipple felt warm and good about it. "Oh, we've got six more of these; I say it's as little as we can do when you come to see us so seldom."

He wouldn't come into the dining room, and Mrs. Whipple passed it off very well. "He's timider than my other two," she said, "He'll just have to get used to you. There isn't everybody He'll make up with, you know how it is with some children, even cousins." Nobody said anything out of the way.

"Just like my Alty here," said the brother's wife. "I sometimes got to lick him to make him shake hands with his own grandmammy."

So that was over, and Mrs. Whipple loaded up a big plate for Him first, before everybody. "I always say He ain't to be slighted, no matter who else goes without," she said, and carried it to Him herself.

"He can chin Himself on the top of the door," said Emly, helping along.

"That's fine. He's getting along fine," said the brother.

They went away after supper. Mrs. Whipple rounded up the dishes, and sent the children to bed and sat down and unlaced her shoes. "You see?" she said to Mr. Whipple. "That's the way my whole family is. Nice and considerate about everything. No out-of-the-way remarks—they have got refinement. I get awfully sick of people's remarks. Wasn't that pig good?"

Mr. Whipple said, "Yes, we're out three hundred pounds of pork, that's all. It's easy to be polite when you come to eat. Who knows what they had in their minds all along?"

"Yes, that's like you," said Mrs. Whipple. "I don't expect anything else from you. You'll be telling me next that my own brother will be saying around that we made Him eat in the kitchen! Oh, my God!" She rocked her head in her hands, a hard pain started in the very middle of her forehead. "Now it's all spoiled, and everything was so nice and easy. All right, you don't like them and you never did—all right, they'll not come here again soon, never you mind! But they can't say He wasn't dressed every lick as good as Adna—oh, honest, sometimes I wish I was dead!"

"I wish you'd let up," said Mr. Whipple. "It's bad enough as it is."

It was a hard winter. It seemed to Mrs. Whipple that they hadn't ever known anything but hard times, and now to cap it all a winter like this. The crops were about half of what they had a right to expect; after the cotton was in it didn't do much more than cover the grocery bill. They swapped off one of the plow horses, and got cheated, for the new one died of the heaves. Mrs. Whipple kept thinking all the time it was terrible to have a man you couldn't depend on not to get cheated. They cut down on everything, but Mrs. Whipple kept saying there are things you can't cut down on, and they cost money. It took a lot of warm clothes for Adna and Emly, who walked four miles to school during the three-months session. "He sets around the fire a lot, He won't need so much," said Mr. Whipple. "That's so," said Mrs. Whipple, "and when He does the outdoor chores He can wear your tarpaullion coat. I can't do no better, that's all."

In February He was taken sick, and lay curled up under His blanket looking very blue in the face and acting as if He would choke. Mr. and Mrs. Whipple did everything they could for Him for two days, and then they were scared and sent for the doctor. The doctor told them they must keep Him warm and give Him plenty of milk and eggs. "He isn't as stout as He looks, I'm afraid," said the doctor. "You've got to watch them when they're like that. You must put more cover onto Him, too."

"I just took off His big blanket to wash," said Mrs. Whipple, ashamed. "1 can't stand dirt."

"Well, you'd better put it back on the minute it's dry," said the doctor, "or He'll have pneumonia."

Mr. and Mrs. Whipple took a blanket off their own bed and put His cot in by the fire. "They can't say we didn't do everything for Him," she said, "even to sleeping cold ourselves on His account."

When the winter broke He seemed to be well again, but He walked as if His feet hurt Him. He was able to run a cotton planter during the season.

"I got it all fixed up with Jim Ferguson about breeding the cow next time," said Mr. Whipple. "I'll pasture the bull this summer and give Jim some fodder in the fall. That's better than paying out money when you haven't got it."

"I hope you didn't say such a thing before Jim Ferguson," said Mrs. Whipple. "You oughtn't to let him know we're so down as all that."

"Godamighty, that ain't saying we're down. A man is got to look ahead sometimes. He can lead the bull over today. I need Adna on the place."

At first Mrs. Whipple felt easy in her mind about sending Him for the bull. Adna was too jumpy and couldn't be trusted. You've got to be steady around animals. After He was gone she started thinking, and after a while she could hardly bear it any longer. She stood in the lane and watched for Him. It was nearly three miles to go and a hot day, but He oughtn't to be so long about it. She shaded her eyes and stared until colored bubbles floated in her eyeballs. It was just like everything else in life, she must always worry and never know a moment's peace about anything. After a long time she saw Him turn into the side lane, limping. He came on very slowly leading the big hulk of an animal by a ring in the nose, twirling a little stick in His hand, never looking back or sideways, but coming on like a sleepwalker with His eyes half shut.

Mrs. Whipple was scared sick of bulls; she had heard awful stories about how they followed on quietly enough, and then suddenly pitched on with a bellow and pawed and gored a body to pieces. Any second now that black monster would come down on Him, my God, He'd never have sense enough to run.

She mustn't make a sound nor a move; she mustn't get the bull started. The bull heaved his head aside and horned the air at a fly. Her voice burst out of her in a shriek, and she screamed at Him to come on, for God's sake. He didn't seem to hear her clamor, but kept on twirling His switch and limping on, and the bull lumbered along behind him as gently as a calf. Mrs. Whipple stopped calling and ran towards the house, praying under her breath: "Lord, don't let anything happen to Him. Lord, you know people will say we oughtn't to have sent Him. You know they'll say we didn't take care of Him. Oh, get Him home, safe home, safe home, and I'll look out for Him better! Amen."

She watched from the window while He led the beast in, and tied him up in the barn. It was no use trying to keep up, Mrs. Whipple couldn't bear another thing. She sat down and rocked and cried with her apron over her head.

From year to year the Whipples were growing poorer and poorer. The place just seemed to run down of itself, no matter how hard they worked. "We're losing our hold," said Mrs. Whipple. "Why can't we do like other people and watch for our best chances? They'll be calling us poor white trash next."

"When I get to be sixteen I'm going to leave," said Adna. "I'm going to get a job in Powell's grocery store. There's money in that. No more farm for me."

"I'm going to be a schoolteacher," said Emly. "But I've got to finish the eighth grade, anyhow. Then I can live in town. I don't see any chances here."

"Emly takes after my family," said Mrs. Whipple. "Ambitious every last one of them, and they don't take second place for anybody."

When fall came Emly got a chance to wait on table in the railroad eating-house in the town near by, and it seemed such a shame not to take it when the wages were good and she could get her food too, that Mrs. Whipple decided to let her take it, and not bother with school until the next session. "You've got plenty of time," she said. "You're young and smart as a whip."

With Adna gone too, Mr. Whipple tried to run the farm with just Him to help. He seemed to get along fine, doing His work and part of Adna's without noticing it. They did well enough until Christmas time, when one morning He slipped on the ice coming up from the barn. Instead of getting up He thrashed round and round, and when Mr. Whipple got to Him, He was having some sort of fit.

They brought Him inside and tried to make Him sit up, but He blubbered and rolled, so they put Him to bed and Mr. Whipple rode to town for the doctor. All the way there and back he worried about where the money was to come from: it sure did look like he had about all the troubles he could carry.

From then on He stayed in bed. His legs swelled up double their size, and the fits kept coming back. After four months, the doctor said, "It's no use, I think you'd better put Him in the County Home for treatment right away. I'll see about it for you. He'll have good care there and be off your hands."

"We don't begrudge Him any care, and I won't let Him out of my sight," said Mrs. Whipple. "I won't have it said I sent my sick child off among strangers."

"I know how you feel," said the doctor. "You can't tell me anything about that, Mrs. Whipple. I've got a boy of my own. But you'd better listen to me. I can't do anything more for Him, that's the truth."

Mr. and Mrs. Whipple talked it over a long time that night after they went to bed. "It's just charity," said Mrs. Whipple, "that's what we've come to, charity! I certainly never looked for this."

"We pay taxes to help support the place just like everybody else," said Mr. Whipple, "and I don't call that taking charity. I think it would be fine to have Him where He'd get the best of everything, and besides, I can't keep up with these doctor bills any longer."

"Maybe that's why the doctor wants us to send Him—he's scared he won't get his money," said Mrs. Whipple.

"Don't talk like that," said Mr. Whipple, feeling pretty sick, "or we won't be able to send Him."

"Oh, but we won't keep Him there long," said Mrs. Whipple. "Soon's He's better, we'll bring Him right back home."

"The doctor has told you and told you time and again He can't ever get better, and you might as well stop talking," said Mr. Whipple.

"Doctors don't know everything," said Mrs. Whipple, feeling almost happy. "But anyhow, in the summer Emly can come home for a vacation, and Adna can get down for Sundays; we'll all work together and get on our feet again, and the children will feel they've got a place to come to."

All at once she saw it full summer again, with the garden going fine, and new white roller shades up all over the house, and Adna and Emly home, so full of life, all of them happy together. Oh, it could happen, things would ease up on them.

They didn't talk before Him much, but they never knew just how much He understood. Finally the doctor set the day and a neighbor who owned a double-seated carryall offered to drive them over. The hospital would have sent an ambulance, but Mrs. Whipple couldn't stand to see Him going away looking so sick as all that. They wrapped Him in blankets, and the neighbor and Mr. Whipple lifted Him into the back seat of the carryall beside Mrs. Whipple, who had on her black shirt waist. She couldn't stand to go looking like charity.

"You'll be all right. I guess I'll stay behind," said Mr. Whipple. "It don't look like everybody ought to leave the place at once."

"Besides, it ain't as if He was going to stay forever," said Mrs. Whipple to the neighbor. "This is only for a little while."

They started away, Mrs. Whipple holding to the edges of the blankets to keep Him from sagging sideways. He sat there blinking and blinking. He worked His hands out and began rubbing His nose with His knuckles, and then with the end of the blanket. Mrs. Whipple couldn't believe what she saw: He was scrubbing away big tears that pulled out of the corners of His eyes. He sniveled and made a gulping noise. Mrs. Whipple kept saying, "Oh, honey, you don't feel so bad, do you? You don't feel so bad, do you?" for He seemed to be accusing her of something. Maybe He remembered that time she boxed His ears, maybe He had been scared that day with the bull, maybe He had slept cold and couldn't tell her about it, maybe He knew they were sending Him away for good and all because they were too poor to keep Him. Whatever it was, Mrs. Whipple couldn't bear to think of it. She began to cry, frightfully, and wrapped her arms tight around Him. His head rolled on her shoulder; she had loved Him as much as she possibly could, there were Adna and Emly who had to be thought of too; there was nothing she could do to make up to Him for His life. Oh, what a mortal pity He was ever born.

They came in sight of the hospital, with the neighbor driving very fast, not daring to look behind him.

Nicolai Gogol

The Overcoat

In the department . . . but perhaps it is just as well not to say in which department. There is nothing more touchy and ill-tempered in the world than departments, regiments, government offices, and indeed any kind of official body. Nowadays every private individual takes a personal insult to be an insult against society at large. I am told that not so very long ago a police commissioner (I don't remember of what town) sent in a petition to the authorities in which he stated in so many words that all Government decrees had been defied and his own sacred name most decidedly taken in vain. And in proof he attached to his petition an enormous volume of some highly romantic work in which a police commissioner figured on almost every tenth page, sometimes in a very drunken state. So to avoid all sorts of unpleasant misunderstandings, we shall refer to the department in question as a certain department.

And so in a *certain department* there served a *certain Civil Servant*, a Civil Servant who cannot by any stretch of the imagination be described as in any way remarkable. He was in fact a somewhat short, somewhat pockmarked, somewhat red-haired man, who looked rather short-sighted and was slightly bald on the top of his head, with wrinkles on both cheeks, and a rather sallow complexion. There is nothing we can do about it: it is all the fault of the St. Petersburg climate. As for his rank (for with us rank is something that must be stated before anything else), he was what is known as a perpetual titular councillor, the ninth rank among the fourteen ranks into which our Civil Service is divided, a rank which, as every one knows, has been sneered at and held up to scorn by all sorts of writers who have the praiseworthy habit of setting upon those who cannot hit back. The Civil Servant's surname was Bashmachkin. From this it can be clearly inferred that it had once upon a time originated from the Russian word *bashmak*, to wit, shoe. But when, at what precise date, and under what circumstances the metamorphosis took place, must for ever remain a mystery. His father, grandfather, and, why, even his brother-in-law as well as all the rest of the Bashmachkins, always walked about in boots, having their soles repaired no more than three times a year. His name and patronymic were Akaky Akakyevich. The reader may think it a little odd; not to say somewhat *recherché*, but we can assure him that we wasted no time in searching for this name and that it happened in the most natural way that no other name could be given to him, and the way it came about is as follows:

Akaky Akakyevich was born, if my memory serves me right, on the night of 23rd March. His mother of blessed memory, the wife of a Civil Servant and a most excellent woman in every respect, took all the necessary steps for the child to be christened. She was still lying in bed, facing the door, and on her right stood the godfather, Ivan Ivanovich Yeroshkin, a most admirable man, who was a head clerk at the Supreme Court, and the godmother, Arina Semyonovna Byelobrushkina, the wife of the district police inspector, a most worthy woman. The mother was presented with the choice of three names, namely, Mokkia, Sossia, or, it was suggested, the child might be called after the martyr Khozdazat. "Oh dear," thought his late mother, "they're all such queer names!" To please her, the calendar was opened to another place, but again the three names that were found were rather uncommon, namely, Trifily, Dula and Varakhassy. "Bother," said the poor woman, "what queer names! I've really never heard such names! Now if it had only been Varadat or Varukh, but it would be Trifily and Varakhassy!" Another page was turned and the names in the calendar were Pavsikakhy and Vakhtissy. "Well," said mother, "I can see that such is the poor innocent infant's fate. If that is so, let him rather be called after his father. His father was Akaky, so let the son be Akaky, too." It was in this way that he came to be called Akaky. He was christened, and during the ceremony he began to cry and pulled such a face that it really seemed as though he had a premonition that he would be a titular councillor one day. Anyway, that is how it all came to pass.

We have told how it had come about at such length because we are anxious that the reader should realise himself it could not have happened otherwise, and that to give any other name was quite out of the question.

When and at what precise date Akaky had entered the department, and who had appointed him to it, is something no one can remember. During all the years he had served in that department many directors and other higher officials had come and gone, but he still remained in exactly the same place, in exactly the same position, in exactly the same job, doing exactly the same kind of work, to wit, copying official documents. Indeed, with time the belief came to be generally held that he must have been born into the world entirely fitted out for his job, in his Civil Servant's uniform and a bald patch on his head. No particular respect was shown him in the department. Not only did the caretakers not get up from their seats when he passed by, but they did not even vouchsafe a glance at him, just as if a common fly had flown through the waiting-room. His superiors treated him in a manner that could be best described as frigidly despotic. Some assistant head clerk would shove a paper under his nose without even saying, "Please copy it," or "Here's an interesting, amusing little case!" or something in a similarly pleasant vein as is the custom in all well-regulated official establishments. And he would accept it without raising his eyes from the paper, without looking up to see who had put it on his desk, or whether indeed he had any right to put it there. He just took it and immediately settled down to copy it. The young clerks laughed and cracked jokes about him, the sort of jokes young clerks could be expected to crack. They told stories about him in his presence, stories that were specially invented about him. They joked about his landlady, an old woman of seventy, who they claimed beat him, or they asked him when he was going to marry her. They also showered bits of torn paper on his head and called them snow. But never a word did Akaky say to it all, as though unaware of the presence of his tormentors in the office. It did not even interfere with his work; for while these rather annoying practical jokes were played on him he never made a single mistake in the document he was copying. It was only when the joke got too unbearable, when somebody jogged his arm and so interfered with his work, that he would say, "Leave me alone, gentlemen. Why do you pester me?" There was a strange note in the words and in the voice in which they were uttered: there was something in it that touched one's heart with pity. Indeed, one young man who had only recently been appointed to the department and who, following the example of the others, tried to have some fun at his expense, stopped abruptly at Akaky's mild expostulation, as though stabbed through the heart; and since then everything seemed to have changed in him and he saw everything in quite a different light. A kind of unseen power made him keep away from his colleagues whom at first he had taken for decent, well-bred men. And for a long time afterwards, in his happiest moments, he would see the shortish Civil Servant with the bald patch on his head, uttering those pathetic words, "Leave me alone! Why do you pester me?" And in those pathetic words he seemed to hear others: "I am your brother." And the poor young man used to bury his face in his hands, and many a time in his life he would shudder when he perceived how much inhumanity there was in man, how much savage brutality there lurked beneath the most refined, cultured manners, and, dear Lord, even in the man the world regarded as upright and honourable . . .

It would be hard to find a man who lived so much for his job. It was not sufficient to say that he worked zealously. No, his work was a labour of love to him. There, in that copying of his, he seemed to see a multifarious and pleasant world of his own. Enjoyment was written on his face; some letters he was particularly fond of, and whenever he had the chance of writing them, he was beside himself with joy, chuckling to himself, winking and helping them on with his lips, so that you could, it seemed, read on his face every letter his pen was forming with such care. If he had been rewarded in accordance with his zeal, he would to his own surprise have got as far as a state councillorship; but, as the office wits expressed it, all he got for his pains was a metal disc in his button-hole and a stitch in his side. Still it would be untrue to say that no one took any notice of him. One director, indeed, being a thoroughly good man and anxious to reward him for his long service, ordered that he should be given some more responsible work than his usual copying, that is to say, he was told to prepare a report for another department of an already concluded case; all he had to do was to alter the title at the top of the document and change some of the verbs from the first to the third person singular. This, however, gave him so much trouble that he was bathed in perspiration and kept mopping his forehead until at last he said, "No, I can't do it. You'd better give me something to copy." Since then they let him carry on with his copying for ever. Outside this copying nothing seemed to exist for him. He never gave a thought to his clothes: his uniform was no longer green, but of some non-descript rusty white. His collar was very short and narrow so that his neck, though it was not at all long, looked as if it stuck a mile out of the collar, like the necks of the plaster kittens with wagging heads, scores of which are carried about on their heads by street-vendors of non-Russian nationality. And something always seemed to cling to his uniform: either a straw or some thread. He possessed, besides, the peculiar knack when walking in the street of passing under a window just at the time when some rubbish was tipped out of it, and for this reason he always carried about on his hat bits of water-melon or melon rind and similar trash. He had never in his life paid the slightest attention to what was going on daily in the street, and in this he was quite unlike his young colleagues in the Civil Service, who are famous as observers of street life, their eagle-eyed curiosity going even so far as to notice that the strap under the trousers of some man on the pavement on the other side of the street has come undone, a thing which never fails to bring a malicious grin to their faces. But even if Akaky did look at anything, he saw nothing but his own neat lines, written out in an even hand, and only if a horse's muzzle, appearing from goodness knows where, came to rest on his shoulder and blew a gale on his cheek from its nostrils, did he become aware of the fact that he was not in the middle of a line, but rather in the middle of the street.

On his arrival home, he would at once sit down at the table, quickly gulp down his cabbage soup, eat a piece of beef with onions without noticing what it tasted like, eating whatever Providence happened to send at the time, flies and all. Noticing that his stomach was beginning to feel full, he would get up from the table, fetch his inkwell and start copying the papers he had brought home with him. If, however, there were no more papers to copy, he would deliberately make another copy for his own pleasure, intending to keep it for himself, especially if the paper was remarkable not so much for the beauty of its style as for the fact of being addressed to some new or important person.

Even at those hours when all the light has faded from the grey St. Petersburg sky, and the Civil Service folk have taken their fill of food and dined each as best he could, according to his salary and his personal taste; when all have had their rest after the departmental scraping of pens, after all the rush and bustle, after their own and other people's indispensable business had been brought to a conclusion and anything else restless man imposes upon himself of his own free will had been done, and even much more than is necessary; when every Civil Servant is hastening to enjoy as best he can the remaining hours of his leisure—one more enterprising rushing off to the theatre, another going for a stroll to stare at some silly women's hats, a third going to a party to waste his time paying compliments to some pretty girl, the star of some small Civil Service circle, while a fourth—as happens in nine cases out of ten—paying a call on a fellow Civil Servant living on the third or fourth floor in a flat of two small rooms with a tiny hall or kitchen with some pretensions to fashion—a lamp or some other article that has cost many self-denying sacrifices, such as doing without dinners or country outings; in short, even when all the Civil Servants have dispersed among the tiny flats of their friends to play a stormy game of whist, sipping tea from glasses and nibbling a penny biscuit, or inhaling the smoke of their long pipes and, while dealing the cards, retelling the latest high society scandal (for every Russian is so devotedly attached to high society that he cannot dispense with it for a moment), or, when there is nothing else to talk about, telling the old chestnut about the fortress commandant who was told that the tail of the horse of Falconnetti's statue of Peter I had been docked—in short, even while every government official in the capital was doing his best to enjoy himself, Akaky Akakyevich made no attempt to woo the fair goddess of mirth and jollity. No one could possibly ever claim to have seen him at a party. Having copied out documents to his heart's content, he went to bed, smiling in anticipation of the pleasures the next day had in store for him and wondering what the good Lord would send him to copy. So passed the peaceful life of a man who knew how to be content with his lot on a salary of four hundred roubles a year; and it might have flowed on as happily to a ripe old age, were it not for the various calamities which beset the lives not only of titular, but also of privy, actual, court and any other councillors, even those who give no counsel to any man, nor take any from anyone, either.

There is in St. Petersburg a great enemy of all those who receive a salary of four hundred roubles a year, or thereabouts. This enemy is none other than our northern frost, though you will hear people say that it is very good for the health. At nine o'clock in the morning, just at the hour when the streets are full of Civil Servants on their way to their departments, he starts giving such mighty and stinging filips to all noses without exception, that the poor fellows simply do not know where to put them. At a time when the foreheads of even those who occupy the highest positions in the State ache with the frost, and tears start to their eyes, the poor titular councillors are sometimes left utterly defenseless. Their only salvation lies in running as fast as they can in their thin, threadbare overcoats through five or six streets and then stamping their feet vigorously in the vestibule, until they succeed in unfreezing their faculties and abilities, frozen on the way, and are once more able to tackle the affairs of State.

Akaky had for some time been feeling that the fierce cold seemed to have no difficulty at all in penetrating to his back and shoulders, however fast he tried to sprint across the legal distance from his home to the department. It occurred to him at length that his overcoat might not be entirely blameless for this state of affairs. On examining it thoroughly at home, he discovered that in two or three places, to wit, on the back and round the shoulders, it looked like some coarse homespun cotton; the cloth had worn out so much that it let through the wind, and the lining had all gone to pieces. It must be mentioned here that Akaky's overcoat, too, had been the butt of the departmental wits; it had been even deprived of the honourable name of overcoat and had been called a *capote*. And indeed it was of a most peculiar cut: its collar had shrunk in size more and more every year, for it was used to patch the other parts. The patching did no credit to the tailor's art and the result was that the final effect was somewhat baggy and far from beautiful. Having discovered what was wrong with his overcoat, Akaky decided that he would have to take it to Petrovich, a tailor who lived somewhere on the fourth floor up some backstairs and who, in spite of the disadvantage of having only one eye and pock marks all over his face, carried on a rather successful trade in mending the trousers and frock-coats of government clerks and other gentlemen whenever, that is to say, he was sober and was not hatching some other scheme in his head.

We really ought not to waste much time over this tailor; since, however, it is now the fashion that the character of every person in a story must be delineated fully, then by all means let us have Petrovich, too. To begin with, he was known simply by his Christian name of Grigory, and had been a serf belonging to some gentleman or other; he began calling himself Petrovich only after he had obtained his freedom, when he started drinking rather heavily every holiday, at first only on the great holidays, and thereafter on any church holiday, on any day, in fact, marked with a cross in the calendar. So far as that went, he was true to the traditions of his forebears and in his altercations with his wife on this subject he would call her a worldly woman and a German. Having mentioned his wife, we had better say a word or two about her also; to our great regret, however, we know very little about her, except that Petrovich had a wife, who wore a bonnet, and not a kerchief; there appears to be some doubt as to whether she was good-looking or not, but on the whole it does not seem likely that she had very much to boast of in that respect; at any rate, only guardsmen were ever known to peer under her bonnet when meeting her in the street, twitching their moustaches and emitting a curious kind of grunt at the same time.

While ascending the stairs leading to Petrovich's flat—the stairs which, to do them justice, were soaked with water and slops and saturated with a strong spirituous smell which irritates the eyes and which, as the whole world knows, is a permanent feature of all the back stairs of St. Petersburg houses—while ascending the stairs, Akaky was already wondering how much Petrovich would ask for mending his overcoat, and made up his mind not to give him more than two roubles. The door of Petrovich's flat was open because his wife had been frying some fish and had filled the whole kitchen with smoke, so that even the cockroaches could no longer be seen. Akaky walked through the kitchen, unnoticed even by Mrs. Petrovich, and, at last, entered the tailor's room where he beheld Petrovich sitting on a large table of unstained wood with his legs crossed under him like a Turkish pasha. His feet, as is the custom of tailors when engaged in their work, were bare. The first thing that caught his eye was Petrovich's big toe, which Akaky knew very well indeed, with its deformed nail as thick and hard as the shell of a tortoise. A skein of silk and cotton thread hung about Petrovich's neck, and on his knees lay some tattered piece of clothing. He had for the last minute or two been trying to thread his needle and, failing every time, he was terribly angry with the dark room and even with the thread itself, muttering under his breath, "Won't you go through, you beast? You'll be the death of me yet, you slut!" Akaky could not help feeling sorry that he had come just at the moment when Petrovich was angry: he liked to place an order with Petrovich only when the tailor was a bit merry, or when he had, as his wife put it, "been swilling his corn-brandy, the one-eyed devil!" When in such a state, Petrovich was as a rule extremely amenable and always gave in and agreed to any price, and even bowed and thanked him. It was true that afterwards his wife would come to see Akaky and tell him with tears in her eyes that her husband had been drunk and had therefore charged him too little; but all Akaky had to do was to add another ten-copeck piece and the thing was settled. But now Petrovich was to all appearances sober as a judge and, consequently, rather bad-tempered, intractable and liable to charge any old price. Akaky realised that and was about, as the saying is, to beat a hasty retreat, but it was too late: Petrovich had already screwed up his only eye and was looking at him steadily. Akaky had willy-nilly to say, "Good morning, Petrovich!" "Good morning, sir. How are you?" said Petrovich, fixing his eye on Akaky's hands in an effort to make out what kind of offering he had brought.

"Well, you see, Petrovich, I—er—have come—er—about that, you know . . ." said Akaky.

It might be as well to explain at once that Akaky mostly talked in prepositions, adverbs, and, lastly, such parts of speech as have no meaning whatsoever. If the matter was rather difficult, he was in the habit of not finishing the sentences, so that often having begun his speech with, "This is—er—you know . . . a bit of that, you know . . ." he left it at that, forgetting to finish the sentence in the belief that he had said all that was necessary.

"What's that you've got there, sir?" said Petrovich, scrutinising at the same time the whole of Akaky's uniform with his one eye, from the collar to the sleeves, back, tails and button-holes, which was all extremely familiar to him, since it was his own handiwork. Such is the immemorial custom among tailors; it is the first thing a tailor does when he meets one of his customers.

"Well, you see, Petrovich, I've come about this here, you know . . . this overcoat of mine. The cloth, you know . . . You see, it's really all right everywhere, in fact, excellent. . . . I mean, it's in fine condition here and—er—all over. Looks a bit dusty, I know, and you might get the impression that it was old, but as a matter of fact it's as good as new, except in one place where it's a bit—er—a bit, you know . . . On the back, I mean, and here on the shoulder . . . Looks as though it was worn through a bit, and on the other shoulder too, just a trifle, you see . . . Well, that's really all. Not much work in it . . ."

Petrovich took the *capote*, first spread it on the table, examined it for a long time, shook his head, and stretched out his hand to the window for his round snuff-box with a portrait of some general, though which particular general it was impossible to say, for the place where the face should have been had been poked in by a finger and then pasted over with a square bit of paper. Having treated himself to a pinch of snuff, Petrovich held the overcoat out in his hands against the light and gave it another thorough examination, and again shook his head; he then turned it with the lining upwards and again shook his head, again took off the lid with the general pasted over with paper, and, filling his nose with snuff, replaced the lid, put away the snuff-box and, at last, said, "No, sir. Impossible to mend it. There's nothing left of it."

Akaky's heart sank at those words. "Why is it impossible, Petrovich?" he said, almost in the imploring voice of a child. "It's only on the shoulders that it's a bit worn, and I suppose you must have bits of cloth somewhere . . ."

"Oh, I've got plenty of bits of cloth, sir, lots of 'em," said Petrovich. "But you see, sir, you can't sew 'em on. The whole coat's rotten. Touch it with a needle and it will fall to pieces."

"Well, if it falls to pieces, all you have to do is to patch it up again."

"Why, bless my soul, sir, and what do you suppose the patches will hold on to? What am I to sew them on to? Can't you see, sir, how badly worn it is? You can't call it cloth any more: one puff of wind and it will be blown away."

"But please strengthen it a bit. I mean, it can't be just—er—really, you know . . ."

"No, sir," said Petrovich firmly, "it can't be done. Too far gone. Nothing to hold it together. All I can advise you to do with it, sir, is to cut it up when winter comes and make some rags to wrap round your feet, for socks, sir, are no damned good at all: there's no real warmth in 'em. It's them Germans, sir, what invented socks to make a lot of money (Petrovich liked to get in a word against the Germans on every occasion). As for your overcoat, sir, I'm afraid you'll have to get a new one."

At the word "new" a mist suddenly spread before Akaky's eyes and everything in the room began swaying giddily. The only thing he could still see clearly was the general's face pasted over with paper on the lid of Petrovich's snuff-box.

"How do you mean, a new one?" he said, still as though speaking in a dream, "Why, I haven't got the money for it."

"Well. sir, all I can say is that you just must get yourself a new one," said Petrovich with callous indifference,

"Well, and if . . . I mean, if I had to get a new one . . . how much, I mean . . ."

"How much will it come to, sir?"

"Yes."

"Well, sir, I suppose you'll have to layout three fifty-rouble notes or more," said Petrovich, pursing his lips significantly.

He had a great fondness for strong effects, Petrovich had. He liked to hit a fellow on the head suddenly and then steal a glance at him to see what kind of a face the stunned person would pull after his words.

"One hundred and fifty roubles for an overcoat!" cried poor Akaky in a loud voice, probably raising his voice to such a pitch for the first time in his life, for he was always distinguished by the softness of his voice.

"Yes, sir," said Petrovich, "And that, too, depends on the kind of coat you have. If you have marten for your collar and a silk lining for your hood, it might cost you two hundred."

"Now look here, Petrovich . . ." said Akaky in a beseeching voice, not hearing, or at any rate doing his best not to hear, what Petrovich was saying, and paying no attention whatever to the effect the tailor was trying to create. "Please, my dear fellow, just mend it somehow, so that I could still use it a bit longer, you know . . ."

"No, sir, it will merely mean a waste of my work and your money," said Petrovich.

After such a verdict Akaky left Petrovich's room feeling completely crushed, while the tailor remained in the same position a long time after he had gone, without going back to his work, his lips pursed significantly. He was greatly pleased that he had neither demeaned himself nor let down the sartorial art.

In the street Akaky felt as though he were in a dream. "So that's how it stands, is it?" he murmured to himself. "I really didn't think that it would turn out like that, you know . . ." Then after a pause he added, "Well, that's that. There's a real surprise for you. . . . I never thought that it would end like that . . ." There followed another long pause, after which he said, "So that's how it is! What a sudden . . . I mean, what a terrible blow! Who could have . . . What an awful business!"

Having delivered himself thus, he walked on, without noticing it, in quite the opposite direction from his home. On the way a chimney-sweep brushed the whole of his sooty side against him and blackened his shoulder; from the top of a house that was being built a whole handful of lime fell upon him. But he was aware of nothing, and only when some time later he knocked against a policeman who, placing his halberd near him, was scattering some snuff from a horn on a calloused fist, did he recover a little, and that, too, only because the policeman said, "Now then, what are you pushing against me for? Can't you see where you're going? Ain't the pavement big enough for you?" This made him look up and retrace his steps.

But it was not until he had returned home that he began to collect his thoughts and saw his position as it really was. He began discussing the matter with himself, not in broken sentences, but frankly and soberly, as though talking to a wise friend with whom it was possible to discuss one's most intimate affairs.

"No, no," said Akaky, "it's pretty clear that it is impossible to talk to Petrovich now. He's a bit, you know . . . Been thrashed by his wife, I shouldn't wonder. I'd better go and see him next Sunday morning, for after all the drink he'll have had on Saturday night he'll still be screwing up his one eye, and he'll be very sleepy and dying for another drink to help him on his feet again, and his wife won't give him any money, so that if I come along and give him ten copecks or a little more he'll be more reasonable and change his mind about the overcoat, and then, you know . . ."

So Akaky reasoned with himself, and he felt greatly reassured.

Sunday came at last and, noticing from a distance that Petrovich's wife had left the house to go somewhere, he went straight in. To be sure, Petrovich did glower after his Saturday night's libations, and he could barely hold up his head, which seemed to be gravitating towards the floor, and he certainly looked very sleepy; and yet, in spite of this condition, no sooner did he hear what Akaky had come for than it seemed as if the devil himself had nudged him.

"Quite impossible, sir," he said. "You'll have to order a new one." Akaky immediately slipped a ten-copeck piece into his hand. "Thank you very much, sir," said Petrovich. "Very kind of you, I'm sure. I'll get a bit o' strength in me body and drink to your health, sir. But if I were you, sir, I'd stop worrying about that overcoat of yours. No good at all. Can't do nothing with it. Mind, I can promise you one thing, though: I'll make you a lovely new overcoat. That I will, sir."

Akaky tried to say something about mending the old one, but Petrovich would not even listen to him and said, "Depend upon it, sir, I'll make you a new one. Do my best for you, I will, sir. Might even while we're about it, sir, and seeing as how it's now the fashion, get a silver-plated clasp for the collar."

It was then that Akaky at last realised that he would have to get a new overcoat, and his heart failed him. And how indeed was he to do it? What with? Where was he to get the money? There was of course the additional holiday pay he could count on; at least there was a good chance of his getting that holiday bonus. But supposing he did get it, all that money had already been divided up and disposed of long ago. There was that new pair of trousers he must get; then there was that long-standing debt he owed the shoe-maker for putting new tops to some old boots; he had, moreover, to order three shirts from the sempstress as well as two pairs of that particular article of underwear which cannot be decently mentioned in print—in short, all the money would have to be spent to the last penny, and even if the director of the department were to be so kind as to give him a holiday bonus of forty-five or even fifty roubles instead of forty, all that would remain of it would be the veriest trifle, which in terms of overcoat finance would be just a drop in the ocean. Though he knew perfectly well, of course, that Petrovich was sometimes mad enough to ask so utterly preposterous a price that even his wife could not refrain from exclaiming, "Gone off his head completely, the silly old fool! One day he accepts work for next to nothing, and now the devil must have made him ask more than he is worth himself!"—though he knew perfectly well, of course, that Petrovich would undertake to make him the overcoat for eighty roubles, the question still remained: where was he to get the eighty roubles? At a pinch he could raise half of it. Yes, he could find half of it all right and perhaps even a little more, but where was he to get the other half? . . .

But first of all the reader had better be told where Akaky hoped to be able to raise the first half.

Akaky was in the habit of putting away a little from every rouble he spent in a box which he kept locked up and which had a little hole in the lid through which money could be dropped. At the end of every six months he counted up the accumulated coppers and changed them into silver. As he had been saving up for a long time, there had accumulated in the course of several years a sum of over forty roubles. So he had half of the required sum in hand; but where was he to get the other half? Where was he to get another forty roubles?

Akaky thought and thought and then he decided that he would have to cut down his ordinary expenses for a year at least: do without a cup of tea in the evenings; stop burning candles in the evening and, if he had some work to do, go to his landlady's room and work by the light of her candle; when walking in the street, try to walk as lightly as possible on the cobbles and flagstones, almost on tiptoe, so as not to wear out the soles of his boots too soon; give his washing to the laundress as seldom as possible, and to make sure that it did not wear out, to take it off as soon as he returned home and wear only his dressing-gown of twilled cotton cloth, a very old garment that time itself had spared. To tell the truth, Akaky at first found it very hard to get used to such economy, but after some time he got used to it all right and everything went with a swing; he did not even mind going hungry in the evenings, for spiritually he was nourished well enough, since his thoughts were full of the great idea of his future overcoat. His whole existence indeed seemed now somehow to have become fuller, as though he had got married, as though there was someone at his side, as though he was never alone, but some agreeable helpmate had consented to share the joys and sorrows of his life, and this sweet helpmate, this dear wife of his, was no other than the selfsame overcoat with its thick padding of cotton-wool and its strong lining that would last a lifetime. He became more cheerful and his character even got a little firmer, like that of a man who knew what he was aiming at and how to achieve that aim. Doubt vanished, as though of its own accord, from his face and from his actions, and so did indecision and, in fact, all the indeterminate and shilly-shallying traits of his character. Sometimes a gleam would appear in his eyes and through his head there would flash the most bold and audacious thought, to wit, whether he should not after all get himself a fur collar of marten. All these thoughts about his new overcoat nearly took his mind off his work at the office, so much so that once, as he was copying out a document, he was just about to make a mistake, and he almost cried out, "Oh dear!" in a loud voice, and crossed himself. He went to see Petrovich at least once a month to discuss his overcoat, where it was best to buy the cloth, and what colour and at what price, and though looking a little worried, he always came back home well satisfied, reflecting that the time was not far off when he would pay for it all and when his overcoat would be ready.

As a matter of fact the whole thing came to pass much quicker than he dreamed. Contrary to all expectations, the director gave Akaky Akakyevich not forty or forty-five, but sixty roubles! Yes, a holiday bonus of sixty roubles. Whether he, too, had been aware that Akaky wanted a new overcoat, or whether it happened by sheer accident, the fact remained that Akaky had an additional twenty roubles. This speeded up the whole course of events. Another two or three months of a life on short commons and Akaky had actually saved up about eighty roubles. His pulse, generally sluggish, began beating fast. The very next day he went with Petrovich to the shops. They bought an excellent piece of cloth, and no wonder! For the matter had been carefully discussed and thought over for almost six months, and scarcely a month had passed without enquiries being made at the shops about prices, so as to make quite sure that the cloth they needed was not too expensive; and the result of all that foresight was that, as Petrovich himself admitted, they could not have got a better cloth. For the lining they chose calico, but of such fine and strong quality that, according to Petrovich, it was much better than silk and was actually much more handsome and glossy. They did not buy marten for a fur collar, for as a matter of fact it was rather expensive, but they chose cat fur instead, the best cat they could find in the shop, cat which from a distance could almost be mistaken for marten. Petrovich took only two weeks over the overcoat, and that, too, because there was so much quilting to be done; otherwise it would have been ready earlier. For his work Petrovich took twelve roubles—less than that was quite out of the question: he had used nothing but silk thread in the sewing of it, and it was sewn with fine, double seams, and Petrovich had gone over each seam with his own teeth afterwards, leaving all sorts of marks on them.

It was . . . It is hard to say on what day precisely it was, but there could be no doubt at all that the day on which Petrovich at last delivered the overcoat was one of the greatest days in Akaky's life. He brought it rather early in the morning, just a short time before Akaky had to leave for the department. At no other time would the overcoat have been so welcome, for the time of rather sharp frosts had just begun, and from all appearances it looked as if the severity of the weather would increase. Petrovich walked in with the overcoat as a good tailor should. His face wore an expression of solemn gravity such as Akaky had never seen on it before. He seemed to be fully conscious of the fact that he had accomplished no mean thing and that he had shown by his own example the gulf that separated the tailors who merely relined a coat or did repairs from those who made new coats. He took the overcoat out of the large handkerchief in which he had brought it. (The handkerchief had just come from the laundress; it was only now that he folded it and put it in his pocket for use.) Having taken out the overcoat, he looked very proudly about him and, holding it in both hands, threw it very smartly over Akaky's shoulders, then he gave it a vigorous pull and, bending down, smoothed it out behind with his hand; then he draped it round Akaky, throwing it open in front a little. Akaky, who was no longer a young man, wanted to try it on with his arms in the sleeves, and Petrovich helped him to put his hands through the sleeves, and—it was all right even when he wore it with his arms in the sleeves. In fact, there could be no doubt at all that the overcoat was a perfect fit. Petrovich did not let this opportunity pass without observing that it was only because he lived in a back street and had no signboard and because he had known Akaky Akakyevich so long that he had charged him so little for making the overcoat. If he had ordered it on Nevsky Avenue, they would have charged him seventy-five roubles for the work alone. Akaky had no desire to discuss the matter with Petrovich and, to tell the truth, he was a little frightened of the big sums which Petrovich was so fond of tossing about with the idea of impressing people. He paid him, thanked him, and left immediately for the department in his new overcoat. Petrovich followed him into the street where he remained standing a long time on one spot, admiring his handiwork from a distance; then he purposely went out of his way so that he could by taking a short-cut by a side street rush out into the street again and have another look at the overcoat, this time from the other side, that is to say, from the front.

Meanwhile Akaky went along as if walking on air. Not for a fraction of a second did he forget that he had a new overcoat on his back, and he could not help smiling to himself from time to time with sheer pleasure at the thought of it. And really it had two advantages: one that it was warm, and the other that it was good. He did not notice the distance and found himself suddenly in the department. He took off the overcoat in the hall, examined it carefully and entrusted it to the special care of the door-keeper. It is not known how the news of Akaky's new overcoat had spread all over the department, but all at once every one knew that Akaky had discarded his *capote* and had a fine new overcoat. They all immediately rushed out into the hall to have a look at Akaky's new overcoat. Congratulations and good wishes were showered upon him. At first Akaky just smiled, then he felt rather embarrassed. But when all surrounded him and began telling him that he ought to celebrate his acquisition of a new overcoat and that the least he could do was to invite them all to a party, Akaky Akakyevich was thrown into utter confusion and did not know what to do, what to say to them all; or how to extricate himself from that very awkward situation. He even tried a few minutes later with the utmost good humour to assure them, blushing to the roots of his hair, that it was not a new overcoat at all, that it was just . . . well, you know . . . just his old overcoat. At last one of the clerks, and, mind, not just any clerk, but no less a person than the assistant head clerk of the office, wishing to show no doubt that he, for one, was not a proud man and did not shun men more humble than himself, said, "So be it! I will give a party instead of Akaky Akakyevich. I invite you all, gentlemen, this evening to tea at my place. As a matter of fact, it happens to be my birthday." The Civil Servants naturally wished him many happy returns of the day and accepted his invitation with alacrity. Akaky tried at first to excuse himself, but everybody told him that it was not done and that he ought to be ashamed of himself, and he just could not wriggle out of it. However, he felt rather pleased afterwards, for it occurred to him that this would give him a chance of taking a walk in the evening in his new overcoat.

That day was to Akaky like a great festival. He came home in a most happy frame of mind, took off his overcoat, hung it with great care on the wall, stood for some time admiring the cloth and lining, and then produced his old overcoat, which had by then gone to pieces completely, just to compare the two. He looked at it and could not help chuckling out loud: what a difference! And he kept smiling to himself all during dinner when he thought of the disgraceful state of his old overcoat. He enjoyed his dinner immensely and did no copying at all afterwards, not one document did he copy, but just indulged himself a little by lying down on his bed until dusk. Then, without dawdling unnecessarily, he dressed, threw the overcoat over his shoulders, and went out into the street.

Unfortunately we cannot say where precisely the Civil Servant who was giving the party lived. Our memory is beginning to fail us rather badly and everything in St. Petersburg, all the streets and houses, has become so blurred and mixed up in our head that we find it very difficult indeed to sort it out properly. Be that as it may, there can be no doubt that the Civil Servant in question lived in one of the best parts of the town, which means of course that he did not live anywhere near Akaky Akakyevich. At first Akaky had to pass through some deserted streets, very poorly lighted, but as he got nearer to the Civil Servant's home the streets became more crowded and more brilliantly illuminated. There certainly were more people in the streets, the women were well dressed and the men even wore beaver collars. There were fewer poor peasant cabmen with their crate-like wooden sledges studded with brass nails; on the contrary, the cabmen were mostly fine fellows in crimson velvet caps with lacquered sledges and bearskin covers, and carriages with sumptuously decorated boxes drove at a great speed through the streets, their wheels crunching on the snow.

Akaky looked at it all as though he had never seen anything like it in his life, and indeed he had not left his room in the evening for several years. He stopped before a lighted shop window and for some minutes looked entranced at a painting of a beautiful woman who was taking off a shoe and showing a bare leg, a very shapely leg, too; and behind her back a gentleman had stuck his head through the door of another room, a gentleman with fine side-whiskers and a handsome imperial on his chin. Akaky shook his head and grinned, and then went on his way. Why did he grin? It might have been because he had seen something he had never seen before, but a liking for which is buried deep down inside every one of us, or because (like many another Civil Servant) he thought to himself, "Oh, those damned Frenchmen! What a people they are, to be sure! If they set their heart on something, something . . . well, something of that kind, you know, then it is something . . . well, something of that kind . . ." But perhaps he never even said anything at all to himself. How indeed is one to delve into a man's mind and find out what he is thinking about? At last he reached the house where the young assistant head clerk of his office lived.

The assistant head clerk lived in great style: there was a lamp burning on the stairs, and his flat was on the second floor. As he entered the hall, Akaky saw on the floor rows upon rows of galoshes. Among them in the middle of the room stood a *samovar*, hissing and letting off clouds of steam. The walls were covered with overcoats and cloaks, some even with beaver collars and velvet revers. A confused buzz of conversation came from the other side of the wall, and it grew very clear and loud when the door opened and a footman came out with a trayful of empty tea-glasses, a jug of cream and a basket of biscuits. It was evident that the Civil Servants had been there for some time and had already finished their first glass of tea.

After hanging up his overcoat himsef, Akaky entered the room, and there flashed upon his sight simultaneously candles, Civil Servants, pipes, card-tables, while his ears were filled with the confused sound of continuous conversation, which came from every corner of the room, and the noise of moving chairs. He stood in the middle of the room, looking rather forlorn and trying desperately to think what he ought to do. But his presence had already been noticed and he was welcomed with loud shouts, and everybody immediately went into the hall to inspect his overcoat anew. Though feeling rather embarrassed at first, Akaky, being of a singularly ingenuous nature, could not help being pleased to hear how everybody praised his overcoat. Then, of course, they forgot all about him and his overcoat and crowded, as was to be expected, round the card-tables set out for whist.

All this—the noise, the talk, and the crowd of people—was very strange and bewildering to Akaky. He simply did not know what to do, where to put his hands and feet, or his whole body; at length he sat down by the card players, looked at the cards, studied the face of one player, then of another, and after a little time began to feel bored and started yawning, particularly as it was getting late and it was long past his bedtime. He tried to take leave of his host, but they would not let him go, saying that they had to drink a glass of champagne in honour of his new overcoat. In about an hour supper was served. It consisted of a mixed salad, cold veal, meat pie, cream pastries and champagne. They made Akaky drink two glasses of champagne, after which he felt that everything got much jollier in the room. However, he could not forget that it was already midnight and that it was high time he went home. To make sure that his host would not detain him on one pretext or another, he stole out of the room and found his overcoat in the hall. The overcoat, he noticed not without a pang of regret, was lying on the floor. He picked it up, shook it, removed every speck of dust from it and, putting it over his shoulders, went down the stairs into the street.

It was still light in the street. A few small grocers' shops, those round-the-clock clubs of all sorts of servants, were still open; from those which were already closed a streak of light still streamed through the crack under the door, showing that there was still some company there, consisting most probably of maids and men-servants who were finishing their talk and gossip, leaving their masters completely at a loss to know where they were. Akaky walked along feeling very happy and even set off running after some lady (goodness knows why) who passed him like a streak of lightning, every part of her body in violent motion. However, he stopped almost at once and went on at a slow pace as before, marvelling himself where that unusual spurt of speed had come from. Soon he came to those never-ending, deserted streets, which even in daytime are not particularly cheerful, let alone at night. Now they looked even more deserted and lonely; there were fewer street lamps and even those he came across were extinguished; the municipal authorities seemed to be sparing of oil. He now came into the district of wooden houses and fences; there was not a soul to be seen anywhere, only the snow gleamed on the streets, and hundreds of dismal, low hovels with closed shutters which seemed to have sunk into a deep sleep, stretched in a long, dark line before him. Soon he approached the spot where the street was intersected by an immense square with houses dimly visible on the other side, a square that looked to him like a dreadful desert.

A long way away—goodness knows where—he could see the glimmer of a light coming from some sentry-box, which seemed to be standing at the edge of the world. Akaky's cheerfulness faded perceptibly as he entered the square. He entered it not without a kind of involuntary sensation of dread, as though feeling in his bones that something untoward was going to happen. He looked back, and then cast a glance at either side of him; it was just as though the sea were all round him. "Much better not to look," he thought to himself, and, shutting his eyes, he walked on, opening them only to have a look how far the end of the square was. But what he saw was a couple of men standing right in front of him, men with moustaches, but what they were he could not make out in the darkness. He felt dazed and his heart began beating violently against his ribs. "Look, here is my overcoat!" one of the men said in a voice of thunder, grabbing him by the collar. Akaky was about to scream, "Help!" but the other man shook his fist in his face, a fist as big as a Civil Servant's head, and said, "You just give a squeak!" All poor Akaky knew was that they took off his overcoat and gave him a kick which sent him sprawling on the snow. He felt nothing at all any more. A few minutes later he recovered sufficiently to get up, but there was not a soul to be seen anywhere. He felt that it was terribly cold in the square and that his overcoat had gone. He began to shout for help, but his voice seemed to be too weak to carry to the end of the square. Feeling desperate and without ceasing to shout, he ran across the square straight to the sentry-box beside which stood a policeman who, leaning on his halberd, seemed to watch the running figure with mild interest, wondering no doubt why the devil a man was running towards him, screaming his head off while still a mile away. Having run up to the police constable, Akaky started shouting at him in a gasping voice that he was asleep and did not even notice that a man had been robbed under his very nose. The policeman said that he saw nothing, or rather that all he did see was that two men had stopped him (Akaky) in the middle of the square, but he supposed that they were his friends; and he advised Akaky, instead of standing there and abusing him for nothing, to go and see the police inspector next morning, for the inspector was quite sure to find the men who had taken his overcoat.

Akaky Akakyevich came running home in a state of utter confusion. His hair, which still grew, though sparsely, over his temples and at the back of his head, was terribly tousled; his chest, arms and trousers were covered with snow. His old landlady, awakened by the loud knocking at the door, jumped hurriedly out of bed and with only one slipper on ran to open the door, modestly clasping her chemise to her bosom with one hand. When she opened the door and saw the terrible state Akaky was in, she fell back with a gasp. He told her what had happened to him, and she threw up her arms in dismay and said that he ought to go straight to the district police commissioner, for the police inspector was quite sure to swindle him, promise him all sorts of things and then leave him in the lurch; it would be much better if he went to the district police commissioner who, it seemed, was known to her, for Anna, the Finnish girl who was once her cook, was now employed by the district commissioner of police as a nurse, and, besides, she had seen him often as he drove past the house, and he even went to church every Sunday and always, while saying his prayers, looked round at everybody very cheerfully, so that, judging from all appearances, he must be a kind-hearted man.

Having listened to that piece of advice, Akaky wandered off sadly to his room, and how he spent that night we leave it to those to judge who can enter into the position of another man. Early next morning he went to see the district police commissioner, but they told him that he was still asleep. He came back at ten o'clock and again they said he was asleep. He came back at eleven o'clock and was told that the police commissioner was not at home. He came back at lunch-time, but the clerks in the waiting-room would not admit him on any account unless he told them first what he had come for and what it was all about and what had happened. So that in the end Akaky felt for the first time in his life that he had to assert himself and he told them bluntly that he had come to see the district commissioner of police personally, that they had no right to refuse to admit him, that he had come from the department on official business, and that if he lodged a complaint against them, they would see what would happen. The clerks dared say nothing to this and one of them went to summon the commissioner.

The police commissioner took rather a curious view of Akaky's story of the loss of his overcoat. Instead of concentrating on the main point of the affair, he began putting all sorts of questions to Akaky which had nothing to do with it, such as why he was coming home so late, and was he sure he had not been to any disorderly house the night before, so that Akaky felt terribly embarrassed and went away wondering whether the police were ever likely to take the necessary steps to retrieve his overcoat.

That day (for the first time in his life) he did not go to the department. Next day he appeared looking very pale and wearing his old *capote*, which was in a worse state than ever. Many of his colleagues seemed moved by the news of the robbery of his overcoat, though there were a few among them who could not help pulling poor Akaky's leg even on so sad an occasion. It was decided to make a special collection for Akaky, but they only succeeded in collecting a trifling sum, for the clerks in his office had already spent a great deal on subscribing to a fund for a portrait of the director and also on some kind of a book, at the suggestion of one of the departmental chiefs, who was a friend of the author. Anyway, the sum collected was a trifling one. One Civil Servant, however, moved by compassion, decided to help Akaky with some good advice at any rate, and he told him that he should not go to the district police inspector, for though it might well happen that the district police inspector, anxious to win the approbation of his superiors, would somehow or other find his overcoat, Akaky would never be able to get it out of the police station unless he could present all the necessary legal proofs that the overcoat belonged to him. It would therefore be much better if Akaky went straight to a certain Very Important Person, for the Very Important Person could, by writing and getting into touch with the right people, give a much quicker turn to the whole matter.

Akaky Akakyevich (what else could he do?) decided to go and see the Very Important Person. What positions the Very Important Person occupied and what his job actually was has never been properly ascertained and still remains unknown. Suffice it to say that the Very Important Person had become a Very Important Person only quite recently, and that until then he was quite an unimportant person. Moreover, his office was not even now considered of much importance as compared with others of greater importance. But there will always be people who regard as important what in the eyes of other people is rather unimportant. However, the Very Important Person did his best to increase his importance in all sorts of ways, to wit, he introduced a rule that his subordinates should meet him on the stairs when he arrived at his office; that no one should be admitted to his office unless he first petitioned for an interview, and that everything should be done according to the strictest order: the collegiate registrar was first to report to the provincial secretary, the provincial secretary to the titular councillor or whomsoever it was he had to report to, and that only by such a procedure should any particular business reach him. In Holy Russia, we are sorry to say, every one seems to be anxious to ape every one else and each man copies and imitates his superior. The story is even told of some titular councillor who, on being made chief of some small office, immediately partitioned off a special room for himself, calling it "the presence chamber," and placed two commissionaires in coats with red collars and galloons at the door with instructions to take hold of the door handle and open the door to any person who came to see him, though there was hardly room in "the presence chamber" for an ordinary writing-desk.

The manners and habits of the Very Important Person were very grand and impressive, but not very subtle. His whole system was based chiefly on strictness. "Strictness, strictness, and again strictness!" he usually declared, and at the penultimate word he usually peered very significantly into the face of the man he was addressing. There seemed to be no particular reason for this strictness, though, for the dozen or so Civil Servants who composed the whole administrative machinery of his office were held in a proper state of fear and trembling, anyhow. Seeing him coming from a distance they all stopped their work immediately and, standing at attention, waited until the chief had walked through the room. His usual conversation with any of his subordinates was saturated with strictness and consisted almost entirely of three phrases: "How dare you, sir? Do you know who you're talking to, sir? Do you realise who is standing before you, sir?" Still, he was really a good fellow at heart, was particularly pleasant with his colleagues, and quite obliging, too; but his new position went to his head. Having received the rank of general, he got all confused, was completely nonplussed and did not know what to do. In the presence of a man equal to him in rank, he was just an ordinary fellow, quite a decent fellow, and in many ways even a far from stupid fellow; but whenever he happened to be in company with men even one rank lower than he, he seemed to be lost; he sat silent and his position was really pitiable, more particularly as he himself felt that he could have spent the time so much more enjoyably. A strong desire could sometimes be read in his eyes to take part in some interesting conversation or join some interesting people, but he was always stopped by the thought: would it not mean going a little too far on his part? Would it not be mistaken for familiarity and would he not thereby lower himself in the estimation of everybody? As a consequence of this reasoning he always found himself in a position where he had to remain silent, delivering himself only from time to time of a few monosyllables, and in this way he won for himself the unenviable reputation of being an awful bore.

It was before this sort of Very Important Person that our Akaky presented himself, and he presented himself at the most inopportune moment he could possibly have chosen, very unfortunate for himself, though not so unfortunate for the Very Important Person. At the time of Akaky's arrival the Very Important Person was in his private office, having a very pleasant talk with an old friend of his, a friend of his childhood, who had only recently arrived in St. Petersburg and whom he had not seen for several years. It was just then that he was informed that a certain Bashmachkin wanted to see him. "Who's that?" he asked abruptly, and he was told, "Some Civil Servant." "Oh," said the Very Important Person, "let him wait. I'm busy now."

Now we believe it is only fair to state here that the Very Important Person had told a thumping lie. He was not busy at all. He had long ago said all he had to say to his old friend, and their present conversation had for some time now been punctuated by long pauses, interrupted by the one or the other slapping his friend on the knee and saying, "Ah, Ivan Abramovich!" or "Yes, yes, quite right, Stepan Varlamovich!" However, he asked the Civil Servant to wait, for he wanted to show his friend, who had left the Civil Service long ago and had been spending all his time at his country house, how long he kept Civil Servants cooling their heels in his anteroom. At last, having talked, or rather kept silent as long as they liked, having enjoyed a cigar in comfortable arm-chairs with sloping backs, he seemed to remember something suddenly and said to his secretary, who was standing at the door with a sheaf of documents in his hand, "Isn't there some Civil Servant waiting to see me? Tell him to come in, please."

Seeing Akaky's humble appearance and old uniform, he turned to him and said shortly, "What do you want?" in an abrupt and firm voice, which he had specially rehearsed in the solitude of his room in front of a looking-glass a week before he received his present post and the rank of general.

Akaky, who had long since been filled with the proper amount of fear and trembling, felt rather abashed and explained as well as he could and as much as his stammering would let him, with the addition of the more than usual number of "wells" and "you knows," that his overcoat was quite a new overcoat, and that he had been robbed in a most shameless fashion, and that he was now applying to his excellency in the hope that his excellency might by putting in a word here and there or doing this or that, or writing to the Commissioner of Police of the Metropolis, or to some other person, get his overcoat back. For some unknown reason the general considered such an approach as too familiar. "What do you mean, sir?" he said in his abrupt voice. "Don't you know the proper procedure? What have you come to me for? Don't you know how things are done? In the first place you should have sent in a petition about it to my office. Your petition, sir, would have been placed before the chief clerk, who would have transferred it to my secretary, and my secretary would have submitted it to me . . ."

"But, your excellency," said Akaky, trying to summon the handful of courage he had (it was not a very big handful, anyway), and feeling at the same time that he was perspiring all over, "I took the liberty, your excellency, of troubling you personally because—er—because, sir, secretaries are, well, you know, rather unreliable people . . ."

"What? What did you say, sir?" said the Very Important Person. "How dare you speak like this, sir? Where did you get the impudence to speak like this, sir? Where did you get these extraordinary ideas from, sir? What's the meaning of this mutinous spirit that is now spreading among young men against their chiefs and superiors?" The Very Important Person did not seem to have noticed that Akaky Akakyevich was well over fifty, and it can only be supposed, therefore, that if he called him a young man he meant it only in a relative sense, that is to say, that compared with a man of seventy Akaky was a young man. "Do you realise, sir, who you are talking to? Do you understand, sir, who is standing before you? Do you understand it, sir? Do you understand it, I ask you?" Here he stamped his foot and raised his voice to so high a pitch that it was not Akaky Akakyevich alone who became terrified. Akaky was on the point of fainting. He staggered, trembled all over, and could not stand on his feet. Had it not been for the door-keepers, who ran up to support him, he would have collapsed on the ground. He was carried out almost unconscious. The Very Important Person, satisfied that the effect he had produced exceeded all expectations and absolutely in raptures over the idea that a word of his could actually throw a man into a faint, glanced at his friend out of the corner of his eye, wondering what impression he had made on him; and he was pleased to see that his friend was rather in an uneasy frame of mind himself and seemed to show quite unmistakable signs of fear.

Akaky could not remember how he had descended the stairs, or how he had got out into the street. He remembered nothing. His hands and feet had gone dead. Never in his life had he been so hauled over the coals by a general, and not his own general at that. He walked along in a blizzard, in the teeth of a howling wind, which was sweeping through the streets, with his mouth agape and constantly stumbling off the pavement; the wind, as is its invariable custom in St. Petersburg, blew from every direction and every side street all at once. His throat became inflamed in no time at all, and when at last he staggered home he was unable to utter a word. He was all swollen, and he took to his bed. So powerful can a real official reprimand be sometimes!

Next day Akaky was in a high fever. Thanks to the most generous assistance of the St. Petersburg climate, his illness made much more rapid progress than could have been expected, and when the doctor arrived he merely felt his pulse and found nothing to do except prescribe a poultice, and that only because he did not want to leave the patient without the beneficent aid of medicine; he did, though, express his opinion then and there that all would be over in a day and a half. After which he turned to the landlady and said, "No need to waste time, my dear lady. You'd better order a deal coffin for him at once, for I don't suppose he can afford an oak coffin, can he?"

Did Akaky Akakyevich hear those fateful words and, if he did hear them, did they produce a shattering effect upon him? Did he at that moment repine at his wretched lot in life? It is quite impossible to say, for the poor man was in a delirium and a high fever. Visions, one stranger than another, haunted him incessantly: one moment he saw Petrovich and ordered him to make an overcoat with special traps for thieves, whom he apparently believed to be hiding under his bed, so that he called to his landlady every minute to get them out of there, and once he even asked her to get a thief from under his blanket; another time he demanded to be told why his old *capote* was hanging on the wall in front of him when he had a new overcoat; then it seemed to him that he was standing before the general and listening to his reprimand, which he so well deserved, saying, "Sorry, your excellency!" and, finally, he let out a stream of obscenities, shouting such frightful words that his dear old landlady kept crossing herself, having never heard him use such words, particularly as they seemed always to follow immediately upon the words, "your excellency." He raved on and no sense could be made of his words, except that it was quite evident that his incoherent words and thoughts all revolved about one and the same overcoat. At length poor Akaky Akakyevich gave up the ghost.

Neither his room nor his belongings were put under seal because, in the first place, he had no heirs, and in the second there was precious little inheritance he left behind, comprising as it did all in all a bundle of quills, a quire of white Government paper, three pairs of socks, a few buttons that had come off his trousers, and the *capote* with which the reader has already made his acquaintance. Who finally came into all this property, goodness only knows, and I must confess that the author of this story was not sufficiently interested to find out. Akaky Akakyevich was taken to the cemetery and buried. And St. Petersburg carried on without Akaky, as though he had never lived there. A human being just disappeared and left no trace, a human being whom no one ever dreamed of protecting, who was not dear to anyone, whom no one thought of taking any interest in, who did not attract the attention even of a naturalist who never fails to stick a pin through an ordinary fly to examine it under the microscope; a man who bore meekly the sneers and insults of his fellow Civil Servants in the department and who went to his grave because of some silly accident, but who before the very end of his life did nevertheless catch a glimpse of a Bright Visitant in the shape of an overcoat, which for a brief moment brought a ray of sunshine into his drab, poverty-stricken life, and upon whose head afterwards disaster had most pitilessly fallen, as it falls upon the heads of the great ones of this earth! . . .

A few days after his death a caretaker was sent to his room from the department to order him to present himself at the office at once: the chief himself wanted to see him! But the caretaker had to return without him, merely reporting that Akaky Akakyevich could not come, and to the question, "Why not?" he merely said, "He can't come, sir, 'cause he's dead. That's why, sir. Been buried these four days, he has, sir." It was in this way that the news of his death reached the department, and on the following day a new clerk was sitting in his place, a much taller man, who did not write letters in Akaky's upright hand, but rather sloping and aslant.

But who could have foreseen that this was not the last of Akaky Akakyevich and that he was destined to be the talk of the town for a few days after his death, as though in recompense for having remained unnoticed all through his life? But so it fell out, and our rather poor story quite unexpectedly acquired a most fantastic ending.

Rumours suddenly spread all over St. Petersburg that a ghost in the shape of a Government clerk had begun appearing near Kalinkin Bridge and much farther afield, too, and that this ghost was looking for some stolen overcoat and, under the pretext of recovering this lost overcoat, was stripping overcoats off the backs of all sorts of people, irrespective of their rank or calling: overcoats with cat fur, overcoats with beaver fur, raccoon, fox and bear-fur coats, in fact, overcoats with every kind of fur or skin that men have ever made use of to cover their own. One of the departmental clerks had seen the ghost with his own eyes and at once recognized Akaky Akakyevich; but that frightened him so much that he took to his heels and was unable to get a better view of the ghost, but merely saw how he shook a finger at him threateningly from a distance. From all sides complaints were incessantly heard to the effect that the backs and shoulders, not only of titular councillors, but also of court councillors, were in imminent danger of catching cold as a result of this frequent pulling off of overcoats. The police received orders to catch the ghost at all costs, dead or alive, and to punish him in the most unmerciful manner as an example to all other ghosts, and they nearly did catch it. A police constable whose beat included Kiryushkin Lane had actually caught the ghost by his collar on the very scene of his latest crime, in the very act of attempting to pull a frieze overcoat off the back of some retired musician who had once upon a time tootled on a flute. Having caught him by the collar, the policeman shouted to two of his comrades to come to his help, and when those arrived he told them to hold the miscreant while he reached for his snuff-box which he kept in one of his boots, to revive his nose which had been frostbitten six times in his life; but the snuff must have been of a kind that even a ghost could not stand. For no sooner had the policeman, closing his right nostril with a finger, inhaled with his left nostril half a handful of snuff than the ghost sneezed so violently that he splashed the eyes of all three. While they were raising their fists to wipe their eyes, the ghost had vanished completely, so that they were not even sure whether he had actually been in their hands. Since that time policemen were in such terror of the dead that they were even afraid to arrest the living, merely shouting from a distance, "Hi, you there, move along, will you?" and the ghost of the Civil Servant began to show himself beyond Kalinkin Bridge, causing alarm and dismay among all law-abiding citizens of timid dispositions.

We seem, however, to have completely forgotten a certain Very Important Person who, as a matter of fact, was the real cause of the fantastic turn this otherwise perfectly true story has taken. To begin with, we think it is only fair to make it absolutely clear that the Very Important Person felt something like a twinge of compunction soon after the departure of poor Akaky Akakyevich, whom he had taken to task so severely. Sympathy for a fellow human being was not alien to him; his heart was open to all kinds of kindly impulses in spite of the fact that his rank often prevented them from coming to the surface. As soon as the friend he had not seen for so long had left, he felt even a little worried about poor Akaky, and since that day he could not get the pale face of the meek little Government clerk out of his head, the poor Civil Servant who could not take an official reprimand like a man. In fact, he worried so much about him that a week later he sent one of his own clerks to Akaky to find out how he was getting on, whether his overcoat had turned up, and whether it was not really possible to help him in any way. When he learnt that Akaky had died suddenly of a fever he was rather upset and all day long his conscience troubled him, and he was in a bad mood. Wishing to distract himself a little and forget the unpleasant incident, he went to spend an evening with one of his friends, where he found quite a large company and, what was even better, they all seemed to be almost of the same rank as he, so that there was nothing at all to disconcert him. This had a most wonderful effect on his state of mind. He let himself go, became a very pleasant fellow to talk to, affable and genial, and spent a very agreeable evening. At dinner he drank a few glasses of champagne, which, as is generally acknowledged, is quite an excellent way of getting rid of gloomy thoughts. The champagne led him to introduce a certain change into his programme for that night, to wit, he decided not to go home at once, but first visit a lady friend of his, a certain Karolina Ivanovna, presumably of German descent, with whom he was on exceedingly friendly terms. It should be explained here that the Very Important Person was not a young man, that he was a good husband and a worthy father of a family. Two sons, one of whom was already in Government service, and a very sweet sixteen-year-old daughter, whose little nose was perhaps a thought too arched, but who was very pretty none the less, came every morning to kiss his hand, saying, "*Bonjour, papa.*" His wife, who was still in the prime of life and not at all bad-looking, first gave him her hand to kiss and then, turning it round, kissed his hand. But the Very Important Person, who was very satisfied indeed with these domestic pleasantries, thought it only right to have a lady friend in another part of the town for purely friendly relations. This lady friend was not a bit younger or better-looking than his wife, but there it is: such is the way of the world, and it is not our business to pass judgment upon it. And so the Very Important Person descended the stairs, sat down in his sledge, said to his coachman, "To Karolina Ivanovna," and, wrapping himself up very snugly in his warm overcoat, gave himself up completely to the enjoyment of his pleasant mood, than which nothing better could happen to a Russian, that is to say, the sort of mood when you do not yourself have to think of anything, while thoughts, one more delightful than another, come racing through your head without even putting you to the trouble of chasing after them or looking for them. Feeling very pleased, he recalled without much effort all the pleasant happenings of the evening, all the witty sayings, which had aroused peals of laughter among the small circle of friends, many of which he even now repeated softly to himself, finding them every bit as funny as they were the first time he heard them, and it is therefore little wonder that he chuckled happily most of the time. The boisterous wind, however, occasionally interfered with his enjoyment, for, rushing out suddenly from heaven knew where and for a reason that was utterly incomprehensible, it cut his face like a knife, covering it with lumps of snow, swelling out his collar like a sail, or suddenly throwing it with supernatural force over his head and so causing him incessant trouble to extricate himself from it. All of a sudden the Very Important Person felt that somebody had seized him very firmly by the collar. Turning round, he saw a small-sized man in an old, threadbare Civil Service uniform, and it was not without horror that he recognized Akaky Akakyevich. The Civil Servant's face was white as snow and looked like that of a dead man. But the horror of the Very Important Person increased considerably when he saw that the mouth of the dead man became twisted and, exhaling the terrible breath of the grave, Akaky's ghost uttered the following words, "Aha! So here you are! I've—er—collared you at last! . . . It's your overcoat I want, sir! You didn't care a rap for mine, did you? Did nothing to get it back for me, and abused me into the bargain! All right, then, give me yours now!" The poor Very Important Person nearly died of fright. Unbending as he was at the office and generally in the presence of his inferiors, and though one look at his manly appearance and figure was enough to make people say, "Ugh, what a Tartar!" nevertheless in this emergency he, like many another man of athletic appearance, was seized with such terror that he began, not without reason, to apprehend a heart attack. He threw off his overcoat himself and shouted to his driver in a panic-stricken voice, "Home, quick!" The driver, recognising the tone which was usually employed in moments of crisis and was quite often accompanied by something more forceful, drew in his head between his shoulders just to be on the safe side, flourished his whip and raced off as swift as an arrow. In a little over six minutes the Very Important Person was already at the entrance of his house. Pale, frightened out of his wits, and without his overcoat, he arrived home instead of going to Karolina Ivanovna's, and somehow or other managed to stagger to his room. He spent a very restless night, so that next morning at breakfast his daughter told him outright, "You look very pale today, Papa!" But Papa made no reply. Not a word did he say to anyone about what had happened to him, where he had been and where he had intended to go.

This incident made a deep impression upon the Very Important Person. It was not so frequently now that his subordinates heard him say, "How dare you, sir? Do you realize who you're talking to, sir?" And if he did say it, it was only after he had heard what it was all about.

But even more remarkable was the fact that since then the appearance of the Civil Servant's ghost had completely ceased. It can only be surmised that he was very pleased with the general's overcoat which must have fitted him perfectly; at least nothing was heard any more of people who had their overcoats pulled off their backs. Not that there were not all sorts of busybodies who would not let well alone and who went on asserting that the ghost of the Civil Servant was still appearing in the more outlying parts of the town. Indeed, a Kolomna policeman saw with his own eyes the ghost appear from behind a house; but having rather a frail constitution—once an ordinary young pig, rushing out of a house, had sent him sprawling, to the great delight of some cabbies who were standing round and whom, for such an insult, he promptly fined two copecks each for snuff—he dared not stop the ghost, but merely followed it in the dark until, at last, it suddenly looked round and, stopping dead in its tracks, asked, "What do *you* want?" at the same time displaying a fist of a size that was never seen among the living. The police constable said, "Nothing," and turned back at once. This ghost, however, was much taller; it had a pair of huge moustachios, and, walking apparently in the direction of Obukhov Bridge, it disappeared into the darkness of the night.

Anton Chekhov

GOOSEBERRIES

The whole sky had been overcast with rain-clouds from early morning; it was a still day, not hot, but heavy, as it is in grey dull weather when the clouds have been hanging over the country for a long while, when one expects rain and it does not come. Ivan Ivanovitch, the veterinary surgeon, and Burkin, the high-school teacher, were already tired from walking, and the fields seemed to them endless. Far ahead of them they could just see the windmills of the village of Mironositskoe; on the right stretched a row of hillocks which disappeared in the distance behind the village, and they both knew that this was the bank of the river, that there were meadows, green willows, homesteads there, and that if one stood on one of the hillocks one could see from it the same vast plain, telegraph-wires, and a train which in the distance looked like a crawling caterpillar, and that in clear weather one could even see the town. Now, in still weather, when all nature seemed mild and dreamy, Ivan Ivanovitch and Burkin were filled with love of that countryside, and both thought how great, how beautiful a land it was.

"Last time we were in Prokofy's barn," said Burkin, "you were about to tell me a story."

"Yes; I meant to tell you about my brother."

Ivan Ivanovitch heaved a deep sigh and lighted a pipe to begin to tell his story, but just at that moment the rain began. And five minutes later heavy rain came down, covering the sky, and it was hard to tell when it would be over. Ivan Ivanovitch and Burkin stopped in hesitation; the dogs, already drenched, stood with their tails between their legs gazing at them feelingly.

"We must take shelter somewhere," said Burkin. "Let us go to Alehin's; it's close by."

"Come along."

They turned aside and walked through mown fields, sometimes going straight forward, sometimes turning to the right, till they came out on the road. Soon they saw poplars, a garden, then the red roofs of barns; there was a gleam of the river, and the view opened on to a broad expanse of water with a windmill and a white bath-house: this was Sofino, where Alehin lived.

The watermill was at work, drowning the sound of the rain; the dam was shaking. Here wet horses with drooping heads were standing near their carts, and men were walking about covered with sacks. It was damp, muddy, and desolate; the water looked cold and malignant. Ivan Ivanovitch and Burkin were already conscious of a feeling of wetness, messiness, and discomfort all over; their feet were heavy with mud, and when, crossing the dam, they went up to the barns, they were silent, as though they were angry with one another.

In one of the barns there was the sound of a winnowing machine, the door was open, and clouds of dust were coming from it. In the doorway was standing Alehin himself, a man of forty, tall and stout, with long hair, more like a professor or an artist than a landowner. He had on a white shirt that badly needed washing, a rope for a belt, drawers instead of trousers, and his boots, too, were plastered up with mud and straw. His eyes and nose were black with dust. He recognized Ivan Ivanovitch and Burkin, and was apparently much delighted to see them.

"Go into the house, gentlemen," he said, smiling; "I'll come directly, this minute."

It was a big two-storeyed house. Alehin lived in the lower storey, with arched ceilings and little windows, where the bailiffs had once lived; here everything was plain, and there was a smell of rye bread, cheap vodka, and harness. He went upstairs into the best rooms only on rare occasions, when visitors came. Ivan Ivanovitch and Burkin were met in the house by a maid-servant, a young woman so beautiful that they both stood still and looked at one another.

"You can't imagine how delighted I am to see you, my friends," said Alehin, going into the hall with them. "It is a surprise! Pelagea," he said, addressing the girl, "give our visitors something to change into. And, by the way, I will change too. Only I must first go and wash, for I almost think I have not washed since spring. Wouldn't you like to come into the bath-house? and meanwhile they will get things ready here."

Beautiful Pelagea, looking so refined and soft, brought them towels and soap, and Alehin went to the bath-house with his guests.

"It's a long time since I had a wash," he said, undressing. "I have got a nice bath-house, as you see—my father built it—but I somehow never have time to wash."

He sat down on the steps and soaped his long hair and his neck, and the water round him turned brown.

"Yes, I must say," said Ivan Ivanovitch meaningly, looking at his head.

"It's a long time since I washed . . ." said Alehin with embarrassment, giving himself a second soaping, and the water near him turned dark blue, like ink.

Ivan Ivanovitch went outside, plunged into the water with a loud splash, and swam in the rain, flinging his arms out wide. He stirred the water into waves which set the white lilies bobbing up and down; he swam to the very middle of the millpond and dived, and came up a minute later in another place, and swam on, and kept on diving, trying to touch the bottom.

"Oh, my goodness!" he repeated continually, enjoying himself thoroughly. "Oh, my goodness!" He swam to the mill, talked to the peasants there, then returned and lay on his back in the middle of the pond, turning his face to the rain. Burkin and Alehin were dressed and ready to go, but he still went on swimming and diving. "Oh, my goodness! . . ." he said. "Oh, Lord, have mercy on me! . . ."

"That's enough!" Burkin shouted to him.

They went back to the house. And only when the lamp was lighted in the big drawing-room upstairs, and Burkin and Ivan Ivanovitch, attired in silk dressing-gowns and warm slippers, were sitting in armchairs; and Alehin, washed and combed, in a new coat, was walking about the drawing-room, evidently enjoying the feeling of warmth, cleanliness, dry clothes, and light shoes; and when lovely Pelagea, stepping noiselessly on the carpet and smiling softly, handed tea and jam on a tray—only then Ivan Ivanovitch began on his story, and it seemed as though not only Burkin and Alehin were listening, but also the ladies, young and old, and the officers who looked down upon them sternly and calmly from their gold frames.

"There are two of us brothers," he began—"I, Ivan Ivanovitch, and my brother, Nikolay Ivanovitch, two years younger. I went in for a learned profession and became a veterinary surgeon, while Nikolay sat in a government office from the time he was nineteen. Our father, Tchimsha-Himalaisky, was a kantonist, but he rose to be an officer and left us a little estate and the rank of nobility. After his death the little estate went in debts and legal expenses; but, anyway, we had spent our childhood running wild in the country. Like peasant children, we passed our days and nights in the fields and the woods, looked after horses, stripped the bark off the trees, fished, and so on . . . And, you know, whoever has once in his life caught perch or has seen the migrating of the thrushes in autumn, watched how they float in flocks over the village on bright, cool days, he will never be a real townsman, and will have a yearning for freedom to the day of his death. My brother was miserable in the government office. Years passed by, and he went on sitting in the same place, went on writing the same papers and thinking of one and the same thing—how to get into the country. And this yearning by degrees passed into a definite desire, into a dream of buying himself a little farm somewhere on the banks of a river or a lake.

"He was a gentle, good-natured fellow, and I was fond of him, but I never sympathized with this desire to shut himself up for the rest of his life in a little farm of his own. It's the correct thing to say that a man needs no more than six feet of earth. But six feet is what a corpse needs, not a man. And they say, too, now, that if our intellectual classes are attracted to the land and yearn for a farm, it's a good thing. But these farms are just the same as six feet of earth. To retreat from town, from the struggle, from the bustle of life, to retreat and bury oneself in one's farm—it's not life, it's egoism, laziness, it's monasticism of a sort, but monasticism without good works. A man does not need six feet of earth or a farm, but the whole globe, all nature, where he can have room to display all the qualities and peculiarities of his free spirit.

"My brother Nikolay, sitting in his government office, dreamed of how he would eat his own cabbages, which would fill the whole yard with such a savoury smell, take his meals on the green grass, sleep in the sun, sit for whole hours on the seat by the gate gazing at the fields and the forest. Gardening books and the agricultural hints in calendars were his delight, his favourite spiritual sustenance; he enjoyed reading newspapers, too, but the only things he read in them were the advertisements of so many acres of arable land and a grass meadow with farm-houses and buildings, a river, a garden, a mill and millponds, for sale. And his imagination pictured the garden-paths, flowers and fruit, starling cotes, the carp in the pond, and all that sort of thing, you know. These imaginary pictures were of different kinds according to the advertisements which he came across, but for some reason in every one of them he had always to have gooseberries. He could not imagine a homestead, he could not picture an idyllic nook, without gooseberries.

"'Country life has its conveniences,' he would sometimes say. 'You sit on the verandah and you drink tea, while your ducks swim on the pond, there is a delicious smell everywhere, and . . . and the gooseberries are growing.'

"He used to draw a map of his property, and in every map there were the same things—(a) house for the family, (b) servants' quarters, (c) kitchen-garden, (d) gooseberry-bushes. He lived parsimoniously, was frugal in food and drink, his clothes were beyond description; he looked like a beggar, but kept on saving and putting money in the bank. He grew fearfully avaricious. I did not like to look at him, and I used to give him something and send him presents for Christmas and Easter, but he used to save that too. Once a man is absorbed by an idea there is no doing anything with him.

"Years passed: he was transferred to another province. He was over forty, and he was still reading the advertisements in the papers and saving up. Then I heard he was married. Still with the same object of buying a farm and having gooseberries, he married an elderly and ugly widow without a trace of feeling for her, simply because she had filthy lucre. He went on living frugally after marrying her, and kept her short of food, while he put her money in the bank in his name.

"Her first husband had been a postmaster, and with him she was accustomed to pies and home-made wines, while with her second husband she did not get enough black bread; she began to pine away with this sort of life, and three years later she gave up her soul to God. And I need hardly say that my brother never for one moment imagined that he was responsible for her death. Money, like vodka, makes a man queer.

In our town there was a merchant who, before he died, ordered a plateful of honey and ate up all his money and lottery tickets with the honey, so that no one might get the benefit of it. While I was inspecting cattle at a railway-station, a cattle-dealer fell under an engine and had his leg cut off. We carried him into the waiting-room, the blood was flowing—it was a horrible thing—and he kept asking them to look for his leg and was very much worried about it; there were twenty roubles in the boot on the leg that had been cut off, and he was afraid they would be lost."

"That's a story from a different opera," said Burkin.

"After his wife's death," Ivan Ivanovitch went on, after thinking for half a minute, "my brother began looking out for an estate for himself. Of course, you may look about for five years and yet end by making a mistake, and buying something quite different from what you have dreamed of. My brother Nikolay bought through an agent a mortgaged estate of three hundred and thirty acres, with a house for the family, with servants' quarters, with a park, but with no orchard, no gooseberry-bushes, and no duck-pond; there was a river, but the water in it was the colour of coffee, because on one side of the estate there was a brickyard and on the other a factory for burning bones. But Nikolay Ivanovitch did not grieve much; he ordered twenty gooseberry-bushes, planted them, and began living as a country gentleman.

"Last year I went to pay him a visit. I thought I would go and see what it was like. In his letters my brother called his estate 'Tchumbaroklov Waste, alias Himalaiskoe.' I reached 'alias Himalaiskoe' in the afternoon. It was hot. Everywhere there were ditches, fences, hedges, fir-trees planted in rows, and there was no knowing how to get to the yard, where to put one's horse. I went up to the house, and was met by a fat red dog that looked like a pig. It wanted to bark, but it was too lazy. The cook, a fat, barefooted woman, came out of the kitchen, and she, too, looked like a pig, and said that her master was resting after dinner. I went in to see my brother. He was sitting up in bed with a quilt over his legs; he had grown older, fatter, wrinkled; his cheeks, his nose, and his mouth all stuck out—he looked as though he might begin grunting into the quilt at any moment.

"We embraced each other, and shed tears of joy and of sadness at the thought that we had once been young and now were both grey-headed and near the grave. He dressed, and led me out to show me the estate.

"'Well, how are you getting on here?' I asked.

"'Oh, all right, thank God; I am getting on very well.'

"He was no more a poor timid clerk, but a real landowner, a gentleman. He was already accustomed to it, had grown used to it, and liked it. He ate a great deal, went to the bath-house, was growing stout, was already at law with the village commune and both factories, and was very much offended when the peasants did not call him 'Your Honour.' And he concerned himself with the salvation of his soul in a substantial, gentlemanly manner, and performed deeds of charity, not simply, but with an air of consequence. And what deeds of charity! He treated the peasants for every sort of disease with soda and castor oil, and on his name-day had a thanksgiving service in the middle of the village, and then treated the peasants to a gallon of vodka—he thought that was the thing to do. Oh, those horrible gallons of vodka! One day the fat landowner hauls the peasants up before the district captain for trespass, and next day, in honour of a holiday, treats them to a gallon of vodka, and they drink and shout 'Hurrah!' and when they are drunk bow down to his feet. A change of life for the better, and being well-fed and idle develop in a Russian the most insolent self-conceit. Nikolay Ivanovitch, who at one time in the government office was afraid to have any views of his own, now could say nothing that was not gospel truth, and uttered such truths in the tone of a prime minister. 'Education is essential, but for the peasants it is premature.' 'Corporal punishment is harmful as a rule, but in some cases it is necessary and there is nothing to take its place.'

"'I know the peasants and understand how to treat them,' he would say. 'The peasants like me. I need only to hold up my little finger and the peasants will do anything I like.'

"And all this, observe, was uttered with a wise, benevolent smile. He repeated twenty times over 'We noblemen,' 'I as a noble'; obviously he did not remember that our grandfather was a peasant, and our father a soldier. Even our surname Tchimsha-Himalaisky, in reality so incongruous, seemed to him now melodious, distinguished, and very agreeable.

"But the point just now is not he, but myself. I want to tell you about the change that took place in me during the brief hours I spent at his country place. In the evening, when we were drinking tea, the cook put on the table a plateful of gooseberries. They were not bought, but his own gooseberries, gathered for the first time since the bushes were planted. Nikolay Ivanovitch laughed and looked for a minute in silence at the gooseberries, with tears in his eyes; he could not speak for excitement. Then he put one gooseberry in his mouth, looked at me with the triumph of a child who has at last received his favourite toy, and said:

"'How delicious!'

"And he ate them greedily, continually repeating, 'Ah, how delicious! Do taste them!'

"They were sour and unripe, but, as Pushkin says:

'Dearer to us the falsehood that exalts than hosts of baser truths.'

"I saw a happy man whose cherished dream was so obviously fulfilled, who had attained his object in life, who had gained what he wanted, who was satisfied with his fate and himself. There is always, for some reason, an element of sadness mingled with my thoughts of human happiness, and, on this occasion, at the sight of a happy man I was overcome by an oppressive feeling that was close upon despair. It was particularly oppressive at night. A bed was made up for me in the room next to my brother's bedroom, and I could hear that he was awake, and that he kept getting up and going to the plate of gooseberries and taking one. I reflected how many satisfied, happy people there really are! What a suffocating force it is! You look at life: the insolence and idleness of the strong, the ignorance and brutishness of the weak, incredible poverty all about us, overcrowding, degeneration, drunkenness, hypocrisy, lying. . . . Yet all is calm and stillness in the houses and in the streets; of the fifty thousand living in a town, there is not one who would cry out, who would give vent to his indignation aloud. We see the people going to market for provisions, eating by day, sleeping by night, talking their silly nonsense, getting married, growing old, serenely escorting their dead to the cemetery; but we do not see and we do not hear those who suffer, and what is terrible in life goes on somewhere behind the scenes . . . Everything is quiet and peaceful, and nothing protests but mute statistics: so many people gone out of their minds, so many gallons of vodka drunk, so many children dead from malnutrition . . . And this order of things is evidently necessary; evidently the happy man only feels at ease because the unhappy bear their burdens in silence, and without that silence happiness would be impossible. It's a case of general hypnotism. There ought to be behind the door of every happy, contented man some one standing with a hammer continually reminding him with a tap that there are unhappy people; that however happy he may be, life will show him her laws sooner or later, trouble will come for him—disease, poverty, losses, and no one will see or hear, just as now he neither sees nor hears others. But there is no man with a hammer; the happy man lives at his ease, and trivial daily cares faintly agitate him like the wind in the aspen-tree—and all goes well.

"That night I realized that I, too, was happy and contented," Ivan Ivanovitch went on, getting up. "I, too, at dinner and at the hunt liked to lay down the law on life and religion, and the way to manage the peasantry. I, too, used to say that science was light, that culture was essential, but for the simple people reading and writing was enough for the time. Freedom is a blessing, I used to say; we can no more do without it than without air, but we must wait a little. Yes, I used to talk like that, and now I ask, 'For what reason are we to wait?'" asked Ivan Ivanovitch, looking angrily at Burkin. "Why wait, I ask you? What grounds have we for waiting? I shall be told, it can't be done all at once; every idea takes shape in life gradually, in its due time. But who is it says that? Where is the proof that it's right? You will fall back upon the natural order of things, the uniformity of phenomena; but is there order and uniformity in the fact that I, a living, thinking man, stand over a chasm and wait for it to close of itself, or to fill up with mud at the very time when perhaps I might leap over it or build a bridge across it? And again, wait for the sake of what? Wait till there's no strength to live? And meanwhile one must live, and one wants to live!

"I went away from my brother's early in the morning, and ever since then it has been unbearable for me to be in town. I am oppressed by its peace and quiet; I am afraid to look at the windows, for there is no spectacle more painful to me now than the sight of a happy family sitting round the table drinking tea. I am old and am not fit for the struggle; I am not even capable of hatred; I can only grieve inwardly, feel irritated and vexed; but at night my head is hot from the rush of ideas, and I cannot sleep . . . Ah, if I were young!"

Ivan Ivanovitch walked backwards and forwards in excitement, and repeated: "If I were young!"

He suddenly went up to Alehin and began pressing first one of his hands and then the other.

"Pavel Konstantinovitch," he said in an imploring voice, "don't be calm and contented, don't let yourself be put to sleep! While you are young, strong, confident, be not weary in well-doing! There is no happiness, and there ought not to be; but if there is a meaning and an object in life, that meaning and object is not our happiness, but something greater and more rational. Do good!"

And all this Ivan Ivanovitch said with a pitiful, imploring smile, as though he were asking him a personal favour.

Then all three sat in arm-chairs at different ends of the drawing-room and were silent. Ivan Ivanovitch's story had not satisfied either Burkin or Alehin. When the generals and ladies gazed down from their gilt frames, looking in the dusk as though they were alive, it was dreary to listen to the story of the poor clerk who ate gooseberries. They felt inclined, for some reason, to talk about elegant people, about women. And their sitting in the drawing-room where everything—the chandeliers in their covers, the arm-chairs, and the carpet under their feet—reminded them that those very people who were now looking down from their frames had once moved about, sat, drunk tea in this room, and the fact that lovely Pelagea was moving noiselessly about was better than any story.

Alehin was fearfully sleepy; he had got up early, before three o'clock in the morning, to look after his work, and now his eyes were closing; but he was afraid his visitors might tell some interesting story after he had gone, and he lingered on. He did not go into the question whether what Ivan Ivanovitch had just said was right and true. His visitors did not talk of groats, nor of hay, nor of tar, but of something that had no direct bearing on his life, and he was glad and wanted them to go on.

"It's bed-time, though," said Burkin, getting up. "Allow me to wish you good-night."

Alehin said good-night and went downstairs to his own domain, while the visitors remained upstairs. They were both taken for the night to a big room where there stood two old wooden beds decorated with carvings, and in the corner was an ivory crucifix. The big cool beds, which had been made by the lovely Pelagea, smelt agreeably of clean linen.

Ivan Ivanovitch undressed in silence and got into bed.

"Lord forgive us sinners!" he said, and put his head under the quilt.

His pipe lying on the table smelt strongly of stale tobacco, and Burkin could not sleep for a long while, and kept wondering where the oppressive smell came from.

The rain was pattering on the window-panes all night.

Jean Rhys

Sleep It Off, Lady

One October afternoon Mrs. Baker was having tea with Miss Verney and talking about the proposed broiler factory in the middle of the village where they both lived. Miss Verney, who had not been listening attentively said, "You know Letty, I've been thinking a great deal about death lately. I hardly ever do, strangely enough."

"No dear," said Mrs. Baker. "It isn't strange at all. It's quite natural. We old people are rather like children, we live in the present as a rule. A merciful dispensation of providence."

"Perhaps," said Miss Verney doubtfully.

Mrs. Baker said "we old people" quite kindly, but could not help knowing that while she herself was only sixty-three and might, with any luck, see many a summer (after many a summer dies the swan, as some man said), Miss Verney, certainly well over seventy, could hardly hope for anything of the sort. Mrs. Baker gripped the arms of her chair. "Many a summer, touch wood and please God," she thought. Then she remarked that it was getting dark so early now and wasn't it extraordinary how time flew.

Miss Verney listened to the sound of the car driving away, went back to her sitting-room and looked out of the window at the flat field, the apple trees, the lilac tree that wouldn't flower again, not for ten years they told her, because lilacs won't stand being pruned. In the distance there was a rise in the ground—you could hardly call it a hill—and three trees so exactly shaped and spaced that they looked artificial. "It would be rather lovely covered in snow," Miss Verney thought. "The snow, so white, so smooth and in the end so boring. Even the hateful shed wouldn't look so bad." But she'd made up her mind to forget the shed.

Miss Verney had decided that it was an eyesore when she came to live in the cottage. Most of the paint had worn off the once-black galvanized iron. Now it was a greenish colour. Part of the roof was loose and flapped noisily in windy weather and a small gate off its hinges leaned up against the entrance. Inside it was astonishingly large, the far end almost dark. "What a waste of space," Miss Verney thought. "That must come down." Strange that she hadn't noticed it before.

Nails festooned with rags protruded from the only wooden rafter. There was a tin bucket with a hold, a huge dustbin. Nettles flourished in one corner but it was the opposite corner which disturbed her. Here was piled a rusty lawnmower, an old chair with a carpet draped over it, several sacks, and the remains of what had once been a bundle of hay. She found herself imagining that a fierce and dangerous animal lived there and called aloud: "Come out, come out, Shredni Vashtar, the beautiful." Then rather alarmed at herself she walked away as quickly as she could.

But she was not unduly worried. The local builder had done several odd jobs for her when she moved in and she would speak to him when she saw him next.

"Want the shed down?" said the builder.

"Yes," said Miss Verney. "It's hideous, and it takes up so much space."

"It's on the large side," the builder said.

"Enormous. Whatever did they use it for?"

"I expect it was the garden shed."

"I don't care what it was," said Miss Verney. "I want it out of the way."

The builder said that he couldn't manage the next week, but the Monday after that he'd look in and see what could be done. Monday came and Miss Verney waited but he didn't arrive. When this had happened twice she realized that he didn't mean to come and wrote to a firm in the nearest town.

A few days later a cheerful young man knocked at the door, explained who he was and asked if she would let him know exactly what she wanted. Miss Verney, who wasn't feeling at all well, pointed, "I want that pulled down. Can you do it?"

The young man inspected the shed, walked round it, then stood looking at it.

"I want it destroyed," said Miss Verney passionately, "utterly destroyed and carted away. I hate the sight of it."

"Quite a job," he said candidly.

And Miss Verney saw what he meant. Long after she was dead and her cottage had vanished it would survive. The tin bucket and the rusty lawnmower, the pieces of rag fluttering in the wind. All would last forever.

Eyeing her rather nervously he became businesslike. "I see what you want, and of course we can let you have an estimate of the cost. But you realize that if you pull the shed down you take away from the value of your cottage?"

"Why?" said Miss Verney.

"Well," he said, "very few people would live here without a car. It could be converted into a garage easily or even used as it is. You can decide of course when you have the estimate whether you think it worth the expense and . . . the trouble. Good day."

Left alone, Miss Verney felt so old, lonely and helpless that she began to cry. No builder would tackle that shed, not for any price she could afford. But crying relieved her and she soon felt quite cheerful again. It was ridiculous to brood, she told herself. She quite liked the cottage. One morning she'd wake up and know what to do about the shed, meanwhile she wouldn't look at the thing. She wouldn't think about it.

But it was astonishing how it haunted her dreams. One night she was standing looking at it changing its shape and becoming a very smart, shiny, dark blue coffin picked out in white. It reminded her of a dress she had once worn. A voice behind her said: "That's the laundry."

"Then oughtn't I to put it away?" said Miss Verney in her dream.

"Not just yet. Soon," said the voice so loudly that she woke up.

She had dragged the large dustbin to the entrance and, because it was too heavy for her to lift, had arranged for it to be carried to the gate every week for the dustmen to collect. Every morning she took a small yellow bin from under the sink and emptied it into the large dustbin, quickly, without lingering or looking around. But on one particular morning the usual cold wind had dropped and she stood wondering if a coat of white paint would improve matters. Paint might look a lot worse, besides, who could she get to do it? Then she saw a cat, as she thought, walking slowly across the far end. The sun shone though a chink in the wall. It was a large rat. Horrified, she watched it disappear under the old chair, dropped the yellow bin, walked as fast as she was able up the road and knocked at the door of a shabby thatched cottage.

"Oh Tom. There are rats in my shed. I've just seen a huge one. I'm so desperately afraid of them. What shall I do?"

When she left Tom's cottage she was still shaken, but calmer. Tom had assured her that he had an infallible rat poison, arrangements had been made, his wife had supplied a strong cup of tea.

He came that same day to put down the poison, and when afterwards he rapped loudly on the door and shouted: "Everything under control?" she answered quite cheerfully, "Yes, I'm fine and thanks for coming."

As one sunny day followed another she almost forgot how much the rat had frightened her. "It's dead or gone away," she assured herself.

When she saw it again she stood and stared disbelieving. It crossed the shed in the same unhurried way and she watched, not able to move. A huge rat, there was no doubt about it.

This time Miss Verney didn't rush to Tom's cottage to be reassured. She managed to get to the kitchen, still holding the empty yellow pail, slammed the door and locked it. Then she shut and bolted all the windows. This done, she took off her shoes, lay down, pulled the blankets over her head and listened to her hammering heart.

I'm the monarch of all I survey.
My right, there is none to dispute.

That was the way the rat walked.

In the close darkness she must have dozed, for suddenly she was sitting at a desk in the sun copying proverbs into a ruled book: "Evil Communications corrupt good manners. Look before you leap. Patience is a virtue, good temper a blessing," all the way to Z. Z would be something to do with zeal or zealous. But how did they manage about X? What about X?

Thinking this, she slept, then woke, put on the light, took two tuinal tablets and slept again, heavily. When she next opened her eyes it was morning, the unwound bedside clock had stopped, but she guessed the time from the light and hurried into the kitchen waiting for Tom's car to pass. The room was stuffy and airless but she didn't dream of opening the window. When she saw the car approaching she ran out into the road and waved it down. It was as if fear had given her wings and once more she moved lightly and quickly.

"Tom. Tom."

He stopped.

"Oh Tom, the rat's still there. I saw it last evening."

He got down stiffly. Not a young man, but surely surely, a kind man? "I put down enough stuff to kill a dozen rats," he said. "Let's 'ave a look."

He walked across to the shed. She followed, several yards behind, and watched him rattling the old lawnmower, kicking the sacks, trampling the hay and nettles.

"No rat 'ere," he said at last.

"Well, there was one," she said.

"Not 'ere."

"It was a huge rat," she said.

Tom had round brown eyes, honest eyes, she'd thought. But now they were sly, mocking, even hostile.

"Are you sure it wasn't a pink rat?" he said.

She knew that the bottles in her dustbin were counted and discussed in the village. But Tom, whom she liked so much?

"No," she managed to say steadily. "An ordinary colour but very large. Don't they say that some rats don't care about poison? Super rats."

Tom laughed. "Nothing of that sort round 'ere."

She said: "I asked Mr. Slade, who cuts the grass, to clear out the shed and he said he would but I think he's forgotten."

"Mr. Slade is a very busy man," said Tom. "He can't clear out the shed just when you tell him. You've got to wait. Do you expect him to leave his work and waste his time looking for what's not there?"

"No," she said, "of course not. But I think it ought to be done." (She stopped herself from saying: "I can't because I'm afraid.")

"Now you go and make yourself a nice cup of tea," Tom said, speaking in a more friendly voice. "There's no rat in your shed." And he went back to his car.

Miss Verney slumped heavily into the kitchen armchair. "He doesn't believe me. I can't stay alone in this place, not with that monster a few yards away. I can't do it." But another cold voice persisted: "Where will you go? With what money? Are you really such a coward as all that?"

After a time Miss Verney got up. She dragged what furniture there was away from the walls so that she would know that nothing lurked in the corners and decided to keep the windows looking onto the shed shut and bolted. The others she opened but only at the top. Then she made a large parcel of all the food that the rat could possibly smell—cheese, bacon, ham, cold meat, practically everything . . . she'd give it to Mrs. Randolph, the cleaning woman, later.

"But no more confidences." Mrs. Randolph would be as skeptical as Tom had been. A nice woman but a gossip, she wouldn't be able to resist telling her cronies about the giant, almost certainly imaginary, rat terrorizing her employer.

Next morning Mrs. Randolph said that a stray dog had upset the large dustbin. She'd had to pick everything up from the floor of the shed. "It wasn't a dog," thought Miss Verney, but she only suggested that two stones on the lid turned the other way up would keep the dog off.

When she saw the size of the stones she nearly said aloud: "I defy any rat to get that lid off."

Miss Verney had always been a careless, not a fussy, woman. Now all that changed. She spent hours every day sweeping, dusting, arranging the cupboards and putting fresh paper into the drawers. She pounced on every speck of dust with a dustpan. She tried to convince herself that as long as she kept her house spotlessly clean the rat would keep to the shed, not to wonder what she would do if after all, she encountered it.

"I'd collapse," she thought, "that's what I'd do."

After this she'd start with fresh energy, again fearfully sweeping under the bed, behind cupboards. Then feeling too tired to eat, she would beat up an egg in cold milk, add a good deal of whisky and sip it slowly. "I don't need a lot of food now." But her work in the house grew slower and slower, her daily walks shorter and shorter. Finally the walks stopped. "Why should I bother?" As she never answered letters, letters ceased to arrive, and when Tom knocked at the door one day to ask how she was: "Oh I'm quite all right," she said and smiled.

He seemed ill at ease and didn't speak about rats or clearing the shed out. Nor did she.

"Not seen you about lately," he said.

"Oh I go the other way now."

When she shut the door after him she thought: "And I imagined I liked him. How very strange."

"No pain?" the doctor asked.

"It's just an odd feeling," said Miss Verney.

The doctor said nothing. He waited.

"It's as if all my blood was running backwards. It's rather horrible really. And then for a while sometimes I can't move. I mean if I'm holding a cup I have to drop it because there's no life in my arm."

"And how long does this last?"

"Not long. Only a few minutes I suppose. It just seems a long time."

"Does it happen often?"

"Twice lately."

The doctor thought he'd better examine her. Eventually he left the room and came back with a bottle half full of pills. "Take these three times a day—don't forget, it's important. Long before they're finished I'll come and see you. I'm going to give you some injections that may help, but I'll have to send away for those."

As Miss Verney was gathering her things together before leaving the surgery he asked in a casual voice: "Are you on the telephone?"

"No," said Miss Verney, "but I have an arrangement with some people."

"You told me. But those people are some way off, aren't they?"

"I'll get a telephone," said Miss Verney making up her mind. "I'll see about it at once."

"Good. You won't be so lonely."

"I suppose not."

"Don't go moving the furniture about, will you? Don't lift heavy weights. Don't . . ." (Oh Lord," she thought, "is he going to say 'Don't drink?'—because that's impossible!) . . . "Don't worry," he said.

When Miss Verney left his surgery she felt relieved but tired and she walked very slowly home. It was quite a long walk for she lived in the less prosperous part of the village, near the row of council houses. She had never minded that. She was protected by tall thick hedges and a tree or two. Of course it had taken her some time to get used to the children's loud shrieking and the women who stood outside their doors to gossip. At first they stared at her with curiosity and some disapproval, she couldn't help feeling, but they'd soon found out that she was harmless.

The child Deena, however, was a different matter.

Most of the village boys were called Jack, Willie, Stan and so on—the girls' first names were more elaborate. Deena's mother had gone one better than anyone else and christened her daughter Undine.

Deena—as everyone called her—was a tall plump girl of about twelve with a pretty, healthy but rather bovine face. She never joined the shrieking games, she never played football with dustbin lids. She apparently spent all her spare time standing at the gate of her mother's house silently, unsmilingly, staring at everyone who passed.

Miss Verney had long ago given up trying to be friendly. So much did the child's cynical eyes depress her that she would cross over the road to avoid her, and sometimes was guilty of the cowardice of making sure Deena wasn't there before setting out.

Now she looked anxiously along the street and was relieved that it was empty. "Of course," she told herself, "it's getting cold. When winter comes they'll all stay indoors."

Not that Deena seemed to mind cold. Only a few days ago, looking out of the window, Miss Verney had seen her standing outside—oblivious of the bitter wind—staring at the front door as though, if she looked hard enough, she could see through the wood and find out what went on in the silent house—what Miss Verney did with herself all day.

One morning soon after her visit to the doctor Miss Verney woke feeling very well and very happy. Also she was not at all certain where she was. She lay luxuriating in the feeling of renewed youth, renewed health and slowly recognized the various pieces of furniture.

"Of course," she thought when she drew the curtains. "What a funny place to end up in."

The sky was pale blue. There was no wind. Watching the still trees she sang softly to herself: "The day of days." She had always sung "The day of days" on her birthday. Poised between two years—last year, next year—she never felt any age at all. Birthdays were a pause, a rest.

In the midst of slow dressing she remembered the rat for the first time. But that seemed something that had happened long ago. "Thank God I didn't tell anybody else how frightened I was. As soon as they give me a telephone I'll ask Letty Baker to tea. She'll know exactly the sensible thing to do."

Out of habit she ate, swept and dusted but even more slowly than usual and with long pauses, when leaning on the handle of her tall, old-fashioned carpet sweeper she stared out at the trees. "Good-bye summer. Good-bye good-bye," she hummed. But in spite of sad songs she never lost the certainty of health, of youth.

All at once she noticed, to her surprise, that it was getting dark. "And I haven't emptied the dustbin."

She got to the shed carrying the small yellow plastic pail and saw that the big dustbin wasn't there. For once Mrs. Randolph must have slipped up and left it outside the gate. Indeed it was so.

She first brought in the lid, easy, then turned the heavy bin onto its side and kicked it along. But this was slow. Growing impatient, she picked it up, carried it into the shed and looked for the stones that had defeated the dog, the rat. They too were missing and she realized that Mrs. Randolph, a hefty young woman in a hurry, must have taken out the bin, stones and all. They would be in the road where the dustmen had thrown them. She went to look and there they were.

She picked up the first stone and, astonished at its weight, immediately dropped it. But she lifted it again and staggered to the shed, then leaned breathless against the cold wall. After a few minutes she breathed more easily, was less exhausted and the determination to prove to herself that she was quite well again drove her into the road to pick up the second stone.

After a few steps she felt that she had been walking for a long time, for years, weighed down by an impossible weight, and now her strength was gone and she couldn't any more. Still, she reached the shed, dropped the stone and said: "That's all now, that's the lot. Only the yellow plastic pail to tackle." She'd fix the stones tomorrow. The yellow pail was light, full of paper, eggshells, stale bread. Miss Verney lifted it . . .

She was sitting on the ground with her back against the dustbin and her legs stretched out, surrounded by torn paper and eggshells. Her skirt had ridden up and there was a slice of stale bread on her bare knee. She felt very cold and it was nearly dark. "What happened," she thought, "did

I faint or something? I must go back to the house." She tried to get up but it was as if she were glued to the ground. "Wait," she thought. "Don't panic. Breathe deeply. Relax." But when she tried again she was lead. "This has happened before. I'll be all right soon," she told herself. But darkness was coming on very quickly.

Some women passed on the road and she called to them. At first: "Could you please . . . I'm so sorry to trouble you . . ." but the wind had got up and was blowing against her and no one heard. "Help!" she called. Still no one heard.

Tightly buttoned up, carrying string bags, heads in head-scarves, they passed and the road was empty.

With her back against the dustbin, shivering with cold, she prayed: "God, don't leave me here. Dear God, let someone come. Let someone come!"

When she opened her eyes she was not at all surprised to see a figure leaning on her gate. "Deena! Deena!" she called, trying to keep the hysterical relief out of her voice.

Deena advanced cautiously, stood a few yards off and contemplated Miss Verney lying near the dustbin with an expressionless face.

"Listen Deena," said Miss Verney. "I'm afraid I'm not very well. Will you please ask your mother—your mum—to telephone to the doctor. He'll come I think. And if only she could help me back into the house. I'm very cold . . ."

Deena said: "It's no good my asking mum. She doesn't like you and she doesn't want to have anything to do with you. She hates stuck-up people. Everybody knows that you shut yourself up to get drunk. People can hear you falling about. 'She ought to take more water with it,' my mum says. Sleep it off, lady," said this horrible child, skipping away.

Miss Verney didn't try to call her back or argue. She knew that it was useless. A numb weak feeling slowly took possession of her. Stronger than cold. Stronger than fear. It was a great unwillingness to do anything more at all—it was almost resignation. Even if someone else came, would she call again for help? Could she? Fighting the cold numbness she made a last tremendous effort to move, at any rate to jerk the bread off her knee, for now her fear of the rat, forgotten all day, began to torment her.

It was impossible.

She strained her eyes to see into the corner where it would certainly appear—the corner with the old chair and carpet, the corner with the bundle of hay. Would it attack at once or would it wait until it was sure that she couldn't move? Sooner or later it would come. So Miss Verney waited in the darkness for the Super Rat.

It was the postman who found her. He had a parcel of books for her and he left them as usual in the passage. But he couldn't help noticing that all the lights were on and all the doors open. Miss Verney was certainly not in the cottage.

"I suppose she's gone out. But so early and such a cold morning?"

Uneasy, he looked back at the gate and saw the bundle of clothes near the shed. He managed to lift her and got her into the kitchen armchair. There was an open bottle of whisky on the table and he tried to force her to drink some, but her teeth were tightly clenched and the whisky spilled all over her face.

He remembered that there was a telephone in the house where he was to deliver next. He must hurry.

In less time than you'd think, considering it was a remote village, the doctor appeared and shortly afterwards the ambulance.

Miss Verney died that evening in the nearest hospital without recovering consciousness. The doctor said she died of shock and cold. He was treating her for a heart condition he said.

"Very widespread now—a heart condition."

3

Discussion of the Short Stories

GRISHA

(Core Conflict: autonomy vs. shame and doubt)

Plot Summary

A 2-year-and-8-month-old toddler is taken out by his nanny for his first walk in the park. He is excited by the new sights and sounds there but does not know how to react, so he does what he would at home, pursuing whatever strikes his fancy. His nanny, interested in her own pleasure, reins him in a bit roughly. She enjoys the attentions of a "tall man with bright buttons," presumably an official, who accompanies them into a sort of restaurant. Once inside, she, the cook, and the soldier exchange pleasantries and embraces. The child becomes overheated, dressed up as he is in the warm room, and overstimulated as well, when to make fun of him the cook gives him a sip of alcohol. Back at home, he tries to communicate his excitement to his mother, but she misunderstands his efforts and gives him a purgative.

(1) *Whose Story? and* (2) *What Problem?*

This story is to some degree a tour de force. How is it possible, after all, to get inside the head of such a young child, equipped only with rudimentary language, and to be able to decipher his thoughts, emotions, and primitive conclusions about what is expected of him? Yet the interactions unfold in the way a child might think of his world. People, animals, and inanimate objects are to some extent interchangeable. The story captures the intensity of the child's perceptions in a way that stimulates adults' recollection of their earliest childhood memories.

Grisha's problem, as the story opens, derives from his innocence and inexperience. His "ungainly appearance and timid, uncertain steps" do not confer deficiency. His room, toys, pet cat, and aunt have been objects of his normal, unbridled curiosity. Though his father has remained vaguely imposing and largely unknown to him, his world has not been a traumatic or deprived one. He is thus able to respond to the larger world outside his home mostly with excitement and enthusiasm—perhaps too much so for his own good. His nanny, though somewhat rough with him, at least protects him from overt harm. Still, he is able to take in much more than he can effectively process. He is therefore vulnerable to overstimulation, especially given the limitations of his ability to express himself verbally and the unresponsiveness of his caregivers to his inadequately verbalized expressions.

(3) *What Happens?*

What happens in the course of the story is that his caregivers, both nanny and mother, let him down. They are so preoccupied with their own pursuits, pleasures, distractions, or needs, that they do not meet him even halfway. They do not try to understand what he is feeling or trying to communicate. Thus, they leave him to struggle with his own inner sensations by himself, and they try to control his enthusiasms and outbursts by getting him to stay in line or to quiet down. Our first hint of his discomfort and inability to protect himself is that he is unable to combat the penetrating sunshine on his own. Then he is frightened at the soldiers' advance, until the nanny's failure to react to them provides him sufficient reassurance.

When he is further distracted, by cats and by oranges, she pulls him back. Finally, his overstimulation becomes nearly unbearable, when he gets overheated in his overstuffed clothes in the stove-heated restaurant and begins to cry. Again, the nanny hushes him up. All these events could still turn out favorably when he returns to his mother, but she, too, fails to understand what he is saying about the "horrid stove" and, lacking a sense of the nanny's limitations or any intuition, herself, about her child, responds to his obvious confusion by imposing yet further control. He has learned that he is on his own in processing the many stimuli the larger world provides and the emotions they provoke.

(4) *What Prognosis?*

Many readers have suggested that Grisha is adequately equipped by both nature and nurture to maintain his general optimism and curiosity, and thus to handle the conflict Erik Erikson calls "autonomy versus shame and doubt." He is lively and appealing, and he learns quickly what are fairly clear demands imposed on his behavior. For example, he lets the appealing, "gleaming" piece of glass lie untouched, once his nanny has chastised him for helping himself to a free sample from the orange-seller. Even if there have been too many demands to take in at once, he will gradually master them, and in the meantime, his irrepressible curiosity is likely to suffer only a little. That he does not respond with humiliation to the teasing offer of alcohol from the cook and its unpleasant effect attests either to his resilience and general ability to carry on or to the protective effect of his youth.

He has had both positive and negative experiences on his first venture out into the larger world. Nothing has happened to shake his trust in his nanny. Nor is his mother's response unkind, even if it is almost completely unresponsive to his need for understanding and comfort. Perhaps the father's unknown and imposing nature imparts some stability and regularity to this middle-class home and ensures its endurance. Grisha's reaching out to the official he and his nanny encounter suggests he is not overly cowed by such figures. Over time one would expect him to continue to test and learn the limits of his curiosity and wonder, and to develop his natural expressive capacities.

Some readers, however, interpret this story much more darkly and emphasize that the environment fails this child at every step. They find his caregivers suffocating every effort he makes to reach out and explore the world. They are unwilling to accept the generalization that throughout human history it is only the exceptional adults who have ever understood the child's sensory-based, rather than language-based, world. They view the mother's response, far from benign or merely insensitive, as harmful and likely to be internalized negatively. Thus, they envision a possibly negative outcome for this child, who they fear might descend into considerable self-doubt, particularly as no such figure as the benign author is likely to come into Grisha's life and translate for him to his caregivers.

(5) *What Would Help Him?*

If we take this as the premorbid history of a child who has developed, say, asthma, following, say, the departure or death of one of his significant caregivers, we can identify with the pediatrician who may have the opportunity to intervene to try to reduce his vulnerability to repeated attacks. Teaching the mother, if she is the one who remains, how to be more responsive, might begin with just such an understanding of her culturally determined expectations of his behavior. She may have been subjected to the same expectations as a child and now, with the loss of one of her supports, will be stressed still further. Thus, any concrete suggestions for accessing available resources may reduce some of the pressure on her, and thereby, on her toddler. An additional issue this story raises is the uncertainty of the habits of children's caregivers generally, a consideration for modern parents in two-worker families. Those taking a more optimistic view of Grisha's premorbid history might, if the resources were available, find him an ideal subject for play therapy.

THE ROCKING-HORSE WINNER

(Core Conflicts: for Paul, initiative vs. guilt and industry vs. inferiority; for Hester, intimacy vs. isolation)

Plot Summary

Paul is a boy of about 5, just beyond the teddy-bear stage but still a preschooler, when this story opens, and he is about 10, almost boarding-school age, when it ends. He realizes early on, with exquisite sensitivity, that his mother is extremely anxious about the family's lack of money and that she is unable to feel love for him and his two sisters. He receives a rocking-horse as a Christmas present and, thanks to the help of the gardener, who is a racing aficionado, begins to bet on horses. Within a year he has managed to parlay a present of 10 shillings from his "lucky" uncle into 300 pounds, which becomes 1500 upon the next win, and shortly thereafter, 10,000. He makes an "anonymous" birthday present of half that amount to his mother late in the second year the story covers, in an effort to erase her debts and silence the ubiquitous clamor for "more money" pervading the house. However, this effort, predictably, fails, as she proceeds to expend even more lavish amounts on home decorations and on preparations for his schooling. To relieve his uncle's uneasiness about his uncanny knack of picking winners, he explains he is sometimes unsure, but his secrecy about how he comes to "know" the winner only adds to his discomfort. Furthermore, he cannot resist the pressure to acquire even more money to satisfy his mother's insatiable need. Finally, she becomes aware of the pressure he is experiencing and begins to worry, at first vaguely, and then more specifically, about what is happening to him. But it is too late: his final success costs such effort as to throw him into a "brain fever," and though he hovers between life and death long enough to taste victory and to reveal his secret, the effort has cost him his life.

(1) *Whose Story? and* (2) *What Problem?*

This story begins in a voice that sounds like that of a parable or fairy tale: "There was a woman who was beautiful, who started with all the advantages, yet she had no luck." It announces that things could not proceed differently than they do. This voice is important in convincing us that the element of the uncanny that it introduces is just barely beyond the realm of the impossible. Words such as *uncanny* and *haunted* enhance this conviction and anchor the events in a warping of reality without a resort to the supernatural: Paul picks winners "as if he had it from heaven," and he "fidgets" when talking about uncanny events, such as the house's "whispering." He even adds a thoroughly plausible detail, namely, that it feels like "people laughing behind your back." His accurate analysis of the family's struggle for status prevents us from interpreting this as a description of a psychotic child. As it marches forward, it takes on the inexorable certainty of classical tragedy, where none of the actors can prevent the inevitable catastrophe.

This story can be viewed either as Paul's or as his mother's. If Paul is the character who changes, this is a story about deterioration and decline. It is about his failed attempt to change his mother, that is, to cure her. His problem is his vulnerability to her anxiety, and his stubborn, valiant unwillingness to let her go. His sisters, though equally aware of her coldness and aloofness, protect themselves by withdrawing into the world of their childhood. They depend on the care provided by their nurse and find their brother peculiar or, worse, vaguely frightening.

(3) *What Happens?*

Paul's struggle between initiative and guilt takes on a perverse cast. Unable to penetrate the shell into which his mother has withdrawn, he turns inward on himself, flashing his close-set, blue eyes at anyone who would disturb him. He grasps desperately for her recognition. He has a plan. He will provide what she claims will make her happy or at least will relieve her anxiety, not recognizing that no new resources can fill the void she feels. Though there are several suggestions that time is moving on, that he is becoming too old for the nursery and for his childhood toys, he does not take the opportunity to grow up. All his efforts to relieve her bitterness and disappointment with life, and also to "compel her attention," fail. His options diminish, one by one, and the pressure mounts to succeed with his last try. He grows increasingly frantic. In his delirium he reveals all his secrets in a final effort to appeal to her, but this revelation is itself ominous: he has no more cover to hide behind. He has come close: in the moment of illumination they are both wearing the same-colored clothing, as if they have fused at last. Surely he has been trying to free himself from his preoccupation, as well, but he has succeeded only in exhausting himself.

(4) *What Prognosis?*

Had he not succumbed to a "brain fever"—described as if it might have been a seizure, an inflammation, or a manic episode—it is still not clear that he would have been able to resume his own, independent development, having already missed out on so much. Early on, his ability to get on well with the gardener, Bassett, and his uncle, Oscar, suggests he may be developing capacities that could serve his own development, toward Erikson's notion of "industry," even if he has no ordinary peers. These two understand his preoccupation, and the latter realizes it is unnatural, but they can only stand by helplessly as the tragedy unfolds. The only hope would have derived from a change in his mother, who, having nearly lost him, might have realized the mortal effect of her isolation and begun in time to assume a different relationship to him.

(5) *What Might Have Helped Him?*

Saving Paul would have required Herculean efforts by a pediatrician or child psychiatrist, working intensively with his mother, better unaware of the terrible odds against success, and benefiting by a good deal of genuine luck. Even so, success would have been unlikely. This story recalled for one reader his reason for choosing against child psychiatry as a career: "It's too painful to see these children, and I get too angry at the parents."

Now we reconsider the story from a different angle:

(1) *Whose Story and* (2) *What Problem?*

If we take Hester, or the mother–child unit, as the character who changes, we can read this story as moving toward some greater awareness on Hester's part of the emptiness of her own life and the destructive misery her coldness and isolation have visited upon her children, and thus toward a somewhat greater capacity for empathic response.

Her problem initially is that she lacks the capacity for generosity or affection. She is reduced to counting on luck. She waits passively for what she desires to come to her, as if it were her destiny, rather than helping procure it for herself through her own efforts. She does not understand her own need for emotional warmth or of the need to give it to her children, so there is nothing she could possibly accept from them. She misunderstands her husband and merely expects things of him, so they have no working relationship. Lacking empathy, she fails to recognize that her children need more from her than the one thing she is capable of offering, namely, a vague anxiety about them. She is failing dramatically in the struggle between intimacy and isolation. The contemporary word for this failure, narcissism, seems hardly adequate to describe the degree of her failure here. Her "great belief in herself" is anything but self-confidence.

(3) *What Happens?*

We wonder whether she will ever move out of her shell of self-absorption and develop some capacity for empathy. When she enters the field of work and discovers she has a talent for drawing advertisements, she succumbs to envy of her employer before she can discover what her talent might lead to. Later, her explosive expenditure of the mysteriously inherited money suggests either a repetition of her customary failure or a bitter renunciation of the luck that had in fact come her way, as if she needed to reject any sweetness from the world, even if, or because, she subliminally suspected its immediate source.

Paul surmises correctly that she will try to interdict his obsession with acquiring money, once she is aware of it. Her reason for insisting he give it up may be a feeling of discomfort, the first manifestation of her concern for him. The first hint of softening toward him may be her concession to allow him to stay on at the house until the upcoming race has been run. She recognizes that they are so close as to be almost interchangeable, however little she may grasp the irony of seeing herself in him. Next, she laughs—an unexpectedly human response—rather than forbid his keeping company with his horse. Further on, she feels an anxiety, that, unlike her accustomed one, which is for herself or for her failure as a mother, is "strange," since it represents the awakening of a genuine concern for Paul. She finds her heart "curiously heavy," as she watches him struggle over the upcoming race, to the point of feeling "almost anguish." She wants to "rush to him at once, and know he was safe." At that moment she is concerned for his privacy, as if she has begun to accept his growing up. Finally, we are called to witness "all her tormented motherhood flooding upon her," so that this time, when her heart grows cold, it may also be breaking.

At the end, she recollects, probably over and over again, rather than hearing her brother's words directly, his admonition that Paul was unfit for the world as he found it. In these words she aches desperately with the recognition and acknowledgment of her tremendous loss. This comment puts the whole conflict between the value of the child and of money into its proper perspective.

Has she changed by opening up to her children's needs and feelings, even if it has cost the death of her first-born? Her two girls have been less damaged, by having been lesser objects of her malignant attention. Joan, the elder daughter, has shown herself a snitch, contemptuous of her brother, and for her it may be too late. For her younger, unnamed sister, however, there may still be time.

Hester's growing awareness of Paul's secret source of "luck" recalls for her the family secret of having been "damaged" by past gambling. This revelation, beyond its suggestive and significant genetic implications, helps us see this as neither Paul's story nor hers, alone, since it is clear that neither is complete without the other, but rather, theirs together, fused as they have become. Perhaps it is the family's altogether, including Hester's brother, Oscar, and the much-diminished father.

(4) *What Prognosis? and* (5) *What Would Help Her?*

Most child psychiatrists find it impossible to treat overwrought children like Paul without focusing their therapeutic efforts on the parents, and even when they do, they usually express little optimism about the outcome of such efforts. Paul's ever-more intense and prolonged riding suggests not merely excessive masturbatory activity but also increasingly prolonged periods of dissociation. Pediatricians see many children like Paul, and their efforts are restricted to attenuating noxious parental pressures either through medication, through referral to protective agencies, or through involving other family resources, such as grandparents, who may be able to exert a mollifying influence. Such clinicians are well aware of the powerful, even terrible, influence adults can have on children by merely what they say to them.

Neither of the benign figures presented in the story itself as potential model clinicians is up to the task of intervening successfully with this mother–son pair or with the family altogether. One of them, Hester's brother, identifies too closely with the family's view of the importance of money, and he, too, is partly at the mercy of the family's genetic vulnerability to gambling. The other, Oscar's former groom and now the family's gardener, Bassett, exerts a benign and affectionate but hardly protective influence on Paul, and he is unlikely, because of his position, to stand up to Hester.

It would be nearly impossible to forge an alliance with Hester, who wields the power in this family. She does not recognize herself as the source of the family's unhappiness and so does not reach out for help. Yet insofar as she is suffering as well, recriminations would not be likely to lead to change. Encouragement of her professional talents might be a good place to start, just to disrupt her enclosed and pessimistic view. Unless at least some of her anguish over status is relieved, she is unlikely to be able to realign her priorities, so as to build some capacity for more positive feelings. Whether the physician is a man or woman, a more authoritative stance that emphasizes a greater perspective might move her toward greater awareness than an accepting one. She might eventually be open to more empathic and emotional exploration, one that could reach the earlier sources of her unhappiness. Even in such a scenario, it would take a considerable amount of luck, once again, either good or bad, to prepare her for an awakening and confrontation of what must surely be terrible feelings of self-loathing.

OYSTERS

(Core Conflict: industry vs. inferiority)

Plot Summary

The narrator looks back to an intense experience that occurred when he was 8 years and 3 months old. His father has been reduced to begging for food, having spent five months looking for clerical work. His son's desperate cry for food awakens him. The boy's senses have been heightened by his desperation, so that he can make out the name of a delicacy, oysters, advertised on the restaurant wall. But he does not know what oysters are. Responding to his father's descriptions, he conjures up, first, an inviting image of seafood soup, and then, of something eaten live, a slimy, aggressive creature that will resist being served up. Nevertheless, his hunger prevails; he cries out for the dish and is invited by the bemused patrons to partake of some. To their great delight, he devours one, shell and all, in his haste, hunger, and ignorance. Later that night, suffering from thirst and indigestion, he awakens to see his father still pacing the floor, famished, ruminating over his indecisiveness.

(1) *Whose Story?* and (2) *What Problem?*

As the story opens, this young boy's problem is not within himself but in the failure of his environment. These first three stories about children evoke strong emotion in readers. In this story, the problem stems from his father's failure to protect him adequately and provide him with food: "*fames*" is Latin for "hunger." He loves his father, perhaps too uncritically, but he lacks neither energy, imagination, nor pluck. At most, perhaps he suffers from guilt, as when, hungry as he is, he inquires whether one can eat oysters even in Lent.

His father, on the other hand, grows increasingly dysfunctional and increasingly distracted as he exhausts his options, from failing to find work, to failing to bring himself to beg for money, to failing even to be able to attend to his son's inquiries or to protect him from humiliation. He is too proud to find the words to express what he needs to say to get food for his son.

(3) *What Happens?*

The boy's perception of his father changes. He comes to realize that he cannot depend on him; rather, he will have to depend on his own resources and probably even to fend for them both. The personal cost has been enormous: he has been reduced to a sort of cannibalism, in which it is necessary to eat the monster alive. Even so, when he awakens, sick, that night, he continues to look to his father for emotional nurturing.

(4) *What Prognosis?*

As he comes to realize he cannot depend on his father, he only grows fonder of him, rather than impatient. Such a response, clearly sustained over time, reveals both depth and strength of character that will serve him well in the future. He is not so much traumatized as merely disillusioned by coming to see his father more clearly, and he is able to take that loss in stride.

The narrator in this story reminded one psychiatric discussion leader of a resident who had great natural skill in dealing with abused children. This young physician, by the time he was 8 or 9, had already surpassed his intellectually limited father, a mailman, for whom his affection had, nevertheless, remained.

(5) *What Would Help Him?*

If they were available, the resources that would help this boy would be concrete ones: food and shelter. The story introduces a common dilemma for modern-day clinicians, even if they have access to such resources—namely, whether the threat to the child arises from parental incompetence, even of a conditional nature, or from outright malice. Both this boy's affection for his father and his own strength of character suggest the former. Thus the resources required might even be time limited, and by no means would they involve child protective services. It should be possible to avoid humiliating this proud but ineffectual father by offering the resources to him for the sake of his son.

Good-bye Marcus, Good-bye Rose

(Core Conflicts: industry vs. inferiority and ego identity vs. role confusion)

Plot Summary

Phoebe, a barely pubescent, 12-year-old girl, finds herself the walking and picnicking companion of a retired sea-captain. She has been told, presumably by her mother, that she should consider herself lucky to be the object of his attention. She is initially attracted to his worldliness, but things change, when he abruptly fondles her just-budding breasts. Thereafter she would prefer not to continue the walks, but she is aware that no one would believe her, should she complain or try to beg off. Therefore, she continues to accompany him during many walks that summer, feeling both attracted and repulsed by his provocative descriptions of the violence and cruelty of the sexual act. His wife, Edith, eventually becomes suspicious and compels him to leave town with her. Blaming herself for her complicity, Phoebe believes that the dreams she has shared with her peers of idealized, future families and children—the Marcus and Rose of the title—are dashed forever.

(1) *Whose Story?*

This is surely Phoebe's story. The sea-captain has presumably indulged in similar exploitative relationships before and may well repeat his behavior in the future. He is so unregenerate anyway as to insist that yielding to temptation is the only way to handle it. His younger wife, Edith, whatever her motives for remaining with him in the face of her unmistakable recognition of his proclivities, gives no hint of moving on. Phoebe's rather absent mother, silent and reserved, appears mostly as a shadowy background figure, who harbors suspicions and imposes expectations but does not listen or respond. Butter, as the saying goes, would not melt in her mouth.

(2) *What Problem?*

Phoebe does not have a problem in the area most crucial to a young adolescent, namely, peer relationships, even feeling, as she does, inferior to them and less desirable. She shares her girlfriends' dreams of the future and is well-enough related to have discussed these with them. What she will make of having been told of her limitations, by contrast with them, in the competitive arena of appealing to a suitor, is unclear, but it does not seem to have left her especially bereft or unsettled. Certainly, she shows no indication of feeling depressed or deprived. She seems typical for her age in wanting to be regarded as more grown-up than she is and in being unaware of the power of her mild flirtatiousness. She appears well behaved and polite, having absorbed the admonitions of her Catholic schooling. She is even quite happy with Captain Cardew's attention, before his inappropriate advances begin.

The only hint of an ongoing problem comes from the glancing descriptions of her mother's character and role. She has told Phoebe "how kind it was of him to bother with a little girl like herself" and has conveyed sufficient distrust that Phoebe anticipates being interrogated as to her complicity in the illicit relationship. There is thus a suggestion that the mother is a dour figure who does not much like men. Nor has she provided a father or father-substitute for Phoebe, who might have taught her a more comfortable and well-rounded view of how to deal with men, older or not.

(3) *What Happens?*

Cardew's abusive act initiates the process of change in Phoebe, throwing her into a "ferment." With that gesture he becomes both debased and exceedingly powerful, an "aged but ageless god." Lacking any friend—adult or peer—with whom to process her reaction, she tries to do so by herself. The child in her is "shocked"; the adolescent, "fascinated." She would like his salacious talk to end, and she would also like it to continue. We know this, because when Edith figures out the game and threatens to interdict it, she feels competitive in response to Edith's competitiveness. Though she is "more than half relieved" when Edith takes Cardew away, Phoebe remains polite, "not quite realizing that she was very unlikely ever to see him again"—that is, missing him after all.

Now she begins to try to figure out what her behavior means about herself and about her future. The stars have lost their luster for her; the words and images of her idealized teacher, their comfort and magic. It is as if she has abruptly switched from being an idealist to being a realist. The guilt the nuns have implanted in her provides fertile ground for further self-deprecation. She applies to herself the dual accusations of a ditty that describes a young girl as neither "pretty . . . [nor] good." Lacking alternatives, she decides that, since she will be taken for bad anyway, she will choose deliberately to be so. If that means forgoing dreams of courtship and children, then so be it. At least, her future life will be "more interesting and more exciting."

(4) *What Prognosis?*

It is obvious that this experience has changed Phoebe, even damaged her. It is not so obvious whether the experience will merely have altered the trajectory of her life—making her "wiser," as she claims—or whether she has been ruined. Once tainted, she believes, she cannot go back. She may either have been liberated, becoming something of an adventuress, or debased, becoming a prostitute or, at least, a difficult character, perhaps enjoying tormenting older men with her sexual power, like Vladimir Nabokov's Lolita. In retrospect she will recognize the power she exerted over Cardew in taking off her hat. It is possible she may bounce back from this experience, if we assess her as being unsullied in either character or self-image. The prognosis will be grimmer if we assess her as having started with a poor self-image and bleak outlook, perhaps even damaged by the loss of her father. Of course, the prognosis will depend also on future events, such as whether she happens to meet an appropriate young man, who appreciates her substantial gifts of pluck and resilience and accepts her for who she is.

Along with the question of her character, the story deliberately leaves unanswered several other tantalizing ones, such as, who was her favorite teacher, since the nun whose words she recalls was her "second favorite," and why the title omits Jack, which was to have been the name of Phoebe's third child.

Some discussion participants have reacted by disclosing episodes of similar abuse from their own adolescence. A future professor of child development volunteered that, upon having her breasts fondled by boys her age, she burned the dress she had been wearing that day. A senior nurse wondered aloud about her motivation in repeatedly subjecting herself to exhibitionistic displays by a man in a local movie house, to which she returned several times.

(5) *What Would Help Her?*

Whether she becomes frankly promiscuous or merely depressed, she might benefit from contact with a physician who might relieve her of her guilt for being sexually attracted to someone inappropriate, a perfectly natural reaction for an adolescent, and one that does not imply that she has invited abuse at the hands of an adult. Adolescent girls are so commonly subjected to experiences of molestation of this kind, or worse, that it would be well for all of us physicians to have the opportunity to examine our reactions to such events and to be prepared to respond without discomfort when we hear about them in our consulting rooms. The risks girls like her undergo when forced by opprobrium into secrecy or flagrant defiance are obvious enough.

Araby

(Core Conflict: ego identity vs. role confusion)

Plot Summary

This story shows a young boy on the cusp of adolescence, experiencing his first love. It begins with the contrast between the drab and repressive world of the school and of neighborhood play, and the glowing and idealized world of sexual attraction. Suddenly all his "child's play" is replaced by passionate longing. All his waking activities are clouded by his focus on the girl, an effort he refers to as "bearing my chalice through a throng of foes." Their first encounter sets in motion plans he does not have the means to realize. He becomes distracted not only from his play and chores but also from his schoolwork. Time, previously generalized to months or weeks, slows, unbearably, in the hours leading up to his visit to the fair, from which he has promised to bring her a souvenir. Neither his aunt nor his uncle is unsympathetic, but they thwart him inadvertently through their self-absorption. His aunt gradually becomes aware of his impatience and urges her husband to let him go his way. The train to the fair creeps forward; the entrance gate threatens to bar his way; the stalls are darkening and shutting down. He is distracted from his goal of picking up a suitable souvenir by coming upon two young men flirting with an attractive salesgirl. He realizes it is too late, and he has too little money, and he must return empty-handed.

(1) *Whose Story? and* (2) *What Problem?*

Other than the intensity of his passions and the acuity of his perceptions, the narrator does not appear different from his companions. These special attributes, assets in most environments, will ultimately catapult him out of his depleted and repressive one, though he has no such confidence that this will be so. What awaits him is only the occasion to compel the confrontation, something worth the effort of struggling to break free, which at his stage of life means something to define himself by.

(3) *What Happens?*

The occasion of his awakening arises so naturally, as it usually does in real life, out of his usual activities and surroundings, as to be almost imperceptible. His first mention of Mangan's sister, a slightly older girl, is of an authority figure to be avoided, like his uncle, who threatens to interrupt the boys' play. Then, at the moment predetermined by the intensity of his feelings, the stultifying drabness of his environment, and the chance play of light, the image of her femininity intrudes and washes over him: "Her dress swung as she moved her body, and the soft rope of her hair tossed from side to side." Like him, we notice that the drab brown of the houses contrasts with the exciting brown of her dress, which, in turn, sets off the whiteness of her neck and petticoat in the lamplight.

He may be looking for a cause to take up without even being aware of doing so, out of a need to break free of the drabness of his world. The past weighs him down, and the future is uncertain. Then love comes along and provides him with what he has been looking for. He does not go far afield: his love-object is closely tied to one of his companions and bears his name rather than her own: "Mangan's sister." Yet in her way, she is as exotic as the bazaar she sends him to and forever out of reach.

These contrasts are then picked up in the action of the story by those between the "blind," "quiet," and "brown" street where the school is located and the young narrator lives, the disconnected relics of the old priest who had occupied his house, and the idealized, illuminated visions of the girl he carries with him wherever he goes.

His abrupt transformation from one of a group to one isolated within himself is unexceptional in someone of his age, even though it is in terms of group values and expectations that he will continue to define himself. His quest to prove himself mirrors the knight's on behalf of his lady: there is to be much devotion and very little intercourse. Pleasure hardly comes into the picture, and the achievement of success is only a passing moment. Denial and suffering nearly become ends in themselves, as if tempering the instrument, rather than putting it to any use at all, were the goal. The intensity of the built-up emotion leads to out-of-body experiences, as when "all [my] senses seemed to desire to veil themselves," and it is necessary to press his hands together to reestablish contact with reality. Real action has slowed so effectively that it is almost surprising that he makes it to the bazaar at all. Yet all of this unfolds as if according to a script familiar to us all.

Even the occasion of their first (and last) conversation is taken up mostly with his private impressions of her: "The light . . . caught the white curve of her neck, lit up her hair that rested there and, falling, lit up the hand upon the railing. It fell over one side of her dress and caught the white border of a petticoat, just visible as she stood at ease." She is half real and half fantasy. We note that this actual impression, itself an elaboration of the first impression of her as a "figure defined by the light," is repeated almost verbatim in a reverie a few days later. In the agony of waiting to fulfill his promise he distances himself from all his pursuits up to these days by calling them "child's play, monotonous child's play," a repudiation that foretells his final self-condemnation.

Like many sensitive boys he fears he will not know what to do in his eagerness when the crucial moment comes: "I felt the house in bad humor and . . . already my heart misgave me." In the few weeks between his first exchange with the girl and the fair, he has become distracted from all his usual pursuits. On the appointed evening, he feels the excruciating precision of the hours. The pawnbroker's widow leaves at 8 p.m., complaining herself of the lateness; at 9 his uncle arrives to give him the money to go; his train arrives at 10 minutes before 10, and the fair has already begun to close down. Adding to his misery, the tone of the salesgirl's voice "is not encouraging," and besides, he has only 8 pence left.

The climax of the story is precipitated, as in several stories across the life cycle, such as "In Dreams Begin Responsibilities," "The Dead," and "Gooseberries," by the narrator's coming face to face with his most intense strivings, which he has been trying mightily to avoid recognizing. The seamier side of his motivation breaks through the idealization, and he feels ashamed of what he sees. In life as in stories, this is the point at which many of us back away. Here the narrator feels himself both a failure for being unable to compel the attention of the annoyed shop girl whose help he needs in order to secure a suitable gift, and a debased creature for desiring what he can no longer deny are sexual favors.

How one reads the meaning of his recognition of being "driven and derided by vanity," and the resultant "shame and anger," determines how one estimates the degree of change that has occurred. Simply put, it depends on whether these immediate reactions are seen as likely to drive him back to boyish pursuits and the collective "we" with which the story begins, or to goad him forward to greater effective mastery of the adult world and clearer self-definition and identity.

(4) *What Prognosis?*

Even if one reads this ending as a setback—indeed, perhaps the more so if one does—it is likely to be only a temporary one. The narrator's capacity to reflect on his actions without casting blame outside, even if he is overly harsh in so doing, is essential for positive change. He hardly overreaches himself at this moment, as all his capacity for absorbing what his environment can offer him has been tuned, refined, and arrayed through his perceptions and reactions over the course of the story. Maturational factors are all on his side, and he can only gain from experience. With his perspicacity and responsiveness, it is only a matter of time before he will get it right, even though further setbacks along the way are likely. A major source of these will be his early tendency to idealize women, to whom this tendency itself will have such initial appeal.

Not all infatuations resolve so felicitously, of course. One discussion participant recalled the agony of an isolated man in early middle age who had remained fixated on the image of a girl who had looked at him once in high school.

(5) *What Would Help Him?*

Such a gifted and essentially independent young man, whatever the vulnerabilities that an early separation or loss of his parents may confer, is unlikely to require the intervention of a specialist. However, a physician commonly encounters similar adolescents with, for example, substance-abuse diatheses, who might well require such a service. It would be possible for these young people to put all their gifts in the service of charming those around them and avoiding self-awareness. Then the physician might well look to the example of the teachers in the Christian Brothers' School, who, far from pressing their greater wisdom on their charges, maintain a very pedestrian approach. They focus only on the everyday performance and the expectation based on past behavior, and care little about the inner workings. Since this young man himself expects little but predictability from the authorities around him, he might do best if approached in a low-key fashion. He would need little encouragement of his substantial talents. Those will eventually provide him an alternative route to personal satisfaction, but he does not ask to be treated as special, and the physician's emphasizing them would be more likely to confuse than to clarify.

The Man Who Was Almost a Man

(Core Conflict: ego identity vs. role confusion)

Plot Summary

Dave is a 17-year-old black adolescent in the rural South. He is polite and responsible, and he works plowing fields for a neighboring white farmer. He longs to be taken seriously, as a man, not as a child, as others tend to regard him. Therefore, he wants to get hold of a gun, which will command respect. Though continually fearful he will be refused or derided for his plan, he manages to hold his ground with a storekeeper, who has a cheap one to sell, and his mother, who reluctantly parts with the money she has held onto from his wages. His attempt to try out the gun ends disastrously, when he inadvertently shoots the farmer's mule in the belly, and she dies. His family, the farmer, and neighbors together see through his cover-up story easily, and he is required to "buy" the mule at the cost of two years' indentured labor. Undeterred, he proceeds to fire the gun again, more cautiously, until he learns to aim it properly. Then, rather than return to face his fate, he hops a freight train to an unknown future.

(1) *Whose Story? and* (2) *What Problem?*

That this is a story about a boy's effort to grow up by getting hold of a gun, rather than by accomplishments in the realms of school, peer activities, and sexual exploration, identifies the context as one of danger for people of his race, even though he is the only one who expresses racial tension explicitly. His mother's acknowledgment that her husband could use a gun implies that it would be for protection against marauders rather than animals, though in the climactic scene after the accidental shooting, the racially mixed crowd laughs at Dave but does not threaten him.

His reference in the first paragraph to a "gun" rather than the expected "fun" as a reward for hard work emphasizes how much he craves respect and feels its lack. Everyone treats him like a child: his fellow workers "can't understan nothing"; the fat, greasy, white storekeeper, Joe, asks if his mother lets him have his own money and calls him "nothing but a boy." Dave falsely asserts to his mother that he has been "talk[ing] wid the boys," when such activity is precisely what he has not been up to. We see how unused he is to scheming when he awkwardly and clumsily knocks a chair to the floor in his hardly contained excitement, and when he is unable to restrain himself from revealing his interest in guns to his father. His parents protect him, as if his impulses were untrustworthy, specifically, that he has "no sense." One of these impulses, to staunch the mule's bleeding by forcing dirt into the bullet-hole, reflects a concreteness that is almost simple-minded.

Yet his ability to plan his moves suggests he is not simple but only, or mostly, unschooled. Even in his shame and humiliation after the accident he has the presence of mind to lie about what he has done with the gun, so as to preserve his options. Furthermore, he is able quickly to calculate the amount of time it will take him to earn $50 at $2 per month, and he is headed for school in the fall.

He is either not fully grown or is small for his age, since he notices that his peers "are biggern [he is]." All of this hurts his pride considerably and makes him angry. But how angry? He has a sweet nature. When he considers taking a pot-shot at his boss's house, his revolver is already empty. No one in his environment fears him or thinks him dangerous in any way. More important, his parents are not angry with him, only frustrated and disappointed. The larger community treats even his major transgression with equanimity and no small dose of humor. Thus, his problem is a lack of pride and self-respect, of adequate capacity for foresight and planning, of knowledge of people or the ways of the world, or, importantly, of the risks he must accept to become a "man."

In Erikson's terms he has not consolidated his ego identity because of a lack of sufficient testing in relation to his peers. He has remained overly dependent on his parents for careful monitoring because he has not yet found his own way, even for someone of his age, and he has therefore not formed any notion of a "career" that would express his desires and needs.

(3) *What Happens?*

However impulsive his actions appear as they unfold, he has clearly been considering his options for some time, prior to the initial events of the story. There is a sense that his healthy assertiveness is what impels him, in spite of his trepidation, to muster the courage to request the catalog and a look at the gun from Joe, the storekeeper, and permission and the money for the gun from his mother. Thereafter, he moves quickly to fire the gun, awkwardly, for the first time; to hold onto it, even after his disaster and subsequent humiliation; and to improve his use of it.

He has learned a partial truth, namely, that one may escape the worst consequences of even a disastrous mistake. He does not realize that another scenario might well have unfolded, were it not for his family's reputation for reliability: his arrest and beating, or worse, injury or even violent death. He has gained confidence, however misplaced, and is determined to escape from what he takes to be his family's overprotectiveness and condescension. He is willing to continue taking risks, as much out of naïveté as out of determination.

What happens next, his final act, is quite unexpected. We are prepared to see Dave put in his place, finally crushed. How is this young man, lacking in all marketable skills other than persistence, ever to command the respect he so desperately seeks? Is he not relieved finally to have learned his lesson? Yet, if the story stopped here, it would not be appropriate for this collection of illustrations of change. It does not. It takes the next step, and shows us another way change can occur, namely, by the character's proceeding as before, even in the face of almost—but not quite—certain defeat, somewhat in the manner of Macbeth's final act of defiance.

Dave will not rest content as the victim of the events he has unleashed. As he jumps on the freight train, he feels himself braver and more willful, for the first time, than at least one of his peers, Bill. At the end his fantasy of finding a place "where he could be a man" is just that: a fantasy, but he is determined to pursue it, wherever it leads him.

(4) *What Prognosis?*

Dave's career may well end soon and badly. A young black man on the loose and brandishing a large pistol, arriving in a rural Southern town where he is not known, may well be shot before being questioned. On the other hand, he might reflect somewhat on his recent experience and rebury his pistol before being caught with it. Then he might even find work, say, in a local store, earning a new reputation for himself, much as any youth has the opportunity to acquire a fresh reputation each time he changes schools. If he keeps his own counsel, he might even be taken simply for the untutored but polite young man he has shown himself mostly to be. But it is likely that even under this more benign scenario, his urge to be respected will eventually get him into trouble, given his limited capacities to command respect by his own actions.

(5) *What Would Help Him?*

Besides a lot of luck he will need help in finding a suitable direction, something his under-resourced rural community does not offer. He needs a mentor who can assess his gifts and limitations and give him increasing responsibility when he earns it. The small-town, emergency room physician he may encounter for a variety of reasons may well know of such an opportunity and may have the connections to steer him toward it. In some large cities, he might be fortunate enough to be remanded to a residential group home for adolescents, if he were to run into trouble and be judged a delinquent. There he might have the experience of a community of peers and more responsive adult supervision, where he could learn to define himself more fully.

He is a likely candidate for the juvenile justice system or, depending on his timing, the correctional system itself. It is not rare for young black men confronting the health care system for a variety of reasons to have a history of such exposure, one that physicians may overlook or prefer not to pursue.

Her First Ball

(Core Conflict: ego identity vs. role confusion)

Plot Summary

Leila, an 18-year-old "country cousin," joins her three city cousins to attend her first ball. She is so excited by the prospect and the advance indications of the event—the accessories her cousins wear, their conversations on the way, the evening lights—that she can hardly contain herself. She does not know what to expect, and yet the event exceeds all her expectations. She even imagines backing out, longing for the peaceful, natural surroundings of her country home, but she perseveres. Several young men do ask her to dance, but in spite of their greater experience with such affairs, they do not seem capable of real interaction with her; rather, they are just going through the motions. Things become worse when a middle-aged, physically quite unattractive man demands his turn. Rather sadistically, he presses himself upon her, presuming upon her innocence and politeness to burden her with the grim prediction that her days of attractiveness are numbered, and that soon enough, she will be as removed from the excitement and swirl as he is, and more appropriate for the role of the aging, withered chaperones than the engaged, desirable participants. Her initial response is to feel crushed, but she regains herself quickly, spurred on by the liveliness of the music. She rejoins the youthful activity, so effectively suppressing her encounter with the older man that, when she accidentally bumps into him, she hardly recalls what has just passed between them.

(1) *Whose Story? and* (2) *What Problem?*

This is a story in which glitter and excitement are everything—or rather, almost everything: there is also the engaging, resilient character of Leila herself. Even the excitement is a reflection of her inner light, which transforms the people and events of the ball into waltzing lampposts, a dancing gas jet, a leaping burst of tuning instruments, and talking colored flags. For the others, the event is, however, nothing new. Their programmed responses to it include calculated boredom, disturbed only momentarily by their incredulity that it could possibly be her first such experience. Her only fault, as the story begins, is a developmental one: her naïveté. She has been more of an observer of life than a participant in it. If anything, she has been strengthened by the opportunity for a slower maturational push fostered and protected by limited social contacts and by enriched ones with nature in her country setting. Even there, in her sheltered, country life, she has learned to dance. There could be some speculation about whether the quantity—but not the quality—of her expectations and reactions exceeds the norm for a late-blooming adolescent girl, just up from the country; however, even if this were so, it would reflect a talent, whatever vulnerability it might confer.

(3) *What Happens?*

Her own anticipatory excitement and the cascade of new sensations bombard and nearly overwhelm her in her first contact with the social whirl. The decorations themselves seem to be alive. Her four city cousins, Meg, Laura, Jose, and Laurie, try to provide both a model and a buffer for her, but even the naturalness and spontaneity of their affectionate interactions raises the bar too high and causes her to hesitate, so much so, that she feels she suffers when comparing herself to them. She regrets her lack of loving brothers and sisters like these. It is only the rush of events that catches her up and sweeps her forward, toward the opening of the ball, and past the crashing disappointment soon to confront her.

As it turns out, she proves competent with her first two partners, young men affecting boredom, whose focus is more on themselves than on her. They merely seem to go through the motions; their hearts are not in the event. When she reaches out to them, tenuously trying to make something of their encounters, they are unable to respond in kind. She retreats to the refreshments, the decorations, and the familiar night sky.

Of course, this only lasts a moment. The action rushes forward with the music, itself much more of a tarantella than a minuet or waltz. The fat, balding, older man, probably in his 50's, and an usher of gloom, who sought her out earlier and persisted in his efforts to place himself on her dance card, now expresses himself in an antiquated fashion: "Is this bright little face known to me of yore?" He comes back to press himself upon her. He, too, is self-absorbed, but unlike the young men, to far more sinister effect. Like his predecessors he is incapable of responding to her openness, although he recognizes her kindness. His sadism is awakened by feeling keenly the loss of youth and grace, if he had any to begin with, and he insists that Leila feel as he does, even as these qualities are flowering in her. His purpose is to extirpate them from her utterly, before she has had a moment to enjoy them. To him, her virginal demeanor is an opportunity for exploitation, as if he could find relief by infusing his bitterness into her.

Has he polished his routine over the years, periodically seeking out vulnerable targets for his predations? Should we judge him to be a failed version of the other chaperones, his contemporaries, whose role, up on the stage, he caricatures? Why has he not taken his proper place among them, content to provide a backdrop to their progeny's youthful exuberance? His condemnation to perennial repetition of his intrusive and unwanted behavior, mirrored in his physical decline, is a fine example of the perils of stagnation, which Erikson has labeled as the failed outcome of his stage of life.

Certainly his message has hit its mark and had its desired effect. He senses he has devastated her and tries to disarm her: "You mustn't take me seriously, little lady." Leila reverts to an attempt at childish irony. She brushes off his remarks, but inside, she is devastated. The little girl she was, such a short time ago, is reduced to tears: "Deep inside her a little girl threw her pinafore over her head and sobbed." But there has been a hint of her inner strength in her refusal to walk outside with this man: she understands his game now and will not expose herself to further humiliation, or perhaps worse. Her inner turmoil is beautifully reflected in the world around her. Outside, the stars have sprouted wings, like bats, and even the natural world is no longer friendly. She has been stripped bare, it seems, and has no recourse. Moments like this, experienced sooner or later in most people's lives, can serve as a test. Until they occur, one does not know what inner strength one possesses. This sort of intrusion prompted one discussion participant to recall her father's devastating remark about her hopes of becoming a ballet dancer, at which she had been working hard, "But you're too big!"

Up to this point in the story, we know about Leila's capacity for idealization but not about her resilience. Will she, too, dissolve into bitterness, as her adversary certainly has? At this point, we are holding our collective breaths. Then the music, "a soft, melting, ravishing tune" starts up again, and she is off with her fourth partner. No further soul-baring will do for her this time. Now she is in control. The surrounding players and props take up their supporting roles. The telling encounter is, once again, with the older man, but she is no longer the vulnerable girl she was, just moments ago. Her transformation is capped off with the description of her as smiling "more radiantly than ever." With a telling insouciance, she "[doesn't] even recognize him again." She has managed to wipe out the impact and even the recollection of their encounter, resuming her rightful place among her peers, in triumph over the threat of backing away into the confusion she had briefly experienced. She has become a participant in the events of her life, rather than an observer.

(4) *What Prognosis?*

As with several of the stories in this collection, we are given a veiled hint about the direction of future developments in the last line, after the action has finished. It is as if the author were saying that the events of the story predicted how a series of crises might unfold for this character.

Leila shows a firm sense of what Erikson calls "identity." If she has the resilience to resume course so deftly in the face of this threat, it is hard to imagine what greater ones will deter her as she continues on through future challenges. Even if the action here is viewed as an avoidance of greater trauma—consider what could have occurred had she not demurred when the older man invited her out for a walk—the impact of his skillful, no doubt practiced and calculated intrusion was traumatic. The comforting cries of the baby owls, her mother's accessibility, and the tranquillity of country life had undoubtedly nurtured what was an adventurous, highly lively, and responsive spirit. Now, this spirit has been tested and proven up to the task of facing significant challenges, and also tempered, such that, if anything, it will be even more able to face similar ones in the future.

This is the effect of surviving manageable traumatic experiences, and the source of the axiomatic admonition to get back up on the horse as quickly as possible, after falling off, in order to avoid a widening of the immediate fear. Leila has proven herself a likely force to be reckoned with, as she continues to mature.

(5) *What Would Help Her?*

Leila's dilemma contains elements of the difficulties so many young women face in their lives. By studying this story and her reactions, we gain insight into the handling of difficulties, such as confronting the new social pressures of college life, where they face abundant pressures to engage in a variety of risk-taking behaviors. Indeed, the majority will present themselves to student-health physicians in the course of their college careers. Some astute college administrators currently express concern over what appears to be a significant increase in the incidence of students' inability to cope with these pressures.

The challenge for the physician confronted with a young woman with Leila's obvious appeal and vulnerability would be to bring about the kind of realization she comes to here about the dangers her enthusiasms expose her to, without subjecting her to further self-doubt or despair. There might be some impulse to bring her down from her idealized expectations too quickly, either out of overprotectiveness or out of the competitive or even erotic feelings she might well arouse.

In Dreams Begin Responsibilities

(Core Conflict: intimacy vs. isolation)

Plot Summary

The narrator imagines the fateful day—for him—on which his father proposes marriage to his mother. It takes place on a quiet Sunday in Brooklyn, with the couple going on an excursion to Coney Island. His father is both rigid and unsure of himself, and is given to illusions of how things should proceed. His mother is more romantic but equally stubborn. Their interactions—on a merry-go-round, at a restaurant, at a photographer's, and finally, at a fortune-teller's—lead to increasing frustration and conflict between them, but his father stumbles into the proposal anyway. The narrator, aware of how these conflicts will ultimately affect him, reacts with increasing horror to these interactions and imagines interrupting their courtship altogether, but chastises himself for doing so and admonishes himself to get on with his own life.

(1) *Whose Story? and* (2) *What Problem?*

This story is told as if it were a dream that occurred on the eve of the narrator's twenty-first birthday. The events, presumably reconstructed from accounts he has heard from family members about his parents' courtship, are set within the frame of an old-fashioned, silent film. Outside the film but still within the dream is the narrator's reaction to these events. When they go smoothly, he relaxes somewhat in the dark of the theater, but when tension between the principals mounts, he becomes increasingly horrified, to the point that he interrupts the film and calls attention to himself, disturbing the theater audience. There are many recognizably dream-like qualities to the events: their periodic interruption by outside action; their ominous overtones, as in a nightmare; their flashes forward in time, as when we learn of the death of the narrator's uncle, that will occur around the time of his birth; and their presentation with the intensity generally associated with dreams or with the life of children.

The timing of the story pointedly marks the transition between adolescence and the assumption of adult responsibilities. Its theme admonishes, in almost finger-wagging fashion, that if you do not give up your obsession with your parents' deficiencies and self-deceptions, you are never going to make that transition. Complaining will not help, and other people are going to lose their patience.

What is it, precisely, that the narrator cannot tolerate about the character of each of his parents and about the combustible mixture they form in his eyes? It cannot be merely his disillusionment with his father's awkwardness and pompousness, his "scornful bluster," or even his failure to appreciate the passionate and romantic nature of his wife-to-be, which, coupled with her insistence on having her way, will ensure that they are doomed to frustrate and disappoint one another. Even the competition that will develop between them, as suggested, for example, by the father's grasping most of the nickel rings she so much desires to take herself, cannot fundamentally be what drives the narrator to want to separate them.

So it must be that the problem lies in the narrator himself, in something within him that he cannot tolerate. It begins but does not end with his generally critical attitude toward his father, something that bodes poorly for their future relationship. This attitude further reflects his difficulty identifying with his father, whose age in the dream he knows he is approaching. It is a difficulty that will present a problem for his image of himself as a potential father. His attitude toward his mother is initially somewhat more favorable, but this, too is problematic, because it leaves him clinging to childish pleasures. When his father is off buying peanuts, he shares her passing merriment at the sea below, as "again and again the pony waves are released," and her sense that freedom and play are about to be left behind, as she notices her bathing-costumed peers happily bathing below the boardwalk. Identifying with her will present problems for his own sexuality, which is here reflected indirectly, in the awesome power of nature, and is thus unpleasant and even terrifying rather than pleasurable.

Furthermore, he cannot bear the "indifference" with which he imagines both his parents confronting the miserable fate they are about to inflict on one another, an assumption that allows him to deny their sexuality altogether. His declaring them so unsuitable reflects the underlying breakdown of parental idealization that usually follows divorce. He displaces this aggressive feeling onto the sun and ocean, which then appear "terrifying." In thus rejecting his parents he is rejecting the rest of the world as well, so that he winds up alone and distraught, even in the crowded theater.

Of course, if he had gotten his wish, several favorable events would never have occurred. His mother, who has had her heart set on this union, would have seen her hopes dashed. His father, fragile to begin with, might have retreated into himself, abandoning his fantasies of being a competent figure like the "big man," President Taft. And of course, the narrator himself would never have been born.

The whole struggle against accepting his parents as they were falls into the category of what Erikson has called the conflict of intimacy versus isolation. As long as he remains masochistically attached to them, like the "child who clings to his sulk when offered the bribe of candy," he cannot move toward intimacy in his own life.

(3) *What Happens?*

The way he tries to resolve his conflict in the course of the story involves as much ebb and flow, progression and interruption, sparkle and blaze, as the sea itself. Change requires such a back and forth progression. There is, first of all, the narrator's faint hope that his parents will realize their incompatibility and call off their courtship. This hope is encouraged by the dissatisfaction of the photographer, who recognizes something flawed in their relationship that resists improvement. The camera itself, in spite of its fantasized resemblance to a Martian, is an instrument for capturing reality. Second, there are the increasingly forceful intrusions of a fellow moviegoer, a woman who tries to comfort him with the thought that it is only a film, after all, and not worth getting upset about, and of an usher in the theater, who admonishes him to get control of himself and calm down. These interruptions perhaps represent the narrator's attempts to come to terms with his parents' shortcomings and accept them. Third, there is the relief of the ending to which he awakens, the reality of a morning simultaneously both "bleak" and "shining." He has succeeded, for the moment, in giving up his fantasy that his parents are the root of his problem. That is, all his deep anxiety has been expressed through a bad dream, leaving him, in the light of day, burdened with nothing more than everyday anxieties.

Another way of framing the course of events is that the narrator moves from a passive stance, observing and reacting to them but remaining outside and thus unable to influence them, to an active one, in which he at least takes responsibility for his own behavior, whether he likes it or not. He acknowledges that he cannot see what he is doing any more than they can.

(4) *What Prognosis?*

At the end, the narrator explicitly announces that his dream is over, and that he has awakened to the reality of the new day. Whether or not he will maintain his victory over past conflicts and move forward with his own life will depend on future events, but he has done what he could for now to put his past behind him. His mother, for example, may reach out to him and try to drag him back, kicking and screaming in protest, to gain leverage in her presumably ongoing conflict with her husband. If he encounters difficulties in his own strivings for intimacy, with which he has had little enough experience, and which will be the more likely if, as he claims, "[his] character is monstrous," he may retreat in the face of rejection. The passionate intensity of his feelings makes him vulnerable to disappointment, as would be the case for the young adolescent in "Araby." Still, if, as is most likely, the pattern of the story predicts his future, then he will continue to progress through a series of agonizing reminiscences, crushing disappointments, and imaginative resolutions.

The story is riddled with stark contrasts, and it flips between them repeatedly: the black and the white horses that his father and mother, respectively, ride on the merry-go-round; the sparkling waves that abruptly become the "terrifying ocean," as his own mood shifts from delight to grim premonition; the warmth of the theater and of June as the dream begins, turning into the harsh, cold light of a January morning. In each of these instances the sea-change takes place within the narrator rather than in the external events themselves. There is something hopeful about the richness of his inner life, which he conveys through a brilliance of language and imagery, even if it is no guarantee of a favorable resolution. He may need several attempts before breaking out of this kind of isolation, and may even receive a lucky and forceful push from the outside.

(5) *What Would Help Him?*

The nearest we come to a glimpse of the kind of physician whom someone like the narrator might seek out is the fussy but determined photographer, who senses that something is wrong with the picture of the parents, even if he is unable to fix it, affirming the narrator's concerns and interposing delay. It is just possible that these same qualities would be helpful in the investigation of the self-deceptions and arrogance of the narrator himself. Moreover, the photographer has artistic integrity: "He is not interested in all of this for the money." Since the narrator is very skeptical, not to say contemptuous, of materialistic values, such integrity is likely to be tested thoroughly in the course of an ongoing relationship.

It would be important to acknowledge and validate his feelings, so that he does not have to scream them out. Even a bit of the clinginess of the fat fortune-teller might be required to keep him from bolting. With luck, such attributes might be successful in awakening him to his more reasonable side, demonstrated by the consoling objectivity of the old lady and the practical admonitions of the usher, so that, perhaps with a resigned sigh, he can move on to the next topic of conflict and disappointment.

There are many reactions that this young man will be likely to provoke, to his detriment. His physician must first of all be able to tolerate a wide range of intense feelings, while being virtually impervious to anxiety. Then, she or he will have to resist being convinced by his intensity and poetic powers of the correctness of his view, even though, since he has considerable insight, he will never be completely wrong. It would be perverse not to agree with many of his judgments or to empathize with his genuine suffering. At the other extreme, the physician will have to avoid being put off by his arrogance, particularly when it is trained, as it inevitably will be, on the physician herself or himself.

My First Marriage

(Core Conflict: intimacy vs. isolation)

Plot Summary

The narrator, a girl of 20 or 21, looks back three years to a relationship that followed soon after her graduation from college in India. She was anticipating an arranged marriage to a young man, Rahul, of her own upper-middle class. Then an older man, identified only as M., poor and impractical but full of grand ideas, showered attention on her. She responded by parroting some of his ideas and running off with him. Her parents, though distraught, continued to shelter her, sending money and visiting the couple. Her father found M. a position, but he lost it by failing to show up for work. Her mother expressed revulsion at his crude habits but continued to visit. Eventually, after a period of withdrawal into introspection and apparently depression, too, he emerged with a vague but more effective message and attracted a following. He remained a malcontent, however, driving off all his followers, not only the beggars but also a wealthy widow who made fairly explicitly sexual overtures to him. Ultimately, he left the narrator to pursue his next whim, admonishing her to return to her parents. Now, two years after his departure, she is once again reconciled to her parents and to her husband-to-be, the ever-patient Rahul.

(1) *Whose Story and* (2) *What Problem?*

The narrator relates the story of her first marriage in a careless and off-hand tone that suggests no awareness that it might have turned out disastrously for her. Her parents have protected and cosseted her so well that she has no awareness of danger. She sounds like an empty vessel, ready to be filled by whoever bothers to do so. She appears to lack self-awareness entirely. She presents herself as merely passing through the world, with no awareness of the irony, clear to us, which her tale reveals—for example, when her husband's cousins, who know his past, criticize his "only talking and never any work," she asserts that "of course, I knew they were only joking."

On the other hand, she has assets, as well. She is not overly dependent on luxury and is adaptable, within limits, to her surroundings. She never feels self-pity or complains about the pain she occasionally feels in spite of being protected by her parents' benign influence. She has confidence in herself, and she is affectionate.

(3) *What Happens?*

Though she never describes her own sexual feelings explicitly, she recounts the elements of what sounds like a sexual obsession: "We stayed in the room, M. and I, and no one came in to disturb us." He fills her impressionable mind with critiques of her upper-middle-class life, its luxury, and its lack of higher values. She has had so little actual experience of life that she is vulnerable. She responds because such notions fill her with a sense of importance and, however illusorily, of independence. "I tried to say no, but I knew I really wanted to go [with him]." She responds to M.'s mood swings and characterological idiosyncrasies with equanimity and admiration, no matter how bizarrely he behaves.

Through all of this, she records, in her bland and casual fashion, the reality of a larger world, its poverty and deprivation, in contrast to the supposedly higher, abstract one that M. has impressed upon her. Her father's indulgence, as he tries to make the best of a bad situation, and her mother's flexibility, however begrudging, show them to possess the wisdom and grace for handling even this nettlesome rebellion, though she gives them no credit for seeing her through it. Just at the point that she learns about M.'s previous wife and has a premonition that she will suffer a similar fate, she writes to her old friend, Rahul, the person with whom she comes most alive. She treats him like a younger brother, admonishing him playfully to do her bidding. Because she bears comfortably fraternal, rather than erotic, feelings for him, she has felt no remorse at abandoning him.

From first to last, M. remains an abstract image that she can never quite visualize, other than when she is looking directly at him. Fortified by him and by her parents, she meanders through their marriage, moving from the sign-painter's house in her native city, to the town where her husband's family lives, back home to the big guest room, to "several places" in the city—the sign-painter's again, a back room at a bookshop, a model house, and finally, a low-rent railway-worker's house, where M. purifies himself and emerges a guru. However irascible and self-centered, M. is not a charlatan, out to take advantage of the vulnerable: he sends her back to her parents upon his departure, conveniently for him, to be sure, but less destructive than he might have been. He has similarly shown himself to be more admirable than a mere opportunist, just prior to this, when he scorns the sexual advances of the plump young widow, one of his persistent followers, who "was going mad with love of God . . . and implored him to relieve her." The marriage ends, as one discussion participant put it, "fortunately, before she gets pregnant and things turn out badly." This has been more of an adventure than a life choice.

The question is what she may have learned from this experience. She has a reasonable sense of who she is, particularly in relation to Rahul, but she has experienced only sexual intimacy with M., who was too self-absorbed to offer more. She has gotten over her infatuation with him, and she is at pains to assert that her life within her family is just as it was before her marriage to him. But the hope of participating in the larger world, rather than idealizing it, as she has always done, still burns within her, and she is left merely "pretend[ing] to be happy." She remembers M., even if the others pretend not to. "But whose face it is I shall see in that hour of happiness—and indeed, whose face it is I look for with such sad longing—is not quite clear to me." That is, M. has remained for her an abstraction, and she may not have learned from this experience how to define her own vision of a life of value.

Nevertheless, it is hard to believe that none of the irony in which her story is steeped does not filter through to her awareness. Even if only in the recounting of her parents' persistent efforts to see her through, she must have sensed what was not clear to her during the living out of it. She has taken much in, while denying its significance, suggesting a greater awareness than she languidly acknowledges.

(4) *What Prognosis?*

Because she is so good at making her peace with those around her, she is likely to do so in her impending marriage with Rahul. Perhaps she will define herself in relation to him, and he is likely to be a most willing subject in her hands. She may even live to some extent through him, putting him up to trying out the work she idealizes but lacks the energy to undertake, herself. Another version of M. may come along, tempting her sorely. On the other hand, she may continue to lead a charmed life: the longing for a fuller one may persist as a sad place in her heart.

(5) *What Would Help Her?*

She does not suffer the pain of her dubious choice, in large part because her support system is so flexible and so good at protecting her from harm. Nor does she experience internal conflict: nothing challenges her belief that hers is the best of all possible worlds, even if it needs a little improving, in ways that seem just barely to elude her. Unless something happens to weaken her supports, she is unlikely to run into difficulties. Her children, however, unless they are as docile as she, may well present a challenge she will not be up to handling. In either of these scenarios, she will need, as always, more resources from without to smooth things over. She is not one who will rise to the occasion alone.

Good Country People

(Core Conflict: intimacy vs. isolation)

Plot Summary

Hulga Hopewell, born Joy, is a 32-year-old woman with a doctorate in philosophy who lives a quiet, isolated life in the rural South. She lost one of her lower legs to a hunting accident when still a child and gets around rather well with her artificial one. However, her life is empty and repetitive: the only people she talks to are her mother and her mother's tenant farmer's wife. Then a traveling Bible salesman drops in on them, and Hulga decides she will seduce him, just to add that experience to her repertoire. Things turn out quite differently from what she expects, when he turns out to be more interested in stealing her treasured artificial leg than her virginity.

(1) *Whose Story?*

As this story opens, all of the characters are stuck—stuck with, and even stuck to, each other. They are not going anywhere. So they are relegated to the game of prying into one another's secrets and guarding their own. Curiosity, or rather, "nosiness," is the name of the game. It is fitting that the opening image is of the tenant farmer's wife, Mrs. Freeman, who has the straightforward look and the methods of a truck. She directs herself to penetrating to the heart of other people's secrets, and the more perverse these are, the more they excite her. They awaken in her a "special fondness."

The main object of her researches, and the only one capable of change, is Joy, a 32-year-old woman who has returned from the university to live with her mother after completing a doctorate in philosophy. She has many secrets, and she employs considerable effort, not to mention a lively wit, keeping them to herself. When she feels they have been penetrated—by Mrs. Freeman, of course, not by her mother, who is incapable of doing so—she blushes. At their heart is how she treasures her artificial leg, at once her defining characteristic and the core of her identity. She takes the leg off and puts it on with the reverence of a religious acolyte performing a ritual, or of a mother cuddling her infant child. Thus, it is devotion, not shame, that she is hiding.

(2) *What Problem?*

Joy's need for secrecy distorts her social relationships, her engagement with the larger world, and her judgment. For example, she tells herself that it is only her weak heart that keeps her down among these "good country people." She does not realize the restriction on her life that comes from her relating only to people she can devalue.

She presents us with an example of someone who is failing at what Erikson calls the struggle for intimacy. Behind such a failure lies a whole range of possible causes, from immaturity to interpersonal anxiety to excessive narcissism. Examples from clinical practice are numerous: the man or woman who cannot make a commitment to a suitable partner because of an overly intense attachment to a parent.

In milder cases of this kind, close friendships and work are not impaired. But Joy's problem is not of this milder kind. It derives from her reaction to the trauma, in which "the leg had been literally blasted off," at the age of 10. Her response to this disfigurement was to deny the emotional pain and eventually to remake herself entirely, through what she considers her "most creative act," renaming herself. The name she chooses, Hulga, though it does not exactly turn ugliness into beauty, at least turns disability into power: it conjures up for her the smith-god Vulcan, "to whom . . . the goddess [i.e., Venus] had to come when called." She takes control of her ugliness by giving it the ugliest name—on this, she and her mother agree—she can find.

This act crystallizes a process of deliberate and determined withdrawal from the world of experience. In adolescence she "had never danced a step or had any normal good times." She has learned to use her considerable power of reason to suppress every feeling but indignation. Still worse, she has no suitable focus for her energy or creativity. She has protected herself from the pain of self-imposed isolation, at the cost of reducing herself to living mostly in an idealized world of fantasy. In this condition she is actually not able to protect herself from the intrusions and, ultimately, predations of the outside world. What remains of her healthy striving for intimacy, cloaked in her fantasy that her first such effort will succeed "without even making up her mind to try," leaves her ripe for exploitation.

(3) *What Happens?*

We can read what happens to her next as essentially a reexperiencing of her initial childhood trauma, and therefore take this as a cautionary story about the dangers of risking change. It is indeed a common experience that when events begin to move forward, they do so too quickly to process. This story moves forward, like its intruder, by lurches: a third of the way through it, when the shift from past to present events occurs, the reader feels jolted to learn abruptly that Hulga and her mother had a visitor for dinner the previous evening.

Guided, or misguided, by the story's title, we are led to believe that this new figure, the Bible salesman, Manley Pointer, is just another good country person. He pops up before us, and before the story's principal characters, much the way opportunity arrives in real life—not exactly in the form we were expecting. It is not clear what he is up to. He knows to begin a relationship by taking in more than he puts out. The mystery here is purposeful in the story, since both we and the characters can endow him with a range of personal fantasies. That is exactly what Mrs. Hopewell and Hulga do, each in her own way.

There is a degree of hopefulness about his and Hulga's interest in one another, though Mrs. Hopewell herself, knowing her daughter, remains skeptical that anything will come of it. His admiration for Hulga is presented as genuine during their first real meeting, where he is described as showing "fascination, like child watching a new fantastic animal at the zoo." His attitude persists into the next morning, too, when they kiss in the hayloft, where he is described as childlike in his kisses and his mumbling, and when the action heats up, he is "astonished" at her atheistic rationalization for her lack of comfortable illusions. This genuineness is not only in Hulga's idealized view of him: to give the devil his due, he has the gift of feeling and expressing admiration, even if he ultimately uses it only to further his exploitative and self-serving designs.

Positive change, unlike trauma, requires some prior preparation, since it is only against such a background that a person can process the new outlook. The extended discussion of the intimate lives of both Mrs. Freeman's daughters may have set the stage. One of them is pregnant already and the other is considering marriage, both thus suggesting intimate activity that will not have escaped Hulga's fertile imagination. Her own sexual desire awakens, and we are given to believe that she has no inhibitions on this score despite her lack of experience. It may even be that she has just had enough of her familiar routines and is ready to break out, whatever the consequences, particularly as she cannot imagine these to be particularly "unexceptional."

Furthermore, she has known the feeling of having her secret laid bare before, by Mrs. Freeman, even if that woman took a much longer time to uncover it than does Manley. But he wants to go further than merely identifying her secret: he wants to see and touch it. She feels no shame about this request, only sensitivity, akin to what "a peacock [feels] about his tail." Nor does the stump to which her artificial leg attaches, actually hurt. She has successfully recovered physically and even, in a narrow sense, psychologically, from the initial trauma, as indicated by her freedom from so-called phantom-limb pain. We know that her desire to be touched is about to overcome her reluctance, and we sense that she is in for a rude awakening.

What is about to occur is that she will give up her protective identity as Hulga and revert back to the more vulnerable Joy, who can, and is about to, be violated. Having initially presented herself to Manley as a girl of 17, the age of the traditional senior prom, she now acknowledges being 30, somewhat closer to the truth. At this age virginity is less the issue for her than an even more primitive vulnerability, one that dates back to her accident. His admiration, reflected in his "delighted child's face," touches her so deeply that she begins to feel connected to him, a first such experience for her. She fantasizes a life together with him, centered on their mutual reverence for the "secret fact" of how her artificial leg attaches. She has fallen in love. At this point the author announces that she is in over her head, with the observation that "she felt as if her heart had stopped and left her mind to pump her blood."

Such a lurch forward is not out of keeping with her character or with this story: everything that has gone before has been preparation. When it happens this way, in literature as in life, it is usually followed by a back-and-forth process of filling in the gaps between the person's prior mode of functioning and the newly acquired one, in an effort to make it feel natural.

Almost as soon as Joy begins to test the mutuality of their fantasies, she confronts their divergence. Nevertheless, it is only in her state of physical helplessness that she can grow emotionally. For a brief moment, at least, her awareness of what is happening is postponed, while she is treated to the display of crudeness and callousness that is Manley's idea of foreplay. Her habitual protective irony deserts her, and she clings to the fantasy that they are both "good country people." He cannot respond in kind to the genuineness of the response he has evoked, and instead he takes it for an insult. Then her anger returns to rescue her from helplessness, and she seems restored to her usual state. But desperation is not the same thing as control: she remains confused, halfway between her prior and new ways of relating. She continues to experience a degree of human relatedness that she has denied for so long. She sees Manley "struggling successfully over the green speckled lake." To her, in both the literal and the religious sense, he appears to walk on water, however shocking her vision of him may appear to us.

If Manley has been successful in accomplishing his purpose, why cannot Joy be similarly so, in her way? Just as she sees more clearly without her glasses, perhaps she can move more gracefully without brandishing her artificial leg. Another way of approaching these questions is to recognize that, although she has just suffered a reenactment of the loss of her leg, she is not entirely the passive victim this time. She has been an active participant in giving it up, however inadvertently. And just possibly, she has gotten something in return. In her new and confused state, the loss of her artificial leg, which paralyzed her reason more than her body, has awakened her emotional capacity to feel for another person.

(4) *What Prognosis?*

What will Joy do at this point? Few of us imagine that she will come to grief alone in the hayloft. So the immediate question becomes, what will she say to her mother and Mrs. Freeman, once she has dragged herself home? It will be difficult to admit her vulnerability, but she can hardly hide the fact that something has happened.

We are free to speculate on what she will do with these newly rediscovered capacities. This story has shown how change might come about, and at what cost, without insisting on a particular eventual outcome. This, in turn, will depend on further acts of fate, as well as upon her basic character. It is the case even with episodes of treatment deemed successful that their future effects are not impervious to the influence of future events. So, it is uncertain, and in a sense, immaterial, whether Joy will merely have a deeper appreciation of the small circle of characters in her rural world, or whether she will indeed return to the university to teach, or whether she will find intimacy with an individual outside her small circle. What is important is the impression we have that, whatever her future course, she has been awakened, not crushed, by this experience. This impression arises from a clear presentation of her strengths of character and imagination, from the complementary virtues—hope and stubbornness—of the supporting characters, and from the unexpected but undeniably suggestive description of Manley's own forward struggle as "successful."

(5) *What Would Help Her?*

Those of us who come away from this story with the sense that Joy has simply been retraumatized will obviously have a different idea of what would have been helpful to her than will those who have a more optimistic sense of her future as a result of her encounter with Manley. All of us will do well to consider what it would take to help her both to recover from this encounter and to integrate it in a useful way.

We have witnessed both her habitual interactions and her yearning to move out from them, so we have considerable information about her ways of relating. Those of us with finer sensibilities may be discomfited by her skepticism, use of irony, and cutting wit, all of which someone like her might use to devalue the clinical interaction, even while she seeks help from it. Some of us might feel the impulse to encourage these defensive sallies on her part, out of a misguided desire to be supportive, or worse, entertained. With her background in philosophy, Joy could provide a wealth of insightful rationales for her behavior. Worse, she might even evoke a competitive response, particularly from those of us who need to prove our knowledge or maintain the upper hand.

To move beyond this static scenario, it will be essential to zero in on what we know to be her sensitive area, namely, precisely how she regards her artificial leg and what she does with it. Mrs. Freeman's and Manley's success in doing this suggest that a passive approach or even active listening will not do. Rather, the neutral but methodical probing of the physician conducting a physical examination will be necessary here. Unlike Mrs. Freeman, who elicits only the general idea, or Manley, whose voyeurism quickly outpaces his curiosity, the helpful physician will have to encourage Joy to describe each detail in her own words, and to enunciate the fantasies accompanying each act she performs. Since she will be highly resistant to doing so, it will take both intuition and clinical judgment to know when to move forward and when to back off, to allow her time to compose herself.

Just as she has established a mildly sadomasochistic relationship with her mother, someone like her will be likely to try to establish a similar one with any physician she submits to, and she will thus evoke feelings of sadism in one who pushes her to reveal herself. Thus it will be critical to be comfortable with our own curiosity. Such a sense is often lacking in those of us without sufficient experience in treating patients who have suffered trauma. We may avoid eliciting the awful details, out of a sense of trepidation for the patients' or our own discomfort. We may thus reinforce their desire to keep the trauma to themselves, rather than revealing it, over time, as a subject like any other. As long as they are permitted to do so, the fact and consequences of the trauma remain an untouched secret that precludes a real relationship with the physician and inhibits their growth. Here, Hulga's artificial leg symbolizes all the crutches we use to avoid walking unaided.

Unlike Mrs. Freeman or Manley, we will do better not to try to penetrate her secret, so much as to invite her to share it freely. That is the way for her to be able to connect it to the rest of her life—in particular, to desires and fantasies about meaningful action and about intimacy with others, that may lead to development of those capacities. In keeping with the way the story has unfolded, this connection is likely to come about suddenly and unexpectedly, after a protracted period of her testing our will and intent. Yet Mrs. Hopewell is not entirely wrong: with a little effort, Joy can still make herself appealing when she wants to. She is willing to take risks to reach out. When she had no perfume at hand, she was willing to give Vapex a try. Joy has not totally transformed herself into Hulga, after all.

Once she starts this process, it will be her inclination to scroll through all her fantasies at once, since she is so lacking in actual experience to provide the links to the next steps she will need to take. This will leave her both confused and defenseless while going about the process. Younger clinicians, with more serviceable ideas of life than she has, certainly, but without her degree in philosophy, may find it difficult to follow her abrupt shifts between intellectual and emotional ways of relating and may feel as awkward as she does. It is fortunate that she blushes easily and thus gives herself away.

There will be many issues to pursue: Who was responsible for shooting off her leg in the first place? Was there a connection between losing her leg and losing her father? What, if anything, is the matter with her heart? From what the story reveals, she is not an easy person to get close to. She is good at keeping others at bay. And there is always the problem for the physician of just how to relate to her artificial leg, which completes and softens her deformity. In the end she must give it up as her defining characteristic, just as any traumatized patient must, and accept that it is only a part of what makes her special.

One colleague, encouraged by the lesson of this story, helped a patient with low self-esteem deriving from a deforming childhood accident to realize his goal of preparing for a high school equivalency examination.

The Dead

(Core Conflict: generativity vs. stagnation)

Plot Summary

Gabriel Conroy, a teacher and freelance journalist in his mid-40s, married and with children, arrives at his elderly aunts' annual Christmas party. He is the perennially favored dinner speaker, and this time his theme is to be the loss of civility that modernity has imposed. Several times during the evening, he becomes flustered and unsure of himself, most notably when another guest and fellow teacher accuses him of indulging in a celebration of modernity himself, to the exclusion of an appreciation of his Irish heritage. Later, he looks forward to a romantic interlude with his wife of many years, in a hotel room that he has engaged. However, stirred by the music she has heard at the party, she is focused on a recollection of her first love affair. When she tells him about it, he is filled with hurt and anger, but somehow, the recollection of the events of the evening moves him to transcend these feelings and experience an unaccustomed tenderness.

(1) *Whose Story and* (2) *What Problem?*

On finishing this story for the first time, we are likely to be puzzled why, if the crucial interactions are to be between Gabriel and his wife Gretta, focused on his failure to understand her feelings until his reverie in the final scene, it was necessary to have such a protracted buildup, such an elaborate party scene, so many characters, so much, as it were, prologue. Our second reading puts all these questions to rest.

When he sets out for the Morkans' annual Christmas dance, Gabriel, along with other gifts and failings, is a middle-aged man capable of admiring his wife—even of adoring her—and of feeling passionately about her after, presumably, a couple of decades of marriage. But he does not yet love her, in the sense of appreciating her as another person in her own right, with her own set of experiences and fantasies that do not all center around or even include him.

Narcissism is the central issue in the psychological treatment of many patients, usually but not necessarily men, coming in mid-life to treatment for long-standing problems in love or work, sometimes accompanied by specific physiological symptoms. Like Gabriel, such men are unaware of their insensitivity to emotional issues and find themselves genuinely bewildered by the intensely negative responses they continually evoke. Like him, they tend to be overly sensitive to sleights and to indulge in constant monitoring of how they are perceived, with what we might incautiously compare to a teenager's degree of self-consciousness. Gabriel is warmly regarded, but he does not feel connected to any of the other guests. He lurches inappropriately toward Lily and Molly, impatient to get through the evening. Such men's (and many women's, too) perpetual and repeated losses arise from their inability to imagine that the other person does not share their feelings. They interpret every gesture or word that can be taken as congruent with their moods as an affirmation, and those that cannot be, as hostile or insensitive or worse, as humiliating—"as if . . . some impalpable and vindictive being was coming against [them]."

We may find it difficult to imagine that his apparent insensitivity is unintentional and may react to him with hostility, considering him self-centered and pompous, paling in contrast to the lush colors of the women in this story, who have considerably more access to their emotional lives than he does. It seems to me, however, that Gabriel goes through most of the story feeling bewildered at how his well-intentioned inquiries can evoke such perfervid outbursts. He appears unable to imagine that other people may harbor emotionally laden experiences of their own, as if he were emotionally illiterate, reduced to interpreting—usually, misinterpreting—through reason what others may be feeling. As for his own emotions, he has little to guide him other than vague generalities, so that he is buffeted by each encounter and forced to modify his discourse repeatedly out of petty motives of revenge or disdain. His outburst to Miss Ivors, that he is "sick of Ireland," suggests more than what he already knows, which is that its current provincialism is stifling to him, as long as he remains out of touch with its past; rather, it reveals that all emotionally charged encounters leave him fumbling, unsure of how to respond, and feeling inadequate. Intermittently he wishes to be away from it all, outside in the cool, night air. He feels at ease only when engaged in some mechanical activity, such as carving, at the head of a table of martially arrayed dishes.

(3) *What Happens?*

To take just one path into the heart of the story: we learn from Lily, the maid, with whom Gabriel is about to have his first run-in, that she gets on well with her three mistresses, because she knows to avoid giving "back answers." Like him, therefore, we are taken aback, a moment later, when, while she is busy greeting the gentlemen guests and helping them off with their coats, she does just that. His infelicitous inquiry into her relationships with young men unleashes a wave of intense feelings from her, which he is unable to comprehend. This encounter will then be repeated and intensified in the one he is soon to have with Molly Ivors, who has uncovered his role as a literary reviewer for a British newspaper and accuses him of neglecting his own country. Again, he is hurt—and this time, not a little irritated, at being called insensitive to a woman's inner life. Without these earlier preparatory encounters, neither Gabriel nor we would be able to process effectively what he elicits in the final scene from Gretta and how he finally manages to respond differently.

By the time the evening is over, and he at last drifts off to sleep, he has relinquished his defensiveness, caught a glimpse of who Gretta is, and seen their relationship in a new and by no means diminished light. This process of awakening, purchased at the cost of many painful misunderstandings and disappointments, may occur rather quickly or take longer. It amounts to a victory over the ordinary variety of narcissism, as here, which makes it possible to love another person as separate from oneself.

On this festive occasion he is not the only one reminiscing. Many of the characters appear to rub one another the wrong way, and perhaps some of them, too, dwell on each encounter. Ignited by Aunt Julia's singing, their perturbations burst forth like fireworks, punctuating the flow of the story. We are startled by Aunt Kate's resentment of the Church's diminished role for women; by Freddy Malins's spirited praise of a black singer then performing at the Theater Royal as the equal of any then about; by Bartell D'Arcy's defense of contemporary voices generally, and of Caruso as being the equal of any of the past greats, even if they sang on the continent and were less known to the Irish; and by D'Arcy's later annoyance at not being able to give a proper demonstration to Miss O'Callaghan; and of course, by Gretta's sad outcry over the recollection of Michael Furey's sacrifice of his life for her. Each of these outbursts throughout the party does its work on Gabriel, awakening him to how intensely the past bears on the present.

In the hotel it seems quite clear that Gabriel is experiencing something entirely new. At the moment that he becomes aware that Gretta's feelings do not echo his own, his tone is "kinder . . . than he had intended." He tries to remain "cold" but "his voice . . . was humble and indifferent." Uncharacteristically, he is listening intently and questioning her, actually paying close attention to her story. Once Gretta has cried herself to sleep, he looks upon her "unresentfully" and is "hardly pained." He is "curious" and filled with "friendly pity." These are terms that could hardly have been used to describe his emotions previously. Then, as he begins to feel connected with those who have gone before, now dead, he is filled with "generous tears." The description of him as never having felt love, as young Michael Furey did, toward any woman, yet recognizing and naming it, leaves open the possibility that the recognition may at last blend with the experience itself. At last, Gabriel feels the deep connection with his cultural past, the link from which, for him as for all of us, guiding affect proceeds. The linking, covering snow, like its effect, is "general."

(4) *What Prognosis?*

It is of course fair to ask whether any single experience, or even a collection of intense experiences condensed in a brief period of time, can lead to genuine change. The events of this story might be considered as having occurred over a longer period of time, with the story representing a condensation of them. We might ask the same question about a course of treatment with any physician: was it a single, defining moment where the change occurred, or was there a pattern of awakening over time, which might then be dramatized or experienced as having occurred all at once? Abraham Kardiner, a famous psychoanalyst, reported that Freud, his own psychoanalyst who was notorious for the brevity of his treatments, replied to him, when he expressed disappointment at being sent off so soon, "You have had the psychoanalysis. If you need some 'working-through,' go see [Dr. Karl] Abraham in Berlin."

He is likely to be severely tested by future events. It will not be easy to move out from under the "shadow" of his "serious and matronly" mother, who in her "sullen" way disparaged his marriage to Gretta. Self-doubt and suspicion will plague him whenever he elicits strong feeling: was it something he said, something he mistook, something he should have known? Did he, after all, need to defend himself? Will he be vulnerable to depression if he abandons his intellectualized defenses, his identification with modernity, and the cosmopolitan lure of the Continent? More specifically, did Gretta tell him the story of her early love simply because the song "Lass of Aughrim" had awakened the memory so intensely in her, or because she at last trusted him enough to tell him, or, as only he might suspect, because she wanted to belittle him? On the other hand, if he will let her, she has much to teach him. He is endowed with the capacity to respond to images and sensations from the world around him and from literature. Importantly, there is for him no going back: he will have to confront Gretta now as a fuller person than he has known before, and his attachment and desire are intense: they have kept him by her side at the crucial moment of revelation.

(5) *What Would Help Him?*

Treatment of such a person as Gabriel, whether by an internist steering him to better control of his potential diabetes or hypertension, given his portliness, or by a pastoral counselor to whom he might bring his personal anguish, given his awakening to his isolation, would require considerable tact and empathy. He would be easily offended by being confronted with almost any realization he had not come to on his own, and he would ruminate over the interpretations of everything the physician said, however well-intentioned, though he might not let on as much. He might well drone on in platitudes that could be mistaken for simple obsessiveness, which is not his fundamental problem. Indeed, his affability and respect for decorum might mislead us practitioners unsuspectingly into assuming that he was engaged in the treatment relationship, an assumption that would be at odds, once he had left the office, with the feeling of emptiness that would remain. Gabriel's role as a teacher is likely to provide innumerable instances of his and his students' mutual misunderstandings. This is no small matter, since the specific struggle to imagine how others may be feeling merges with his further need, if he is to succeed at regenerating himself, to refresh his work as well. Locating and identifying his enduring concerns, above and beyond his reputation, would take some digging. Yet in them is where his heart and his warmer emotional life lie.

On the favorable side, we have the example of the story itself. The same self-centeredness that is reflected in his efforts to determine how he might have provoked every painful encounter will also enable him to reflect on each of the possibilities, in turn, and to come to his own judgment as to the more likely origin of the response. He can connect to his cultural past, from which he derives a set of enduring values that can serve him well. And he is a good judge of character, with more persistence than his moment-to-moment vacillation would suggest. He has managed, after all, to choose an appropriate partner, of humor and grace, who has, it appears, little difficulty expressing her own emotional needs, however much he has surely tried her patience over the years. She reads him well, while managing to avoid the conflicts he provokes so easily.

Over time he might well develop self-awareness and make good use of it. He might report fresh impressions of those around him in terms other than those based on his expectations of them. He might pursue, for example, new diet and exercise regimens on his own, without having to be directed. His sense of humor might deepen to include a lighter and, ironically, less critical view of himself. In identifying with such an ideal physician, he might begin to listen to his own "thought-tormented music," at last, before his chance slips away.

THE ADULTEROUS WOMAN

(Core Conflict: generativity vs. stagnation)

Plot Summary

A woman in her early 40s, married since graduating high school but childless, agrees reluctantly to accompany her merchant husband on a selling trip south into the cold Algerian plateau. They take an uncomfortable journey by bus, during which she is aware of the attentions of one of the few other European passengers, a legionnaire. Arriving at an oasis, she is confronted with a different, more ancient world than her familiar one on the coast. There, as her rather phlegmatic husband warms to the process of selling, she begins to respond to the unfamiliar sights and sounds, at first passively, then actively, as she begins to recall the hopes and ambitions she had as an adolescent girl. She persuades her husband to accompany her to the parapet around the oasis, so that she can get a better view of the surrounding desert. Seeing the far-off nomads stimulates thoughts of the authenticity of their lives. Later that night, she returns to the parapet alone, to have an encounter in which she reaches out and has a fulfilling spiritual and physical connection with the night sky and the nomadic culture below.

(1) *Whose Story?*

This is certainly Janine's story. She sees, hears, smells, tastes, and, above all, feels every sensual object in the cold, hard, foreboding and yet inviting landscape where it takes place. The author treats her with such affection and respect that he appears to be sharing the experience with her, rather than standing outside and observing. He does not intrude as a character himself in the role of narrator, even though he presents the story in the third person and at one point notes that "perhaps" she was thinking this or that. He implicitly admires her intelligence and rich vocabulary, as when she refers to Arab shopkeepers as "Olympian." She has a sense of humor, as when she responds to her husband at dinner by considering "the victory of the cooks over the prophets." Most important, she has the gift of a soaring lyrical imagination. The ability of a man (the author) to experience the world as a woman experiences it, both in mind and in body, is instructive to us physicians, who might question the possibility of such an empathic leap.

Like her husband Marcel, the other characters move toward her, only to disappear. Why do the jackal-soldier, the tall Arab in the blue burnoose, and later, the young men on bicycles, not make any effort to intrude further? She is certainly excited by their advances, as she makes clear by her quick glances—foreplay of the eyes, one discussion participant called it—to make certain that Marcel is preoccupied. It is as if they were only part of the landscape, serving to draw her ever further out of herself.

(2) *What Problem?*

Janine recounts her problem over and over, in both philosophical and physical terms: she suffers from "a weight in the region of her heart . . . a knot tightened by the years, habit, and boredom." Like so many women obliged by their circumstances, she has buried her hopes and longings, "the girl she had once been." This emotional narrowing has caused physical deterioration. Her once supple body has grown ponderous; she feels "heavy," and she suffers from swollen ankles. Her stamina is sapped by an asthmatic condition. Worse, she has abandoned responsibility for providing for her emotional needs. "For what is not the most elementary need [i.e., beyond basic material support], how to provide?" she asks. Sometimes she describes her problem as childlessness or fear of death or of growing old alone. She realizes that even a man like Marcel, who she knows loves her, will make love to a woman "without desire, burying himself in her flesh." She has consented to accompany him on his trip south only "because it would have taken too much energy to refuse." In short, given her habitual renunciation of all expectations, she has anticipated this brief interruption of her usual routine as a way to help ensure its continuation, rather than as a way out of it.

She says that she has, so to speak, made her bed and is content to lie in it. She is too much in touch with herself to settle for blame-casting, as some in her situation might be tempted to do, finding Marcel an easy target. She does not regret having chosen marriage over an independent life twenty-five years earlier, or even the disappointment over the unfulfilled expectation she had of Marcel's professional career. Rather, she feels disappointed in herself, that she has given up the hopes of the young girl she was when she left school, that she has allowed herself to be buried in her secure and comfortable but isolated life. When this feeling of alienation intensifies, she feels she has no place at all in this world and "would have liked to take up less space."

Many people, having established a relationship, satisfactory or otherwise, to their cultural and sociopolitical environment and to the important people in their lives, ask themselves at this stage of life whether there is not more to expect, that is, whether some sort of renewal is possible. Erikson labels this the conflict over generativity versus stagnation, and its successful resolution is the main issue confronting those in their 40s and 50s. It will begin, not with looking outward, but with looking inward. Coming to grips with our youthful expectations is the beginning of this process. Formulating what we have learned and beginning to pass it on is the next step. This story offers one way to go about that search.

Janine recalls the hopeful and supple young woman she was as an adolescent. She has deliberately chosen to give up her own pursuits in order to enter into intimacy with Marcel. She is gratified to feel "needed" and not alone, but this decision, essential at an earlier stage in her life, has now left her spiritually empty—in Erikson's terms, stagnating. What has survived is a confidence in her sensuousness and attractiveness to men, and it is this she uses to enact her "adulterous" fantasies, to bring herself back in touch with what she has missed out on, including, but not limited to, her sexuality. She is not put off by Marcel's disparagement of what he considers Arab pretentiousness; on the contrary, she remains attracted by his "crestfallen" look of disappointment on encountering each new manifestation of it. And he has continued to live up to her expectations: he can stop in his tracks and alter course to please her, as he does when he consents to accompany her to the parapet of the fort for the first time, in spite of his desire to rest.

(3) *What Happens?*

It is essential that the reader be clear about what happens at the climax of this story, about the nature of the "adulterous" act predicted by the title, and with whom Janine finally connects. There are many hints of the more usual sort of liaison, from the "jackal-soldier," to the tall, gloved Arab in the blue burnoose, even to the herd of late-night cyclists. She certainly has many opportunities to stray, since her husband, Marcel, so often has his back toward her and his mind on his work. Still, how she finally reaches out is of another order, something altogether magnificent and original, arising from within her to define the wonderful and unique person she is.

Once we understand the climactic moment, the events leading up to it fall nicely into place. This single day has been for Janine what the evening's party has been for Gabriel Conroy in "The Dead," a cascade of intensely evocative events that has enabled each of them to reawaken emotions and expectations that had long lain dormant, ones that were crucial to their spiritual lives, to their sense of wholeness and purpose. She reconnects to the spiritual and emotional life she nurtured as an adolescent.

The change that overtakes her begins, without her awareness, on the dull, monotonous bus ride, proceeds through a series of intense disappointments and awakenings, and continues through the ecstatic experience on her second visit to the parapet. Although she initially identifies with the trapped and aimlessly drifting fly, she begins to open up, even in the closed space of the bus, to awareness of the more harmonious world into which she is drifting. She has a series of encounters with men, but it is we more than she who expect her liberation to come about through the usual form of adultery. Singly and in throngs they stride or pedal toward and around her, only to turn mysteriously and tantalizingly away. She responds with the awakening of her sensuality, but she realizes that she is not at first ready to join in what they offer; she is still, as she says, "too tall, too thick, too white."

Her transformation has already begun by the time she descends from the bus. Her sensuous dreams "of the erect and flexible palm trees and of the girl she had once been" begin to awaken her, even as she sways, half-asleep on her feet, alone in her hotel room. Then her body, which during the years of her marriage had betrayed her, begins to reveal a wisdom of its own: she is made sick by eating pork, as if she were becoming less French and more Arab. She stands aside at the first shop to let in the light, trying to regain some of her lost agility. Then, as Marcel warms to the enjoyment of successful selling, and the sky brightens, she responds increasingly to her surroundings.

Her awakening does not proceed smoothly: abrupt shifts of mood follow one another. Stunned by the "stupid arrogance" of the Arab in the sky-blue burnoose who strides past her and Marcel, and feeling as if their trip has been a loss, she abruptly recalls the chance suggestion of the innkeeper that she visit the parapet of the fort to gain a view of the surrounding desert. Creative impulses like this frequently arrive at our moments of greatest disappointment. We underestimate the role of chance in creating opportunities in life.

Ascending the parapet for the first time, she has what could be called a transcendental experience. Taking in the blend of human, animal, and natural forms, the visible and the imagined, she breaks free of the constraints of time and space, so that she enters, at least for an instant, "This kingdom [that] had been promised her, yet that would never be hers." The figures she glimpses and takes in at the boundary of the horizon are those of people who can tolerate the loneliness and, by contrast with her own experience, all the adventure and diversity of human experience. They suggest to her, if only for this one moment, a vision of what she had hoped, many years earlier, to encounter and participate in. "Life was suspended—except in her heart, where, at the same moment, someone was weeping with affliction and wonder."

Even at this point it seems that she is doomed to be torn between her husband's impassivity and her passivity, dragging herself toward death. But she summons up the inner strength to initiate, at last, the adulterous act that fulfills the story's title. The altered state of consciousness between sleep and waking allows for a refiguring of all the stimulation of the day, so that, paradoxically, the weight of the years becomes a goad to action. She will not let her last chance slip away.

What remains for her is to give herself entirely to this newly discovered world. It is something she must do alone, without Marcel at her side. She awakens during the night to complete her unfinished business. Interpreting each gesture her sleeping husband makes, she carries on a dialogue with herself that recapitulates all their interactions and conflicts over the years. Then, on the wind, comes the call from the south, "where desert and night mingled now under the again unchanging sky, where life stopped, where no one would ever age or die any more." It is a call that she cannot resist.

What happens to her is so profound and dramatic—moving, in the deepest sense of the word, that it is hard to keep in mind that the action of this story all takes place during a single day and night. It is significant that she is not the sort of woman who needs time to process her experiences; they burst upon her fully formed and instantly meaningful. It is important to keep this in mind about her, even though it is clear that she has plenty of time to herself, and that being responsive to her husband is at best a fleeting and intermittent task. Her whole life has been patterned by a series of long hours and days of isolation, interspersed with moments of disappointment or passion.

Her route back to the parapet that night, as he sleeps, allows one last exposure to the more conventional sort of adultery: she is surrounded in the dark by a group of Arabs on bicycles, and there is a momentary hint of possible assault, echoing her fears about the first group of Arab shepherds who surrounded the broken-down bus. But by now we do not anticipate anything that fits the ordinary definition, even though we can hardly anticipate what is coming. Now, at night, only the starry sky is visible; everything else exists only in her imagination. But that is enough: her dizziness beneath the whirling, falling constellations and her familiarity with the parapet itself allow her to open herself at last. She actively precipitates her orgasm as her inner and outer experiences fuse.

The explicit terms in which this last experience is described leave little room for doubt about what has occurred: the gyrations, her opening, the pressing of her belly against the parapet, the waters filling her [with] wave after wave, her moans, the sky stretching over her [with her having] fallen on her back, and finally her release in tears. As one colleague put it so succinctly: "She has an orgasm with the universe." She has moved out of herself to take in this vastly comforting, self-sufficient world of men and nature, which she has entered through her own efforts. This self-creating act puts her in touch with the night sky, described in such lyrical terms that the reader, too, may be suffused by it.

Has she been unfaithful to Marcel? Yes and no. Only his fatigue and self-absorption relieve her of the necessity of stealing back into their hotel room. Her delicacy and reassurance, when he briefly awakens, are aimed only at avoiding disturbing his sleep. She has certainly had a nighttime encounter, but it has been with the night itself. She has managed to fulfill her dreams through the creative force of her own imagination and the power of her longing. She is weeping with relief. Now she can face her loneliness and come to terms with the solitude of the human condition and its ineluctable voyage toward old age and death, unafraid.

(4) *What Prognosis?*

Was this single event insufficient, or will she fall back, dragged down by her familiar routines? Once she returns to her home on the coast, her life is likely to be changed, but whether only internally or externally as well, in terms of new pursuits, will depend on factors yet unknown. Whether she will reach out to acquaintances in a different way, or even to the Arab community she had known previously only at a distance, is not the point. What she will have available to her is the girl she once was, with her confidence and awareness restored. Her sexuality has been reawakened. We may differ in our expectations as to whether she will enjoy more sexual pleasure with Marcel than before.

Her active search for this second encounter with the desert, this time at night, provides a strong suggestion that she will continue to enlarge her expectations in other ways. Connected now with both her inner desires and with a larger world from which she has held herself back, she will have many routes to escape the boredom she had previously used as an anodyne. We have become used to her making much of little and shaping it to her needs.

(5) *What Would Help Her?*

In life, someone like Janine or only slightly less resourceful might find herself at her gynecologist's, complaining of vague physical discomfort, instead of making this trip with her husband. Experienced clinicians are well aware of the narratives that underlie a new presentation of symptoms at this stage of life. Premenopausal symptoms might well be present. What clues might suggest the real origin of her discomfort, and how might these be dissected and resolved?

One imposing obstacle, in spite of her clear intelligence, would be her modesty, her reluctance to speak of her rich, inner life. She would not be easy to get to know, since she would not be accustomed to sharing it. We might even have to be on guard not to be put off by her passive demeanor and to underestimate her. Fortunately for us, she would come to life when asked the standard questions about her youth and adolescence. But the significant clues as to her alertness and capacity for change could not be elicited quickly; they would have to be gathered patiently by allowing her to utilize her great bursts of intuition, imagination, and synthesis. It would be intrusive to encourage her. With only a few clues of the physician's needs and interests to go on, she would become a most empathic and responsive listener and even provider of exactly what was required—not at all what her own growth demanded. Quite likely she would begin to notice themes and connections common to herself and to us.

To be helpful, physicians would have to be comfortable with the erotic feelings she would be likely to evoke. Much would depend on the interpretation of her boredom, as a prelude either to closing down or to renewal. Here again, the story provides some clues. A figure along Marcel's lines, laconic and persistent, rather than active and inspired, would be more likely to allow her own regenerative powers to emerge. What would at least permit patience and restraint would be her low level of demand for any intervention at all.

He

(Core Conflict: generativity vs. stagnation)

Plot Summary

A poor farm couple in the rural South, the Whipples, have three children, the second of whom is developmentally disabled. The elder son, Adna, and the daughter, Emly, are quite normal, and thus the objects of their parents' benign neglect, while the disabled one, referred to only as He or Him, as if with religious awe, is the focus of their attention. At great cost the wife is preoccupied with keeping up the appearance of his—and the family's—normality before neighbors and family. Indeed he is affectionate and seems happy with his life. The farmer recognizes both his limitations and his usefulness as an extra farm hand, but his wife recognizes only his assets, such as his lack of fear with dangerous farm animals. She sends him to tear the suckling piglet from its protective mother sow, so that it can be served up to her brother's family when they visit. When her husband sends him to fetch the neighbor's dangerous bull, she both fears for his safety and anticipates criticism for not being protective enough. The family's fortunes continue to deteriorate. He nearly dies of pneumonia but his parents pull him through. His siblings leave for more promising jobs elsewhere, so he is left as his father's only farmhand. Then he slips on the ice and sustains a severe head injury, leaving him with seizures and unable to walk. The doctor makes a grim prognosis and recommends transfer to the local state asylum. As she accompanies him there, for what she knows will be his last trip, he begins to cry, knowing somehow that he is being sent away. She realizes, for the first time, that he is aware of what is happening, and she wonders if she has not mistreated him all along.

(1) *Whose Story? and 2) What Problem?*

This is Mrs. Whipple's story. The other members of the family, including Him, accept the harsh realities of their lives and try to make the best of it. Their problems are those of poverty and of an impoverished community. Even the burden of caring for the disabled child is only one among many.

Mrs. Whipple's response to these exigencies has been quite different from the others'. She lives in a fantasy world in which things are as they should be, appearances are what matters, and people are polite and straightforward in their motives. What belies this approach is that she suffers continual anxiety that the reality will break through. She is hard on her husband for seeing things straight. Thus the story is about the limits of her pride and denial, about what causes her to give up this posture, and about what she stands to gain by doing so.

(3) *What Happens?*

Even before physical calamities overtake her "simple-minded" son, she has been given to putting a good face on her family's constrained resources. His handicap offers her the opportunity to take her face-saving efforts even further. She treats his limitations—fearlessness, acceptance of cold and hunger, unquestioning obedience—as assets. Indeed this approach enables her to feel proud of him and enables him, at least for a time, to have a productive life that might otherwise not have been possible. She and her husband present him with tasks that their other children could not manage and borrow from Him to provide scarce resources for them.

Workshop participants have emphasized the important issue of reciprocity that is so essential in the relationship between a handicapped member and the rest of the family. The effort cannot be one-sided only, lest it lead to exhaustion. Mr. Whipple provides a benchmark for the realistic exercise of this reciprocity. He is able to make considerable sacrifices and in return makes realistic demands. His wife, on the other hand loves her son excessively—"more than her other children together, and her husband and mother thrown in for good measure," she announces, early on, in the closest approach of anyone's to humor. As a result, she is visited with such anxiety over what harm may befall him, and of the opprobrium this would evoke from the community, that she is bereft of pleasure in his accomplishments. Furthermore, this denial comes at a cost: when it breaks down, it leaves her, and ultimately him, devastated. There has been no prior confrontation with reality that would have allowed preparation for such a development.

Such a breakdown, though not necessarily inevitable, was highly likely, given the hard luck continually visited on this family. As vulnerable to injury as the disabled son was, under a difference scenario he might have lived out his life on the farm, at least until his parents aged. But a bout of pneumonia left him weakened, and the fall on the ice, leading to what sounds like a subdural hematoma, with consequent paraplegia and seizures, incapacitated him beyond their ability to care for him.

How we take the terms of this ultimate confrontation with reality determines our understanding of the outcome of this story. There is no doubt that it is precipitated by his awareness that something calamitous is happening, leading to his first expression of unhappiness ever and his first tears. Seeing this response, Mrs. Whipple is forced to confront his feelings and to see him as an individual for the first time. The thoughts racing through her mind, her usual self-recriminations, suggest she is not yet ready to accept this new view of him; however, it is hard to imagine that she will be able to maintain her denial. The tragedy of this story lies in the gap between her pride, buttressed by her good intentions, and their ultimate inadequacy.

(4) *What Prognosis?*

Her realization that she can no longer protect her son causes her to give up her denial. It comes in the same moment for both of them. She is aware, or will soon be, that she will never see him again, and that he is unlikely to survive in the institution. She will have great difficulty overcoming her guilt at having denied his reality and then failed to protect him from its consequences. Only if she does, will she be able to move beyond illusions of family reunion with her other children and invest in them and in her husband what she had been withholding from them.

(5) *What Would Help Her?*

As the well-intentioned but under-resourced country doctor in the story understood, what this family needed was not advice but resources. His suggestions for managing the earlier pneumonia and for the referral to the asylum, in the face of his accurate prognosis for the son, were all appropriate. But in the face of the departure of all the children, some sort of further intervention may be required to ensure that the family survives. Mr. Whipple will have difficulty enough managing the farm on his own. Helping her to accept the virtue, if not the wisdom, of her approach to her son, in having allowed him to have a meaningful life might be a first step.

But there is surely a larger question here, namely, how does the pediatrician, family physician, or even specialist deal with the questions any family might have on confronting a child's significant disability? Being able to offer the greater understanding and especially, enriched resources available today in some settings might make the task somewhat easier, but such assets might only mask more fundamental issues. Do we recommend mainstreaming this child insofar as possible, accepting the inherent risks of disappointment that are likely, devoting the family's efforts to protecting him, or do we recommend institutionalization early, so as to conserve resources needed or better devoted elsewhere? The lack of simple answers to these questions is complicated by the inevitable onslaught of the communities of advocates for each category of the handicapped, each of which will invite or command the family to hand over its child to their care. But issues such as the siblings' likely attachment to the disabled sibling need to be anticipated and addressed. This story shows that focusing on the family's pride is an excellent place to begin.

The Overcoat

(Core Conflict: for Akaky as well as for his middle-aged fellow-citizens, generativity vs. stagnation)

Plot Summary

This story chronicles the life and untimely death of Akaky Bashmachkin, a lowly copy clerk in his 50s, buried in the ranks of St. Petersburg's civil servants and noteworthy mostly for being so nondescript as to be virtually unrecognizable. He receives attention only as the butt of office jokes. He is an easy target because he is so unaware of slights and so unable to defend himself from them. One kindly exception among the ranks of civil servants hears in his protestations the plaintive cry, "I am your brother," a theme that grows slowly throughout the story. Far from being driven to despair or even melancholy, however, Akaky is more than content to be left to his copying, which provides him with continuous delight. However, the bitter cold of the Russian winter and the limited durability of the overcoat that was his only defense against it intrude upon him. When his tailor, Petrovich, insists the old rag is too threadbare to be repaired, and that he will make a new and splendid replacement for it, a new chapter opens. Under Petrovich's stern tutelage, the clerk begins to imagine for himself what is nothing less than a new life, symbolized and graced by the overcoat-to-be. To pay for it, he saves up money by introducing still further deprivations into his constrained life, comforted by the reward that awaits him. For once the bell turns out to be worth the candle: not only are both he and his tailor delighted with the result, but even his fellow clerks cannot help but take notice. For the first time they acknowledge his presence as one of them. They propose an evening celebration, en route to which Akaky takes note, also for the first time, not only of the range of civil society but even of some of its attractions, such as pretty women. After some perfunctory congratulations on his new acquisition, however, the more worldly clerks return to their customary amusements, leaving Akaky to his own devices, and slightly intoxicated at that. He departs for home, but now the streets are more deserted and threatening. As he attempts to traverse an especially large and foreboding square, he is accosted by a pair of muggers, apparently, who steal his overcoat. A watchman witnessing the encounter from the far side of the square notes nothing untoward. His advice to pursue the matter in the morning introduces the next and penultimate chapter, which concerns Akaky's efforts to have the authorities investigate the theft and return his overcoat. Thus it is that he comes before the third major character in the story, besides himself and the tailor, the Very Important Person. This official, gently and ironically caricatured like everyone else in the story, contains within himself the range of vices of officialdom. He is pompous, vain, and bullying, believing such a posture is expected of him, but there is some suggestion of another side as well, perhaps reflective of his having learned something on the way up. Unfortunately, Akaky's fate is to be the victim of the former side. Upon being summarily dismissed, he returns home in despair, managing to catch his death of cold on the way. He expires, and that is the end of him—or so it seems. The final chapter describes what happens to the Very Important Person and to the citizenry of St. Petersburg, as a result of the spreading fame of the story of the unfortunate clerk who was their brother. The ghost or vision of the clerk begins accosting overcoat-wearers throughout the city, finally descending upon the Very Important Person, as he is on his way to partake of the comforts of his mistress. Having had his better side stirred by some pity and not a little guilt, and thus chastened and subdued, he hurries home to more mundane domestic routines. That is the end of Akaky's ghost. However, as if to make the point that his life and death are not to be forgotten, another ghost, this one distinguished by his enormous size and his huge mustachios, just as described by Akaky in his first reports of the muggers to the authorities, comes to haunt the easily forgetful citizenry of St. Petersburg.

(1) *Whose Story? and* (2) *What Problem?*

One reading of this story places Akaky, the copy-clerk, at its center. A man "well over fifty," his problem is that he is so single-mindedly devoted to the pleasures of his work and oblivious to the rest of the world, including any prospect of his own advancement, that he is treated by his superiors with a "frigidly despotic" attitude, as if he were no more than a "common fly," and by his peers as the butt of their sly jokes. Certainly he never makes an "attempt to woo the fair goddess of mirth and jollity." He has chosen for himself a life of withdrawal from common humanity.

(3) *What Happens?*

The story then focuses on how he approaches the task of regenerating himself, one that must strike the reader as almost beyond the realm of possibility. In this reading, the tailor Petrovich enters the scene to become the agent of change. Petrovich, a former serf, now aggrandized by professional success and by drink, is both an irascible authority, demanding appeasement of his easily offended pride, and an encouraging, stern taskmaster, confident of the ultimate success of his ministrations. He drags Akaky, reluctantly at first, into the circle of his optimistic, one-eyed vision. At first the latter is unable to imagine any change in the routine of his life that will permit him to obtain the means to pay for it, but even within his customary, limited vision he is able to deny himself yet more, and once he has a purpose outside himself, he begins to dream of new possibilities, until "his whole existence seemed now somehow to have got fuller, as though he had got married, as though there was someone at his side, as though he was never alone, but some agreeable helpmate had consented to share the joys and sorrows of his life, and this sweet helpmate, this dear wife of his, was no other than the selfsame overcoat with its thick padding of cotton-wool and its strong lining that would last a lifetime."

The enhanced stature he experiences under Petrovich's tutelage stimulates other latent capacities to notice and to be moved by the larger world. On the way to the party celebrating his newly achieved status, he experiences a sexual awakening, "a liking for which is buried inside every one of us." At the same instant we get a glimpse of the former Akaky, when he tells himself, having just glimpsed the painting of the gentleman's leering at the woman's shapely leg that had drawn his attention and stopped him, so to speak, in his tracks, he dismisses the look of desire as something foreign to himself, characteristic only of "those damned Frenchmen!" The opposition of those emotions is highlighted by the author's aside to us, "how indeed is one to delve into a man's mind and find out what he is thinking about."

This will turn out to be the high point of Akaky's change. His comrades make only a momentary show of recognizing him in his new incarnation before they return to their customary amusements and leave him alone again, to his. From this point on, everything goes downhill, except perhaps for the fleeting moment on his way home when, disinhibited by drink, "he even set off running after some lady, who passed him like a streak of lightning, every part of her body in violent motion," or when, the next morning, he "felt for the first time in his life that he had to assert himself" and did not go to work, or in the grandiose ravings of his final delirium. Whatever Akaky has achieved, he loses again on the way home, and his futile efforts at reinstatement are doomed to the same official dismissal as his former life had been, but this time, with fatal consequences.

(4) *What Prognosis?*

According to this reading, his strenuous efforts to obtain satisfaction might perhaps be seen as a demonstration of newly awakened desires for recognition. Then it would be possible to see him as capable of regenerative change, if only his environment, or a kinder fate, would have let him. Even with such a reading, there is the question of what to make of the final events of this story, which follow his death. As one discussant put it: "I was so anticipating the change in Akaky, that I was disappointed when he died and couldn't enjoy the change longer."

(5) *What Would Have Helped Him?*

The tailor Petrovich provides us with the model of the sort of physician capable of helping this withdrawn, self-contained man. Encouragement, such as that offered by one of Akaky's benign supervisors, was of no avail. Only the direct demand for a higher level of output, with the bar set at precisely the right level, would do. The issue, which Petrovich demonstrates so adeptly, is to make the desired goal one that enhances the esteem of each party in the doctor–patient dyad, rather than a contest of wills. This story helped a colleague engage a patient whose unusual brain tumor caused him to ingest harmful foreign bodies, such that his life was focused on unrealistic demands that he avoid doing so, in a discussion of the risks and benefits of surgery that ultimately cured him.

This story can be considered from another angle:

(1) *Whose Story? and* (2) *What Problem?*

There is another possible reading of this story, which places the citizenry of St. Petersburg, eventually focused on the character of the Very Important Person, but by no means limited to him, at the center of the story and makes Akaky the agent of their change rather than the one who changes. All his colleagues, of whatever rank and disposition, and not only those but also the officials and others who were capable of resonating with his story—indeed "all law-abiding citizens of timid dispositions," become its principal subjects. Nor does such a reading demand that it be seen as a simple morality tale, reinforcing the admonition to recognize that we are one another's brothers. Whatever their particular stages of life and thus core Eriksonian conflicts, they are brought closer to the possibility of successful resolution by opening themselves up to the greater self-awareness that his cautionary tale confers.

(3) *What Happens?*

Each of them is compelled to take notice of one among them whom they had not had to notice before. That is, part of their conception of him has been that he has been incapable of commanding their attention, something his steadfast prior refusals to respond to their provocations has encouraged and reinforced. They have been lulled into the comfortable belief that they knew all there was to know about him, and thus that they were free to elaborate as they wished, for example, with the jokes about his being about to marry the landlady who reputedly also beat him. Those who are described as kindlier are merely those who have imagined their kinship with him sooner than others. Perhaps, too, their memories of how recently they have acquired their elevated status are slightly more acute than their fellows'. Just as when Akaky strolled through the streets of his native city, taking them in with all their social stratification and allure for the first time, "as though he had never seen anything like it in his life," so his exemplary rise and fall was to afford his fellow citizens the opportunity to do likewise, in theirs: "He was to be the talk of the town for a few days after his death," and of much fear and trembling, thereafter.

Though presented only briefly, the story of the transformation of the Very Important Person is carefully prepared. He has had misgivings about his treatment of the clerk; he has attended a comfortable gathering of peers, which, along with alcohol, has caused him to lower his guard; and he has felt so effusive as to imagine himself deserving of further, if illicit, reward. In this state of heightened expectation he is abruptly visited by the recollection, or ghost, of Akaky—it does not much matter which, since in response to the image he throws off his own overcoat. Thereafter, he is a changed man, one who admonishes less, and listens more, to those bringing their suits before him. "It was not so frequently now that his subordinates heard him say, 'How dare you, sir? Do you realize who you're talking to, sir?' And if he did say it, it was only after he had heard what it was all about."

(4) *What Prognosis?*

With this act on the part of the Very Important Person, Akaky's memory can finally be put to rest, dissolving into the lingering effects of the general superstition of local officials, who continually look to ghosts to remind themselves that their authority is not without limits.

(5) *What Would Help Them?*

It is interesting to speculate on how public health officials might go about changing the behavior of a whole class of people. Some certainly have, and with considerable success, if one looks at the example of how significantly the incidence of teen-age smoking has been reduced in the United States, apparently by taking a similar approach to that adopted by the tobacco companies in the first place, namely positive, rather than negative, advertising. Before such a campaign could be undertaken, it had to be imagined. Similar efforts, less widely known, have been used to promote condom use among homeless and frequently HIV-infected men, where good-humored group discussion that includes condom-donning practice sessions leads, at least according to self-report, to diminished risk-taking behavior.

Akaky provides us with one kind of model for the successful health commissioner. He does not intrude into many aspects of the citizens' lives but maintains a single focus. He does not attempt to instill fear about their dangerous lifestyle practices but allows them to draw their own conclusions about where they are headed. Clearly, he admonishes by personal example, even offering himself as the least capable of change. If I can reach out beyond myself and take you into my life, he implies, how much easier must it be for you, who are considerably more sophisticated, to do the same for me. Like Bill Wilson, another kind of model, himself a physician and the founder of Alcoholics Anonymous, he knew whereof he spoke. Like Wilson's, Akaky's story is particularly encouraging in contrast to the repeated failure of the many directive and blame-casting approaches that preceded them.

Gooseberries

(Core Conflict: ego integrity vs. despair)

Plot Summary

Ivan, a veterinary surgeon, and his somewhat younger friend Burkin, a schoolteacher, are out walking through familiar countryside. Ivan begins to recount a story about his brother that he has been anxious to tell for some time, but it begins to rain. They repair to the estate of a younger, mutual friend, Alehin, who operates a mill. On arrival there Alehin greets them and washes himself, while Ivan revels in a long swim in the mill-pond. A beautiful servant-girl, Pelagea, brings them towels and robes. They settle into chairs in a comfortable living room, used only for special occasions, and Ivan at last tells his story. It concerns the search for happiness and the question of how one can enjoy it in the face of the suffering and brutality suffered by the vast numbers of poor serfs. His brother, Nikolay, has found his, through brutish means and at the cost of a brutish existence. All that matters to him is owning land where he can grow his beloved gooseberries. Ivan acknowledges to his two friends that he has harbored the same elitist impulses, but, as an intellectual, unlike his brother, he feels the need to justify his own desire for pleasure. He is inspired with the idea of "doing good," and as he believes it is too late for him, he admonishes his friends to do so. Alehin, exhausted from the day's work and pleased that his home has been blessed with this intellectual discussion, goes off to sleep, but Burkin, unperturbed up to this point, lies awake, troubled by what he has heard.

(1) *Whose Story? and* (2) *What Problem?*

This must be primarily Ivan's story. Though various details about events in his brother's life and their respective age difference would put his age somewhere in his mid-50s, his description of himself as "old and not fit for the struggle" suggests he is in the last stage of life. Some of the change he undergoes has already taken place during his prior reflections on his brother's situation, and more occurs here, in the recounting to his friends. His problem, particularly acute, now that he is "gray-headed and near the grave," derives from his being so self-absorbed. All his life, he has indulged in speculation rather than action, the typical intellectual's problem, and he has been pretentious, as well. He does not seem to know much about life except in theory. The immediate focus of his attention is the question of how to achieve happiness; more specifically, how one may feel free to enjoy the sensuous pleasures of life, even while being aware that most people—particularly the poor serfs—suffer because of the world's surfeit of greed, exploitation, meanness, and general want. He is unaware how difficult this would be to accomplish. This is not a problem for Nikolay, who can simply turn his back on suffering and, indeed, add to it with impunity.

Another way to frame Ivan's problem is to put it in interpersonal terms: he is envious of his brother's solution to the problem and acknowledges that he is so. In spite of his aesthetic revulsion at all the elements of his brother's life, both inward and outward, he has realized that he has, without acknowledging it to himself, shared an elitist view that would enable him to distance himself from the serfs who make country living possible for landowners. Like us he can see that Alehin has resolved at least a part of the problem much more successfully: he works alongside the mill-hands, has retained a breathtakingly lovely servant-girl, and has made room, literally and figuratively, for occasional intellectual distractions. Nevertheless, Ivan makes no effort to understand Alehin's view and can only admonish him with his own, which is the necessity somehow to "do good."

As a result of this problem, he is on the verge of what Erikson terms despair. He is perturbed and has not learned much about issues of importance to him. Furthermore, he is unable to request help from his friends, either by inquiring or by listening. He is left casting about, impulsively clutching at generalities. Within Freud's schema and without Erikson's, it would have seemed unlikely that change could occur so late in life, or that habits so long in forming could ever yield to new approaches to an issue he could no longer evade.

But Ivan is not totally without resources. He has been engaged in the practice of veterinary surgery, after all, which has kept him in touch with the life of the larger world, even if he has not delved deeply enough into it. He is capable of enjoying sensuous pleasure as well, not only of his pipe, which he takes out each time he begins his tale, and of the loveliness of women, but of the physical sensations of his own body, as when he swims exuberantly in the mill-pond. Thus he is ready for this confrontation between his ideals and reality, even if he has delayed it too long, for one reason or another, just as the telling of his story has been interrupted and postponed.

(3) *What Happens?*

This is a story about pursuing our passions to the point that they express our deepest longings, and the regrets we face if we fail to do so. It opens with several alternations of intense feeling. First, the weather is heavy with rain that does not come. When it bursts forth, Ivan and Burkin are discomfited by the messiness and mud and shift from "love of countryside" to "anger with one another." Next, they stand amazed at the sight of the servant-girl's beauty. Then Ivan is snobbishly put off by the various colors of dirt washing off his younger friend, Alehin, even though the latter has acquired it by hard work. Next comes a feeling that will become central to the story's theme, namely, sensual pleasure. Ivan becomes so distracted by his enjoyment in swimming around the mill-pond that Burkin must call him in to tea. At last, the scene is set for the telling of his story, but again, what should unfold as a tranquil and pleasant moment turns into disappointment for the listeners, among whom are the departed, who are watching from their picture frames on the wall.

Though he begins coherently enough, he cannot help diverging from the description of his brother's selfish pursuit of happiness, in order to moralize on mankind in general. He eventually wanders off into two related anecdotes of monetary greed not involving his brother's story at all, so that Burkin must call him back again to the task which, after all, he had set for himself. Ivan returns to his account of his brother, and finds him, his cook, and his dog to be like pigs, and his estate, "alias Himalaiskoe," to be a pigsty. Unlike his imagined ideal estate and unlike Alehin's real one, Nikolay's actual estate does not even have a pond but only a muddy stream. The story overall is a recitation of the intellectual's reasons for holding the materialist in contempt, including a rather contemptuous view of the latter's self-deceptions. Even the brother's pride and joy, his gooseberries, turn out to be "sour and unripe." Ivan invokes the poet Pushkin's understanding of how we would all prefer flattery to hearing the truth about ourselves, but misses, at first, the irony of how it applies to himself: he does not want to acknowledge his envy of his brother's happiness. That visit moves him closer to the real problem with the realization that he shares his brother's ability to deny the destructiveness of greed and reality of suffering, but without his ability to pursue pleasure. Thus he has at least become somewhat more tolerant.

However, this realization initiates a new conflict for him, one that breaks through his denial and leaves him discontent, whether in town or in the countryside. The worst is that the very sight of others' happiness has become "painful." He announces, "There ought to be behind the door of every happy, contented man some one standing with a hammer continually reminding him with a tap that there are unhappy people." He comes to the conclusion many reach in the last period of their lives, when they believe they have managed things badly and wish for the chance to return to an earlier period for another try. He is back to the point when the current story opens and still none the better off for having finally had the opportunity to recount his brother's story. His conclusion at this point, namely, that happiness is impossible but that doing good is not, proves satisfying to none of his listeners, who, presumably, have been striving for both. Nor is he any more satisfied. He leaves Alehin with an admonition to do good, omitting the one to pursue happiness along with it.

In the course of finally telling his brother's story and admitting his own similar prejudices, Ivan has succeeded in moving out from himself. Furthermore, the current story is not yet over. As all three sit in silence, each with his own thoughts, the room itself, with its many comforts, suggests another conclusion to what it has just witnessed. Alehin, exhausted from the day's labors, is pleased simply that abstract issues have been discussed on his premises, taking him away from the practicalities of his daily life. What Burkin is considering, we do not yet quite know. But Ivan, if true to his earlier about-face after visiting his brother, is perhaps coming to a more satisfying realization. As earlier, when, overcome with the pleasure of swimming, he had to ask the Lord's forgiveness, so once again he does so, as he lies down to sleep. Might he be able at last to accept the pleasure of such an encounter, even if he has not fully earned it by living a more dedicated life than his own has been? Is acceptance, rather than a retreat into denial, why he is able to fall asleep so easily?

At this moment, Burkin, considerably less tormented and much more firmly grounded than his friend, experiences an unpleasant reaction to Ivan's pipe. Is he, too, becoming aware of contradictions in his own life, and if so, in time to resolve them? The rain comes again, releasing them all from tension. One colleague, moved by Burkin's more practical style, suggested that a balance between personal and professional life offers a way out of the dilemma that consumes Ivan.

There is a sort of medical insight that underlies the basic theme of this story. If the pleasure of life can be summed up in its sensuousness, then the sensuousness can be summed up in the intense pleasure of a particular taste. The Romans acknowledged the idiosyncrasy of taste and created an aphorism enjoining us not to quibble over it. We note that it goes beyond associations to perhaps a more biological basis: Ivan does not share his brother's love of gooseberries, though they shared a common love of the countryside in their youth.

(4) *What Prognosis?*

We may conclude that Ivan is so conflicted, so out of touch with others generally, and so removed from the world of meaningful action, that he must be incapable of meaningful change. Or we may come to a more hopeful conclusion, based on the practical value of his professional work, on his ability to enjoy the pleasures of women and of the exercise of his own body, and on his general emotional intensity and willingness to struggle, however much he avoids or belittles the emotions of others. Ivan has access to the recollections of the freedom he and his brother enjoyed in childhood, which may yet inspire him to rediscover it anew, even this late in life. Thus the question is whether he will continue what he has begun. Just as he has been able to enjoy the sensuousness Pelagea suggests without having to torment himself by lusting after her, perhaps he may also be capable of overcoming his selfishness and envy, and with them, some of his discontent. He has become more self-aware in the telling of his brother's story, and in the transformation that has occurred in the process of the telling. Insofar as he can accept his own contradictions, he may have begun to identify with suffering and to engage in it without guilt. The process has been cathartic for him and awakened the beginnings of empathy, though he has not had a chance yet to develop very far.

(5) *What Would Help Him?*

Physicians commonly see elderly patients with problems like Ivan's. Typical afflictions of this age include chronic conditions such as hypertension, diabetes, and arthritis, and even in the absence of these, a general difficulty accepting physical limitations. Even worse, some may come to realizations similar to Ivan's only when confronted with life-threatening illnesses. If there is validity in general wisdom that aging tends to accentuate basic personality characteristics, then the conflicts and dissatisfactions of such patients will play into their symptoms, if we are willing to take a look at them. Since these are chronic conditions, we will have contact with such patients over an extended period of time, and with it, the opportunity to suggest new ways of looking at these issues.

In simplest terms the process of enhancing ego integrity comes down to that of accepting both what one has achieved and has failed to achieve over the course of a lifetime, in the context of a realistic sense of one's limitations. Initiating new activities has a different meaning and value from doing so at an earlier stage of life, yet so may still contribute to the favorable resolution of conflict at this age. Thus, for example, were Ivan indeed to throw himself into activities he would consider "doing good," he would be redefining the value of his life to that point. He would also benefit from a consideration of whether the ultimate basis of his sense of incompleteness lies elsewhere, in a deeper understanding of his role in his society and his relationships to others, and thus, from a change in his perspective.

We have a fairly serviceable model in Burkin for the kind of physician who might be helpful to him in this process. As noted above, Burkin's role has been to keep him from getting sidetracked, as he follows his impulses out to their frequently unexpected conclusions. This is no mean feat, since Ivan tends to get distracted so easily, following as he characteristically does the emotion behind his ideas. It requires firmness, authority, and a willingness to intrude. Perhaps even more, as Burkin shows, what is required is a willingness to share the experience along with the patient and be moved along with him; not all guilt, it turns out, is irrational.

Sleep It Off, Lady

(Core Conflict: ego integrity vs. despair)

Plot Summary

Miss Verney is a woman "well over 70," who has just begun to find herself preoccupied with her own death, for reasons that are unclear. She announces her preoccupation to a friend, who shudders inwardly. Miss Verney has many premonitions. Some of these are benign enough, such as a lilac whose future flowering she is unlikely to live long enough to witness, and some are more nagging and persistent, such as tasks she is less and less able to accomplish. Her old, run-down shed comes to remind her of her grave or coffin. She fears that it is inhabited by a large rat, which first she merely imagines, then sees or thinks she sees, and then cannot get off her mind. She tries to engage a builder to remove the shed but becomes discouraged when he points out difficulties. She calls upon a kindly neighbor to get rid of the rat, but he gives up without success and seems hostile in her eyes when he accuses her of hallucinating the rat because of her drinking. She cannot rely on her cleaning woman's discretion, so she keeps her fears more and more to herself. As she withdraws from people, she retreats within herself, restricting her intake of food though not of alcohol. She experiences temporary episodes of partial paralysis. Her doctor suspects a heart condition and suggests she have a phone installed so as to be able to keep in touch, sensing her underlying fear and withdrawal, but he does not intervene actively. Finally, her fears focus on a neighbor's child, Deena, who displaces the rat as the main source of her terror. She imagines the child looking through her, ferreting out both her secrets and her secretiveness. One morning, having disobeyed the doctor's orders to avoid straining herself, she is afflicted with a much more prolonged episode of paralysis and collapses out in her shed, unable to stir but still fully awake and communicative. She hopes that Deena will summon help, but the child relishes her helplessness and spits out a venomous condemnation, "Sleep it off, lady." Covered with rat-attracting garbage, she is left to die of exposure, of a true stroke, or of the predicted heart attack, literally frightened to death.

(1) *Whose Story?* and (2) *What Problem?*

Miss Verney clearly suffers from the physiological disorders of alcoholism and cardiovascular fragility. She also appears to suffer from characterological issues, which have left her apparently without family and social supports, although we only infer this from their exclusion from the story. Her friend Letty, younger by a decade or so, still lives "in the present," blissfully avoiding, most of the time, contemplation of the inevitable. Miss Verney's world may be interpersonally impoverished, or it may only seem so in her eyes. Her perceptions alternate among the real, the dream, the fantasy, and the illusion, and she remains up to the end only barely able to distinguish among these.

(3) *What Happens?*

This is a story of change for the worse. It tells how the fear of death can be experienced as a gradual closing in. Miss Verney's grip on reality weakens, as she progressively fails, first in her plans, then in the reliability of her few human contacts, and finally, in her ability to maintain even her physical integrity. She eats and exercises less, and she drinks, if anything, more. Her plan to tear down the old shed appears less of an improvement project than a futile struggle against decline. She is able intermittently to gather her wits and settle herself, but she sees herself as increasingly bereft of resources. During this process, which appears to extend over a matter of months, she gives in to despair.

Alcohol plays a large role in her deterioration, first because it clouds her ongoing perceptions and causes memory lapses, in which she cannot reconstruct how she got into a particular situation (so-called blackouts), and second because it provides a convenient excuse for those content to abandon her to her distress—first the kindly neighbor, Tom, and then the malicious one, Deena. Even her tearfulness may be a manifestation of the emotional lability that alcoholic deterioration confers. On the other hand, in a sense alcohol is her only reliable source of comfort, one that her doctor tactfully chooses not to interdict.

But this process of increasing helplessness is not merely an acceleration of what happens during the ordinary experience of physical decline or even a version of how the dementias must feel from the inside. It is also an account of how aging feels to this particular woman, who was not merely independent by choice but also isolated, somehow, by character. Life will not, in all likelihood, end in this way for her friend Letty, for example, who uses magical thinking constructively to ward off, rather than intensify, her fear of death. The tenuousness of her human relationships is revealed in how quickly they sour. Even her appreciation of her cottage is suddenly tarnished by the perception of her shed as an "eyesore," although it had not previously disturbed her and is still seen by a young man from a building firm as a potential asset, perhaps converted into a garage. Long-unnoticed debris abruptly threatens her, as if harboring her persecutor, the rat, which has come to symbolize for her the angel of death. She demonstrates resilience up to a point, gathering and settling herself temporarily, but she succeeds in focusing her thoughts only to plan for the solution to what are mostly illusory concerns. There is nothing from her past life, apparently—neither family nor friends nor memories—that she can turn to for comfort and security.

(4) *What Prognosis?*

Even if she had not died at this point, her prognosis for dying either similarly or worse is clear: the trajectory is steadily downward. Without a persistent and beneficent intervention from outside, she might go on hovering above disaster for a time, but the frightening outcome would be the same.

(5) *What Would Help Her?*

Older readers can find the story disturbing, reminding them as it does of what lies not too far ahead in their own lives, and of what they may have witnessed with their parents'. Younger readers, too, might need to distance themselves from this experience; there is a time-honored tradition of medical staff humor regarding the elderly that reflects such a reaction. For one senior physician this story recalled the unsettling experience, early in her training, of coming upon a ward of elderly patients, all attached to intravenous lines, each one alone, including among them a well-known physician, plagued with bedsores. For a nurse, it was the recollection of a dying friend who told her, "You just don't want to leave the party."

Next, clinicians would have to be quite comfortable with intruding into the patient's life, trusting their hunch as to what was unfolding, and acting upon it. Respecting the patient's pride and independence does not mean waiting to be asked. Our standard might be what we would want for someone in our family, including their wishes not to be reformed, as one colleague reminded us.

Finally, the clinician's goal need not be to reverse the process—here, reducing the risks to which Miss Verney's underlying cardiovascular fragility exposes her. It is rather to support the lifestyle that she has chosen, while reducing the fear of loneliness and isolation that makes her chosen lifestyle intolerable—not to mention dangerous. Such an active intervention might lead her, in turn, to make other choices for herself.

[illegible]

4

Applying Short Stories to Clinical Work

If you have come this far with me, you have already engaged in considerable dialogue over the discussions of these stories and taken not a few leaps of faith. First among these is that writers can speak to us rather directly about our patients, and that we can begin to see our patients as characters in these stories, even though diagnoses and treatments have a more objective and scientific basis than do literary discussions. Another is that if we want to learn to engage patients in this way, we can do so, effectively and efficiently, even within the exigencies of our training and practice. Not all readers will grant me this, but I obviously believe it can be done, if we will let the great writers guide us. I believe they can be with us in our consulting rooms, just as much as they have been with us in our living rooms and bedrooms.

You have also figured out that I am a certain kind of physician—not all that unusual, but not representative of all of us, either. I believe that each clinical encounter—and even more, a series of them over time—offers us an opportunity to promote growth and positive change, and that we need to be looking for such opportunities all the time, though we will fail frequently. It is not enough to offer recommendations and then stand by and observe what happens; such a plan often leaves us blaming the patient for failure to improve, rather than sharing the blame.

I readily accept the characterization of this approach as interventionist or activist, but reject that I am imposing my personal values on patients. It would not be possible to do so, anyway. Patients readily grasp our intent, and they regularly refashion any fumbling attempts at suggestions for change, either into eloquent affirmations of suggestions they embrace, or into polite (or contemptuous) rejections of these, when we are off the mark. The starting point in these exchanges, as in the discussion of the stories, is a willingness to accept partial and subjective understanding—what the poet Keats, who studied medicine before beginning to write poetry, called the capacity for "negative capability," meaning, "when a man is capable of being in uncertainties, mysteries, doubts, without any irritable reaching after fact and reason."

Nor do final, objectively correct answers exist anyway to the most important clinical questions. To give one common, concrete example: I recently inquired of a group of expert psychopharmacologists how to manage a particular side effect caused by an otherwise highly effective medication for a serious mental condition. They split evenly over whether to try a substitute medication or to encourage lifestyle changes to ameliorate the side effect, giving cogent—but divergent—reasons for these suggestions. The challenge to me then was to apply these objective and thus necessarily general solutions to this particular patient.

I do not turn to stories for help if the case is unfolding as I would expect, whether it is going well or not. If our rapport is adequate, and the patient is engaged in her or his care and willing at least to consider necessary lifestyle changes, I proceed in a routine fashion. But when I run into persistent difficulties, I turn to stories for help.

The first way to use these stories to illuminate clinical situations follows from the way we have read them: every bit of information must fit together seamlessly. If the patient's lab values have begun to deteriorate without obvious cause, then we have overlooked or failed to integrate a determining piece of historical information. The same goes for a treatment intervention that should work but does not: a piece of the explanation is missing, and we will need either to figure it out from what we know or acquire further information.

Like any useful resource, short stories contribute to medical practice by improving clinical outcomes. They can routinely help us as physicians conceptualize the issues of a particular case and frequently can do so for patients, as well. Failure to face and resolve life issues eventually proves exhausting, and it contributes to a range of physiological disturbances, such as hypertension and reduced immunity, either directly or through the intermediary step of harmful behaviors. These may include lifestyle issues, such as poor diet and exercise, or other poor health habits, such as smoking. Success, on the other hand, includes patients' contributions to the management of their chronic illnesses, including adherence to medication regimens and participation in decisions regarding treatment interventions. Primary care physicians, in particular, who maintain relationships with their patients over an extended period of time, eventually have many opportunities to intervene around harmful behaviors, even within the constraints of their necessarily brief individual contacts.

The general approach to any patient struggling to resolve a clinical issue is to offer a story from the appropriate stage of the life cycle and to add another one that deals with the patient's specific problem. For example, a colleague reported resisting elective surgery to release tendon contractures in both his hands and asked how a reading of stories might help him to decide. He believed the characters came from overindulgence in exercise following his retirement. He was able to use the approaches illustrated in "Gooseberries," about coming to terms with what Erikson calls "our one and only life cycle," and one by Joseph Conrad, "The Secret Sharer," about embracing one's competitive strivings constructively, to overcome his hesitation and self-doubt.

I routinely introduce such an intervention at a point in the treatment where the patterns are sufficiently clear both to the patient and to me. I begin by reflecting on a story illustrating the patient's age-appropriate conflict or of the character in a story closest in temperament or situation to the patient. Then, I describe the fictional situation and suggest how it relates to the patient's in whole or in part. I ask if the patient would like a copy of the story to read. In future visits I listen for or inquire into whether the patient has read the story and whether it seems to apply. She or he might describe the story differently from me, but that level of engagement with the story already implies a greater degree of self-awareness or reformulation of the problem for us both. For example, a patient who reacted with extreme sensitivity to being slighted even by long-standing friends, found herself increasingly isolated. She was comforted by Jorge Luis Borges's story, "Funes the Memorious," which describes a character in this respect like her, who remembers too much and suffers from those remembrances, recalling "every leaf on every tree," such that he could no longer see things whole. She was comforted to know that her responses were not unique.

Another use of stories is to make up quickly for my lack of familiarity with the culture of a given patient. For example, as I undertook the treatment of a woman from the Philippines, I was uncertain what aspects of her behavior might simply be culturally determined rather than idiosyncratic to her. I asked her for a recommendation for short stories that would introduce me to her culture. Through them I learned of the ongoing group closeness in adulthood that was common there, because of the frequency of delayed marriages.

The next step is to talk to patients about their struggles to improve lifestyle habits or patterns of relationships in terms of these stories, which point the way to finding creative solutions. Patient and physician can step back from their individual perspectives and view the issues through a neutral intermediary. Seeing precisely how others in similar predicaments have resolved these issues leads to discussions of interventions suited to the individual patient. Note that, as far back as Sophocles, failings appear in literature as extensions of character, rather than as poor choices. Thus they focus the discussions on how to move forward rather than on recriminations for past behavior.

I also offer stories to patients in specific clinical situations to illuminate particular aspects of their behavior and how they might move forward toward change. A patient who acknowledged his difficulties with empathy and understood well their origins in his early life experiences was skeptical that he could change his long-ingrained habit of taking all questioning as criticism. Having had a mother similar to Gabriel Conroy's, he was puzzled but encouraged by the latter's experience of late awakening to new sources of inspiration and strength in his wider culture, outside his immediate family.

When stories are successful in helping patients in this way, it is because they raise the discourse above the individual concern and illustrate its universal features. The characters in the story have become models for the patient, just as they have been for me, a part of our repertoires.

Our patients, coming from across town or from across the country to consult with us, are not different from Grisha or Joy or Gabriel or Ivan.

The authors who have created them for us have told us everything we need to know about them. I have discussed how they strike me, and how they fit into Erikson's framework, so you can agree or disagree and thus come to your own conclusions and come to know these characters at least as well as I do. Go ahead: sit down with them, enjoy their company. They enrich our personal and professional lives, just as much as do any of our most satisfying or most troubling cases.

Appendix: Some Other Stories Illustrating Change (listed with their special topics)

"Silent Snow, Secret Snow" by Conrad Aiken (first descent into psychosis)
"Flying Home" by Ralph Ellison (race)
"The Sheriff's Children" by Charles Chesnutt (race)
"Bartleby, the Scrivener" by Herman Melville (managing the eccentric person)
"The Secret Sharer" by Joseph Conrad (taming one's aggressive impulses)
"The Short Happy Life of Francis Macomber" by Ernest Hemingway (overcoming passivity)
"Mario and the Magician" by Thomas Mann (overcoming passivity)
"Brokeback Mountain" by Annie Proulx (acknowledging homosexuality)
"How I Contemplated the World from the Detroit House of Correction and Began My Life Over Again" by Joyce Carol Oates (the value of idealization)
"The Ledge" by Lawrence Sargent Hall (the value and dangers of denial)

"Martha, Martha" by Zadie Smith (race and class)
"All the Days of My Life" by Sheila Kohler (resolving trauma and loss)
"The Use of Force" by William Carlos Williams (integrating sexual and aggressive impulses into the healing process)
"The Magic Barrel" by Bernard Malamud (overcoming narcissism)
"The Kiss" by Anton Chekhov (retreat from intimacy)
"The Beast in the Jungle" by Henry James (failure to accept intimacy)
"The Use of Force" by William Carlos Williams (acknowledging sadism and erotic feelings toward patients)
"Second Opinion" by R. K. Narayan (intergenerational rapprochement)
"Enormous Changes at the Last Minute" by Grace Paley (seizing opportunity)
"The A & P" by John Cheever (identity through commitment)
"Paul's Case" by Willa Cather (the danger of narcissism)

Printed in the United States
By Bookmasters